# Parallel Distributed Processing

# Parallel Distributed Processing

## Implications for Psychology and Neurobiology

Edited by

## R. G. M. MORRIS

*University of Edinburgh*

CLARENDON PRESS · OXFORD

1989

Oxford University Press, Walton Street, Oxford OX2 6DP

Oxford New York Toronto
Delhi Bombay Calcutta Madras Karachi
Petaling Jaya Singapore Hong Kong Tokyo
Nairobi Dar es Salaam Cape Town
Melbourne Auckland
and associated companies in
Berlin Ibadan

Oxford is a trade mark of Oxford University Press

Published in the United States
by Oxford University Press, New York

British Library Cataloguing in Publication Data
Parallel distributed processing: implications for
psychology and neurobiology.
1. Man. Cognition. Neuropsychological aspects
I. Morris, R. G. M.
153.4
ISBN 0-19-852178-2

Library of Congress Cataloging in Publication Data
Parallel distributed processing: implications for psychology and
neurobiology/edited by R. G. M. Morris.
Based on a conference organized by the Experimental Psychology
Society and held at the University of Oxford on July 1, 1987.
Includes bibliographies and indexes.
1. Cognition—Congresses. 2. Parallel processing (Electronic
computers)—Congresses. 3. Electronic data processing—Distributed
processing—Congresses. 4. Neural circuitry—Congresses.
5 Neurobiology—Congresses. 6. Human information processing—
Congresses. I. Morris, R. G. M. (Richard G. M.) II. Experimental
Psychology Society.
[DNLM: 1. Cognition—congresses. 2. Mental Processes—congresses.
3. Models, Psychological—congresses. 4. Nervous System—
physiology—congresses. WL 102 P2215 1987]
BF311.P3133 1989
153—dc20
89-8699
ISBN 0-19-852178-2

Typeset by
Cotswold Typesetting Limited, Gloucester
Printed in Great Britain by
Alden Press Ltd, Oxford

# Preface

Recent years have witnessed a substantial growth of interest in 'Parallel distributed processing', 'connectionist', or 'neural network' models of cognitive function. Such models have been in existence for many years, but the publication of Hinton and Anderson's (1981) book *Parallel models of associative memory* (Lawrence Erlbaum Associates), followed, in 1986, by the two-volume book by Rumelhart, McClelland, and their colleagues entitled *Parallel distributed processing: explorations in the microstructure of cognition* (Bradford Books, MIT Press) did much to attract the attention of experimental psychologists. Beginning in 1987, PDP 'workshops' sprang up in several British and North American Universities, with the participants working their way through the chapters in these books and discussing their implications.

Throughout the 1970s and 1980s, many neurobiologists also developed an interest in trying to understand how complex networks of real neurons perform various tasks. The early papers of David Marr, discussing the cerebellum, archicortex and neocortex, are perhaps the best-known examples of this approach (e.g. 'Simple memory: a theory for archicortex', *Philosophical Transactions of the Royal Society*, 1971, **262**, 23–81). However, in his 1982 book *Vision*, Marr expressed some intellectual disappointment with this early work, worrying that these models failed to grasp the complexities of the algorithms being computed by complex networks. In its place, he outlined an approach which, while emphasizing the importance of different levels of explanation for the neurosciences, also stressed the need for these different levels to be bridged. Sadly, David Marr did not live to see the promise of his new approach fulfilled. Many neurobiologists now hope that current developments in the formal analysis of neural networks will provide just such a bridge between psychological accounts of cognitive function and accounts couched at the level of real neurons. In addition, new tract-tracing, immunocytochemical and recording techniques make it possible to describe the detailed course and topography of neural interconnections within discrete networks, the neurotransmitters used, and the capacities of specific pathways for synaptic plasticity in sufficient detail to make modelling worthwhile.

The central aim of the present volume is to ask the question: 'What are the implications of these new parallel distributed processing (PDP) models?' Or, to put it another way, should those experimental psychologists and neurobiologists interested in cognitive function set about their experiments differently in the light of these developments? Clearly, this is an issue on which there is a tremendous difference of opinion. Some see the PDP approach as representing a great step forward in the effort to build neurally realistic models of sufficient sophistication to capture the detailed microstructure of cognition. Others worry that the explanations offered are deceptive. In particular, some neurobiologists worry that just because neurons are arranged in large parallel networks is no reason in itself to suppose that they are carrying out their processing using algorithms like back-propagation which are presently the focus of so much attention as models of cognitive function.

This book has emerged out of a one-day conference organized by the Experimental Psychology Society and held at the University of Oxford on 1 July 1987. That meeting was organized into a morning session devoted to work on human perception, memory, and language function, and an afternoon session devoted to psychological and neurobiological work on animals. The organization of the book is slightly different, partly to emphasize the different levels of explanation characterized by the psychological and neurobiological approach. There are three sections. Part I is concerned with *formal models*. It introduces the approach and discusses the all-important assumptions and algorithms of PDP models. Part II is concerned with *implications for psychology* and covers both human and animal research. This section describes the attempts of three different groups of experimenters to consider the relevance of PDP-type models, but also includes one chapter critical of the approach. Part III is concerned with *implications for neurobiology*. Here also, three authors are impressed by the force of the neural network approach, one is more cautious. Each of the sections of the book is introduced by a short chapter sketching out some of the issues discussed and alluded to in the main chapters that follow. Some readers may find it helpful to read these three chapters first to get an idea of the scope of the book.

Organizing the meeting in Oxford and putting this book together has been both a privilege and a pleasure, but are two tasks which would not have been possible without the help of others. I am particularly grateful to Drs Brian Rogers and Peter McLeod, both of the Department of Experimental Psychology in Oxford, who made all the necessary preparations, including a television relay into an adjoining lecture theatre—such was the interest in the meeting. I am also grateful to Professor L. Weiskrantz for his permission to use the facilities of his Department. Professor N. S. Sutherland and Dr David Willshaw acted as Chairmen for the morning and afternoon sessions and kept things running smoothly and to time. The contributors to the book tolerated and, in all cases, accepted my requests for minor changes in their manuscripts for the sake of continuity and consistency in the book. They also kindly agreed to offer their support to a fund recently set up by the Experimental Psychology Society to support research by postgraduate students. Two of the chapters have been published previously. Geoffrey Hinton's chapter has previously appeared in a volume published by Lawrence Erlbaum; while Steven Pinker's chapter, originally written for the present book, has also appeared in *Trends in*

*Neuroscience.* I am grateful to Erlbaum Associates and Elsevier for allowing the present reprinting. Finally, I am grateful to Leslie Chapman for her assistance with the Index and to the staff of the Oxford University Press who have supported the project from the outset and who have so ably seen it through to completion.

*University of Edinburgh*                                                    R.G.M.M.
October 1988

# Contents

x  Contents

# Contributors

**Richard Granger** Centre for the Neurobiology of Learning and Memory, University of California, Irvine, California, 92717 USA

**Robert D. Hawkins** Centre for Neurobiology and Behaviour, Columbia University, 722 West 168th Street, New York, New York 10032 USA

**Geoffrey E. Hinton** The Canadian Institute for Advanced Research and Departments of Computer Science and Psychology, University of Toronto, Toronto M5S 1A4, Canada

**Glyn W. Humphreys** Cognitive Science Research Centre, School of Psychology, University of Birmingham, PO Box 363, Birmingham B15, England

**Helen Kaye** Department of Experimental Psychology, University of Cambridge, Downing Street, Cambridge, CB2 3EB, England

**H. Christopher Longuet-Higgins, F.R.S.** Laboratory of Experimental Psychology, University of Sussex, Brighton, BN1 9QG, England

**Gary S. Lynch** Centre for the Neurobiology of Learning and Memory, University of California, Irvine, California, 92717, USA

**Nicholas J. Mackintosh, F.R.S.** Department of Experimental Psychology, University of Cambridge, Downing Street, Cambridge, CB2 3EB, England

**Ian P. L. McLaren** Department of Experimental Psychology, University of Cambridge, Downing Street, Cambridge, CB2 3EB, England

**James L. McClelland** Department of Psychology, Carnegie-Mellon University, Pittsburgh, Pennsylvania, 15213 USA

**Richard G. M. Morris** Department of Pharmacology, University of Edinburgh Medical School, 1 George Square, Edinburgh, EH8 9JZ, Scotland

**Karalyn Patterson** MRC Applied Psychology Unit, 15 Chaucer Road, Cambridge, CB2 3EF, England

**Steven Pinker** Department of Brain and Cognitive Sciences, Massachusetts Institute of Technology, Cambridge, Massachusetts 02139, USA

**Alan Prince** Program in Linguistics and Cognitive Science, Brandeis University, 415 South Street, Waltham, Massachusetts 02154, USA

**Edmund T. Rolls** Department of Experimental Psychology, University of Oxford, South Parks Road, Oxford, OX1 3UD, England

**Mark S. Seidenberg** Department of Psychology, McGill University, Montreal, H3A 2T5, Canada

**Bruce A. Whittlesea** Department of Psychology, Mount-Allison University, Sackville, New Brunswick, E0A 3C0, Canada

# Part I

Formal models

# 1

# Network models of the mind
## H. CHRISTOPHER LONGUET-HIGGINS

**The association of ideas**

The fact that people can associate ideas, such as names and faces, or sounds and symbols, is too obvious to need documentation. If there were a limited number of possible ideas, the developing brain could allocate a separate neurone to each, and connect every pair of such neurones by a modifiable synapses, to be facilitated if and only if the two ideas occurred in association. Ideas can, however, be very complicated, so the number of possible ideas is enormous—far too large for each to be assigned a neurone on the off-chance of it turning up. Complex ideas, 'patterns', must therefore be indexed by the association of simpler ones, 'features', to which neurones can be allocated without extravagance. By recording the pairwise associations between the features of a pattern we can set up a simple associative memory (Marr 1969), from which the pattern can be recovered by activating enough of its features and allowing these to activate the remainder. Memories of this kind not only solve the problems of 'store allocation' and 'content-addressability', but are also relatively robust against partial corruption of the contents.

Becoming more ambitious, we may attempt to use an associative net for storing not just one but several patterns (Willshaw, Buneman, and Longuet-Higgins 1969). If two such patterns share any features, there is a possibility of 'cross-talk' between them when either pattern is retrieved. This can be regarded either as a nuisance or as a bonus, according to intellectual taste: the convergent thinker will see it as a limitation on the accuracy of recall, the divergent as a source of creative generalization. But in its powers of generalization the associative net is subject to the same sort of limitations as the one-layer perceptron (Rosenblatt 1962), since it is essentially a battery of such perceptrons working in parallel on the same set of input elements. Not that this is a crippling disability; associative nets can learn to reason inductively (Willshaw 1972) and to supply the best completion of any pattern picked from an ensemble in which the accessible elements of a pattern supply *independent* clues about the inaccessible elements (Minsky and Papert 1969; Hinton and Sejnowski 1983). But a number of vital cognitive skills such as concept formation and language acquisition are known to lie beyond the competence of the associative net (Hinton and Anderson 1981), so the question arises whether all parallel distributed processing (PDP) networks of this general type are subject to similar limitations.

## Two different questions

There are two questions to be asked about a PDP network or, indeed, any model of mental or cerebral activity:

1. What tasks can such a network be designed to perform?
2. Which of these tasks can the network learn to perform?

The questions must be distinguished, since most machines, however well they perform their intended functions, cannot learn anything at all. For the perceptron (i.e. the one-layer perceptron, unless otherwise stated) and the associative net, ancestors of the PDP network, the answers to both questions are known.

The perceptron is, in essence, a device for dividing bit-patterns into two classes. Each element of the pattern is registered by a separate unit, and these units are directly connected by lines of modifiable 'weight' to an output unit with an adjustable threshold. Whether or not the output unit fires depends on whether the sum of the weights on the lines from the 'active' units—those which register a 1 rather than a 0—does or does not exceed the output threshold. If and only if there exists some plane, in the space of possible patterns, that separates the patterns of one class from those of the other, then a suitable choice of weights and output threshold will ensure that the perceptron correctly distinguishes between patterns of the two kinds. Thus one can make a perceptron that distinguishes the 2-bit pattern (0,0) from any other 2-bit pattern, but no choice of weights and threshold will enable the patterns (0,1) and (1,0) to be distinguished from either of the other two, because there is no straight line in 2D separating the points (0,1) and (1,0) from the points (0,0) and (1,1). It is in this sense that the perceptron cannot solve the 'exclusive or' problem—that of telling when just one of the two input elements, but not both, has the value 1.

Remarkably enough, if a given task can be performed by a suitably prepared perceptron, then an unprepared perceptron of similar architecture can learn to perform the task. This result follows directly from the perceptron convergence theorem (Minsky and Papert 1969). It also holds for the associative net because, as already remarked, such a net is nothing more than a battery of perceptrons working in parallel, with every output unit directly connected to every input unit. It must be emphasized, however, that the restriction to 'linear' tasks, coupled with the proven ability to learn any such task, applies only to the one-layer perceptron and to its offspring the associative net.

For PDP networks with hidden units the two questions posed above remain largely unanswered, but one useful result is available, namely that a two-layer perceptron—one with a single layer of hidden units between the input layer and the output unit—can, if suitably prepared, compute any Boolean function of the input vector. Thus the 'exclusive or' predicate, the Waterloo of the one-layer perceptron, can easily be evaluated by a two-layer perceptron if the number of units and the weights of the various connections are suitably chosen (Rumelhart and McClelland 1986). The generalization of this result to PDP networks is the proposition that any mapping whatever between Boolean input vectors and output vectors can be achieved by a network with a single layer of hidden units. Unfortunately, neither result is of much practical importance, because, for an arbitrary Boolean function and a sizeable number of input units, the number of hidden units required would be quite absurdly large.

As yet, no result equivalent to the perceptron convergence theorem has been established for the multilayer perceptron, but the recently invented 'back-propagation' procedure of Rumelhart, Hinton, and Williams (1986) is a natural generalization of the perceptron learning algorithm. It has been applied with impressive results to a number of learning tasks, and in the other two chapters of this section two more such tasks crumble beneath the same steam roller.

## Glimmerings of intelligence

In the good old days of the von Neumann computer (the one on your desk) one could either theorize about the correctness of programs or actually write programs to impress the onlooker with the wonders of artificial intelligence. What should have been the program to end all such programs was the general problem solver, GPS for short, of Newell, Shaw, and Simon. It used to remind one of the patent beetle killer consisting of two wooden blocks with the directions: 'Place beetle on block A and strike smartly with block B'. Perhaps there is a message here for anybody who expects PDP networks to solve all our computing problems: the representation of the problem, the choice of architecture for the network and the control of its activity may well be the most challenging parts of the enterprise.

The chapters by Hinton and by McClelland are, in their separate ways, pioneering studies in PDP modelling. It is worth reflecting why an associative net without hidden units could never learn the two family trees that Hinton's network appears to master. It would, for example, be unable to 'notice' (becuase of its incompetence with the 'exclusive or') that person 1 and person 2 always belong to the same subset of the individuals mentioned (the English family or the Italian family), never to alternative subsets. Hinton is well aware that a considerable element of intuition is involved in the design of a PDP network to solve a given learning task; but as he points out, rule-governed network design is unlikely to become a reality until we have a good mathematical theory of learning tasks in general.

McClelland's chapter gives substance to Piaget's notion of 'the equilibration of structures' in the mind of the developing child. The scientific status of this concept has always seemed a little precarious: how could one submit it to logical or experimental test? McClelland's PDP model for Siegler's balance beam task meets the case admirably, and interprets in detail a number of striking facts about the stages through which children pass in learning the task. Were that all, one might feel inclined merely to add it to the growing list of successful PDP models; but McClelland has succeeded in distilling from the back-propagation algorithm used by the model a learning principle that he states in the following terms:

Adjust the parameters of the mind in proportion to the extent to which their adjustment can produce a reduction in the discrepancy between expected and observed events.

Such adjustments are, as he points out, exactly what are called for by the back-propagation algorithm, which Hinton explains in his chapter and also uses in his relationship-learning network.

**Where we are**

Everyone seems to agree that we would dearly like to have more theorems about what can or cannot be learned by PDP networks, and what architectures are required for the acquisition of given sorts of skill. In the past the computational modelling of cognitive skills (Longuet-Higgins 1987) has been carried out in languages designed for serial rather than parallel computers, but such work is not necessarily outdated by a shift of emphasis in the direction of PDP. The issue is, in any case, less a matter of principle than of implementation. In the meantime it is surely to be hoped that the art of PDP modelling will soon mature into a computational technique at least as reliable and versatile as more conventional methods of cognitive modelling.

**Acknowledgements**

My thanks are due to Stuart Sutherland and David Willshaw for useful comments, and to the Royal Society and the Science and Engineering Research Council for research support.

## References

Hinton, G. E. and Anderson, J. A. (eds.) (1981). *Parallel models of associative memory.* Erlbaum, Hillsdale, N.J.

Hinton, G. E. and Sejnowski, T. J. (1983). Optimal perceptual inference. *Proceedings of the IEEE Conference on Computer Vision Pattern Recognition*, 448–53. IEEE Computer Society Press, Silver Spring, Maryland.

Longuet-Higgins, H. C. (1987). *Mental processes: studies in cognitive science.* MIT Press, Cambridge, Mass.

Marr, D. (1969). A theory of cerebellar cortex. *Journal of Physiology (Lond)* **202**, 437.

Minsky, M. and Papert, S. (1969). *Perceptrons.* MIT Press, Cambridge, Mass.

Newell, A., Shaw, J. C. and Simon, H. A. (1960). A variety of intelligent learning in a general problem solver. In *Self-organizing systems*, (eds. M. C. Yovits and S. Cameron) pp. 153–189. Pergamon Press, London.

Rosenblatt, F. (1962). *Principles of neurodynamics.* Spartan, New York.

Rumelhart, D. E. and McClelland, J. L. (1986). *Parallel distributed processing.* MIT Press, Cambridge, Mass.

Rumelhart, D. E., Hinton, G. E., and Williams, R. J. (1986). *Nature (Lond.)* **323**, 533.

Willshaw, D., Buneman, O. P., and Longuet-Higgins, H. C. (1969). A non-holographic model of associative memory. *Nature (Lond.)* **222**, 960–67.

Willshaw, D. J. (1972). A simple network capable of inductive generalization. *Proceedings of the Royal Society of London B* **182**, 233–47.

# 2

## Parallel distributed processing: implications for cognition and development[1]
### JAMES L. McCLELLAND

### Introduction

What kind of processing mechanism is the mind? Is it a sequential information processing machine, like the von Neumann computer? Or is it a massively parallel processor? The fact that human thought takes place in a device consisting of some tens of billions of neurons seems to support the parallel view. Yet until recently, there has been little attention to this fact among those who study the higher mental processes, and little convergence in the study of mind and brain.

Feldman (1981) has pointed out that the human brain places constraints on the methods that might be used to implement human thought. Neurons are relatively sluggish, noisy processing devices, compared to today's computers. Yet people can perceive a visual scene at a glance and recognize an object in about half a second. Feldman estimates that this leaves time for perhaps a hundred processing steps; but sequential algorithms for perception generally require hundreds of thousands. The facts imply that we exploit the brain's obvious capacity for parallel processing.

In view of this, researchers have begun to work toward theories of mental processes that rely on these parallel capabilities. These models are variously known as parallel distributed processing (PDP) models, neural models, or, perhaps most generally, connectionist models. Work is proceeding in several directions. Cognitive scientists seeking to provide a characterization of the nature of human thought have turned to building computational models in which a number of interconnected processors work in concert in performing some information processing task. Meanwhile, neuroscientists seeking to understand the functional properties of neural circuits are also building computational models, exploring the collective properties of ensembles of neuron-like processing units. These enterprises often have somewhat different goals; yet each informs and enriches the other, and each is pursued with the hope that someday these two directions of research will converge upon a shared understanding of brain and mind.

In this chapter, I take primarily a congitive perspective. First, I review the connectionist framework, stressing how basic aspects of cognition—representation, processing, knowledge, and learning—are captured in the connectionist framework. Next, the framework is applied to fundamental questions about the development of human thought, and some of the implications that the framework has for basic questions about cognition and development are illustrated.

## The connectionist framework

The term 'connectionist models' was introduced by Feldman (1981; Feldman and Ballard 1982). In these papers, the term was used to refer to a class of models that compute by way of connections among simple processing units. Another phrase often used to describe some connectionist models is *parallel distributed processing* or PDP models (Rumelhart, McClelland, and the PDP Research Group 1986; McClelland, Rumelhart, and the PDP Research Group 1986). PDP models are instances of connectionist models that stress the notion that processing activity results from the processing interactions occurring among rather large numbers of processing units.

In this article I intend the phrase 'the connectionist framework' to encompass all kinds of connectionist models. The framework may be thought of as providing a set of general assumptions about basic aspects of information processing, and a set of soft constraints on the range of specific assumptions that might be made. In what follows I consider each of several aspects of an information processing system. I describe the general assumptions connectionist models make about these aspects and I characterize some of the specific assumptions that might be made. The presentation draws heavily on Rumelhart, Hinton, and McClelland (1986), which can be consulted for further details.

## Primitives and their organization

Like all cognitive models, connectionist models must propose some building blocks and some organization of these building blocks. In connectionist models, the primitives are *units* and *connections*. Units are simple processing devices which take on activation values based on a weighted sum of their inputs from the environment and from other units. Connections provide the medium whereby the units interact with each other; they are weighted, and the weights may be positive or negative, so that a particular input will tend to excite or inhibit the unit that receives it, depending on the sign of the weight (we shall return to these matters when we consider the dynamics of processing below).

Any particular connectionist model will make assumptions about the number of units, their pattern of connectivity to other units, and their interactions with the environment. These assumptions define the architecture of a connectionist model. The set of units and their connections is typically called a *network*.

It should be noted that a very wide variety of architectures is possible. Two are shown in Figs 2.1 and 2.2. One of these, in Fig. 2.1 (from the distributed

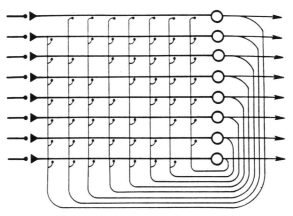

**Fig. 2.1**  A fully connected autoassociator network, with connections from each unit to every other unit. Each unit receives input from outside the network, and sends output outside the network. All connections may be either positive or negative in this very general formulation. (From J. L. McClelland and D. E. Rumelhart, 1985, 'Distributed memory and the representation of general and specific information', *Journal of Experimental Psychology: General*, **114**, 162. Copyright 1985 by the American Psychological Association. Reprinted by Permission.)

model of memory examined by McClelland and Rumelhart 1985) shows a set of completely interconnected units, each receiving input from the environment, and each projecting back to the environment. In some sense, the network in this diagram is the most general possible connectionist architecture, in that all others involve restrictions of this general case. For example, some units may receive no input from the environment; some may send no output outside the net; and some of the interconnections among units in the network may be deleted. There may, furthermore, be restrictions on the values of some of the connections. In the general case, each may be positive or negative, but the architecture may prescribe, for example, that a certain group of units have mutually inhibitory connections of fixed strength.

Figure 2.2 gives an example of a more restricted architecture, from the interactive activation model of visual word recognition (McClelland and Rumelhart 1981). In this model, units stand for hypotheses about displays of letter strings at each of three levels of description: a feature level, a letter level, and a word level. There are excitatory connections (in both directions)

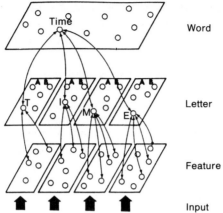

**Fig. 2.2**   A sketch of the network used in the interactive activation model of visual word recognition (McClelland and Rumelhart 1981). Units within the same rectangle stand for incompatible alternative hypotheses about an input pattern, and are mutually inhibitory. Bi-directional excitatory connections between levels are indicated for one word and its constituents. (From J. L. McClelland, 1985, 'Putting knowledge in its place: a scheme for programming parallel processing structures on the fly', *Cognitive Science*, **9**, 115. Copyright 1985 by Ablex Publishing. Reprinted by permission.)

between mutually consistent units on adjacent levels, and inhibitory connections between mutually inconsistent units within the same level. Thus the unit for T in the first letter position excites and is excited by the units for features of the letter T, as well as the units for words that begin with T. This unit also inhibits, and is inhibited by, units for other letters in the same letter position.

### Active representation

Representations in connectionist models are patterns of activation over the units in the network. In some ways, these kinds of patterns are similar to representations in other frameworks; after all, representations in a computer are ultimately patterns of 0s and 1s. There are differences, however. For one thing it is quite natural for connectionist representations to be graded, in the sense that each unit's activation need not be one of two binary values. In some models, activations are restricted to binary or some other number of discrete values, but more typically each unit may take on a continuous activation value between some maximum and minimum. A more important difference is this: connectionist representations are truly active, in the sense that *they give rise to further processing activity directly*, without any need for a central processor or production-matching-and-application mechanism that examines them and takes action on the basis of the results of this examination.

Models differ in terms of the extent to which individual processing units can be identified with particular conceptual objects, such as letters, words, concepts, etc. The models illustrated in Figs 2.1 and 2.2 represent endpoints on a continuum. In the distributed model of memory, each conceptual object is thought of as a pattern of activation over a number of simple processing units. In the interactive activation model of word perception, on the other hand, each unit stands for a primitive conceptual object, such as a letter, a word, or a distinct visual feature. A large number of models lie between these two extremes (see Hinton, McClelland, and Rumelhart 1986, and Feldman 1988, for general discussions of the issue of distributed representation).

**Processing**

Processing in connectionist models occurs through the evolution of patterns of activation over time. This process is governed by assumptions about the exact way in which the activations of units are updated, as a function of their inputs. Updating can be synchronous (all units updated simultaneously) or asynchronous (units updated in random order). Updating generally occurs as follows. First, a *net input* is computed for each unit to be updated. The net input is the sum of the activations of all of the units that project to it, with each contributing activation weighted by the weight on the connection from the contributing unit to the receiving unit.[2] The net input may also include a *bias* term associated with the unit, as well as a term for input arising from outside the network. Thus for unit $i$, the net input is given by:

$$net_i = \sum_j w_{ij}a_j + bias_i + input_i.$$

Here $j$ runs over all the units with connections projecting to unit $i$. The net input can then be used to set the new activation of the unit according to some monotonic but non-linear function such as the one shown in Fig. 2.3. Alternatively, the net input can be used to set the activation of the unit probabilistically to one of two discrete values (usually 1 or 0). Another possibility is that the net input may act as a force, tending to drive the activation of the unit up or down a small amount in each time step.[3]

It is typical to use some form of non-linear activation function, so that the activation of a unit is not simply set equal to the net input or some weighted average of the net input and the previous activation of the unit. Non-linearities are typically necessary for two reasons. 1. Linear networks are subject to explosive growth of activation due to positive feedback loops unless the weights are severely constrained (see Shrager, Hogg, and Huberman 1987). 2. Many computations require a layer of non-linear units between input and output. Without non-linearities, multiple layers of units add no additional

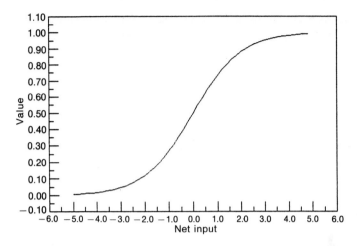

**Fig. 2.3**    The logistic function, a smooth non-linear function that is frequently used in relating activations of units to their net inputs. This function is often used to set the activation of a unit to a value between 0 and 1, or to set the activation of the unit to 1 or 0 probabilistically, with the probability determined by the value of the function.

computational power over that offered by a single layer (see Rumelhart, Hinton, and McClelland 1986, for further explanation).

## Knowledge

Crucial to the very idea of cognition is the notion that information processing is guided by knowledge. We recognize the word THE as a definite article because of knowledge we have about the relation between letter strings and linguistic forms. We infer that a spoon may have been used if we hear 'the man stirred the coffee' because of knowledge we have about the kinds of instruments that are used for stirring. In many models, these kinds of knowledge would be stored in tables. For example, information about THE would be stored in a table called a lexicon, listing correspondences of letter strings and the linguistic objects they represent.

In connectionist models, knowledge is stored in the connections among the processing units. This assumption works together with the assumptions that connectionist models make about representations. An active representation on a set of units, together with the knowledge stored in connections, will give rise to new patterns of activation on the same or on other units.

Typically in connectionist models, connection strengths are real-valued. In models whose connections are set by assumption, it is typical to assume homogeneity of connection strengths as much as possible, to avoid excessive degrees of freedom. In models that learn, however, connection strengths are typically allowed to take on whatever values the learning process gives them; parsimony arises from the use of a homogeneous principle of learning.

**Learning**

If knowledge is in the connection weights, learning must occur through the adjustment of these weights. This weight adjustment process is assumed to occur as a by-product of processing activity. Some knowledge can in fact be built into connectionist models, in the form of initial connection strengths, before there has been any learning, but it is common to explore the limits of what can be acquired through connection strength adjustment with minimal pre-wiring. The initial architecture of the network serves to impose constraints on the learning process; these can in many cases greatly facilitate learning and generalization, if these constraints are appropriate to the problem the network is given to learn.

A wide variety of 'learning rules' for tuning connections has been proposed. A recent review is provided by Hinton (in press). Generally, these rules state that the adjustment that is made to each connection should be based on the product of a 'pre-synaptic' term, associated with the unit that is sending input through the connection, and a 'post-synaptic' term, associated with the unit that is receiving input through the connection. For example, the *Hebb rule*, as used by Anderson (1977), makes the change in the strength of a connection proportional to the product of the activation of the sending unit and the receiving unit.[4] Learning through connection strength adjustment is very different from learning processes in most other types of models. It is governed by simple mathematical expressions, and results in knowledge that is completely implicit, in that it is embedded inextricably in the machinery of processing, and is completely inaccessible to introspection or report. However, it should be noted, that while the connection changes themselves are not accessible, the patterns of activation whose construction they make possible can be accessible to other parts of the processing system.

**The environment**

Though it has been implicit in what I have said already, there is another aspect of connectionist models that deserves comment, namely their *environment*. The environment consists of an ensemble of possible patterns that might be presented to the network. In most cases, these patterns are thought of as separate events; each one presented when the network is in a resting state, then left on until processing is complete. However, input patterns can have a richer temporal structure, or course; each event may consist of a sequence of events, or of a graded progression of input activations.

For networks with fixed connections, the environment simply defines the domain of inputs on which the network might be tested. For networks in which the connections are adjusted as a result of processing experience, however, the environment plays a crucial role in determining exactly what is learned. Thus models that aim to capture aspects of cognitive development through connectionist learning include among their assumptions a specification of the details of the experience that gives rise to the resulting developmental sequence. In many cases, these assumptions play a major role in determining the success or failure of the modelling effort.

## The spirit of the thing

The connectionist framework is cast, not as a list of specific detailed assumptions, but as a set of *general principles* and some guidelines that provide weak constraints on the range of variants that fall within the scope of these principles. Indeed, as Rumelhart, Hinton, and McClelland (1986) noted, it is possible to build a von Neumann computer out of connectionist primitives, if they are organized in accordance with the von Neumann architecture. It thus becomes important to focus on the spirit of the connectionist framework. Generally, connectionist models of cognitive processes have been constructed expressly to exploit the capability for parallelism inherent in the approach, to make use of the graded capabilities of patterns of activation, and to capture the incremental nature of human learning in many tasks through the adjustment of connection strengths based on signals arising in the course of processing.

## The microstructure of cognition

Finally, it is worth pointing out that the connectionist framework is not incompatible with other levels of description in cognitive science. Thus, there is nothing inconsistent with connectionist models in the claim that a cognitive system may traverse a sequence of states in a temporally extended cognitive task such as solving an arithmetic problem. According to the connectionist approach one would tend to view each such step in the process of solving the problem as a new state of the processing network. Indeed, Rumelhart *et al.* (1986) describe a network that performs a mental tic-tac-toe simulation, settling into a sequence of states representing the results of the successive mentally simulated moves made by each player.

There are important differences between conventional and connectionist models of sequential behaviour. In connectionist models, the states need not be so discrete as they generally are in other models (Rumelhart and Norman 1982; Jordan 1986; Smolensky 1986). Furthermore, the powerful constraint–satisfaction characteristics inherent in the connectionist framework are not typically exploited by conventional models of sequential processing. The idea that each step is a sequential process involves a massively parallel constraint–satisfaction process seems like a promising starting place for a new way of thinking about the macrostructure of cognition.

The point that connectionist models characterize the microstructure of cognition applies not only in respect of time, but also in respect of the structure of the processing system and in respect of the description of the computational operations that the system is performing. Structurally, a processing system may consist of many parts, and for some purposes it may be adequate to describe its structure in terms of these parts and the flow of information between them. Computationally, too, it may often be useful and illuminating to describe what a part of such a system computes without referring specifically to the role in this computation that is played by the specific units and connections. The claim is, though, that it will be necessary to delve more deeply than this to provide a full description of the mechanisms of cognition.

**Are connectionist models mere implementations?**

In allowing that there may be a macrostructure to thought, connectionists may seem to suggest that their models merely describe the implementation details of a processing system that would be best characterized more abstractly. However, we simply do not know exactly what level of description is the appropriate one for characterizing many behavioural phenomena. Many who have turned to connectionist models have done so because these models have seemed to provide exactly the right level of description for characterizing certain kinds of cognitive processes. Just where the bounds of usefulness of the connectionist framework may lie seems at this point to be one of the very open questions. Since there is little in cognitive psychology that we understand perfectly at present, we are not in a position to say which aspects of cognition might be explainable without recourse to a model of the microstructure.

**Connectionist models and cognitive development**

In the preceding part of this chapter, I have tried to give an overview of the connectionist framework for cognitive modelling. Here, I consider the question: Does the connectionist framework have any implications for the answers that we give to basic questions about human cognition? I will argue that it does. The questions are ones that arise within the field of cognitive development; they are motivated by dramatic behavioural phenomena. Several different kinds of answers have been given to these questions. We will see how the connectionist framework opens them anew and suggests what may be different answers in many cases.

## The phenomena

The field of cognitive development is replete with examples of dramatic changes in children's thinking as they grow older. Here I give three examples: (1) failures of conservation and compensation; (2) progressive differentiation of knowledge about different kinds of things; and (3) U-shaped learning curves in language acquisition.

### *Failures of conservation and compensation*

Perhaps the best-known phenomena in cognitive development are the dramatic failures of conservation that Piaget has reported in a wide range of different domains. One domain is the domain of liquid quantity. A child of 3 years is shown two glasses of water. The glasses are the same, and each contains the same amount of water, and the child sees that the amount is the same. But when the contents of one of the glasses is poured into a wider container, the child will say that there is less liquid in the wider container.

It is typical to say that this answer given by the young child reflects a failure to recognize two things: (1) that quantity is conserved under the transformation of pouring from one container to another; and (2) that greater width can compensate for less height. Many tasks are specifically designed to tap into the child's ability to cope with these kinds of compensation relations between variables.

One such task developed by Inhelder and Piaget (1958), the so-called *balance-beam task*, is illustrated in Fig. 2.4. In this task, the child is shown a

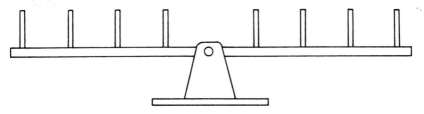

**Fig. 2.4** Balance beam of the kind first used by Inhelder and Piaget (1958), and later used extensively by Siegler (1976, 1981; Siegler and Klahr 1982). (Reprinted from Siegler 1976, Fig. 1, with permission.)

balance beam with pegs placed at evenly spaced intervals to left and right of a fulcrum. On one peg on the left are several weights; on one peg on the right are several weights. The beam is immobilized, and the child is asked to judge which side will go down, or whether they will balance. We will have occasion to examine performance in this task at length below; for now it suffices to note that young children (up to about 6 or 7 years in this case) typically respond as if the distance from the fulcrum was completely irrelevant. They will say the beam should balance if the weight is the same on both sides, regardless of distance. Otherwise they say the side with the greater weight will go down. These children, then, appear to miss the fact that lesser weight can be compensated for by greater distance. Typically by the age of 11 years or so children have some appreciation for this trade off; the details of the developmental progression are quite interesting, as we shall see below.

*Progressive differentiation of ontological categories*

Other researchers, studying different domains, have noticed other kinds of developmental progressions. Keil (1979) studied children's judgements about whether you could say things like 'A rabbit is an hour long'. He supposed such judgements tapped children's knowledge about different kinds of things. In these judgements, Keil was interested not in whether the child saw a sentence as true or false, but in whether the child felt that one could make certain kinds of predictions (e.g. that something is an hour long) when the something is a member of a certain 'ontological category' (e.g. living thing). Keil found that children were much more permissive in their acceptance of statements than adults were, but their permissiveness was not simply random. Rather, children would accept statements that overextended predicates to categories near the ones that they typically apply to, but would not extend them further. Thus some children will accept predications like 'The rock is asleep', but not 'The rock is an hour long'. It was as though children's knowledge of what predicates apply to particular categories becomes progressively more and more differentiated, as illustrated in Fig. 2.5.

*U-Shaped learning curves in language development*

Early on, children often get certain kinds of linguistic constructions correct which they later get wrong; only much later do they recover their former correct performance. One example is the passive construction, applied to semantically biased materials, such as 'The man was bitten by the dog'. (See Bever, 1970, for a discussion of the development of the use of the passive construction.) Early in development, children correctly interpret such sentences; they appear to be using information about what roles the different

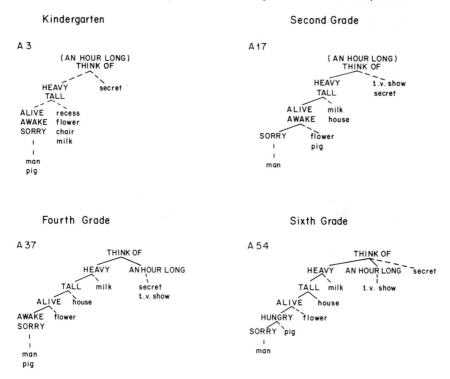

**Fig. 2.5**   Four different 'predictability trees' illustrating the progressive differentiation of concepts as a function of age. Terms in capitals at internal nodes in the trees represent predicates, and terms in lower case at terminal nodes in the trees represent concepts that are spanned by all the predicates written on nodes that dominate the terminal. A predicate spans a concept if the child reports that it is not silly to apply either the predicate or its negation or both to the concept. Thus the first tree indicates that the child will accept 'The man is (not) alive', and 'The chair is (not) tall', but will not accept 'The chair is (not) alive'. Parentheses indicate uncertainty about the application of a predicate. (Redrawn from Keil, 1979, Appendix C, with permission.)

nouns typically play in the action described by the verb, since they tend to be correct only when the correct interpretation assigns the nouns to their typical roles. At an older age, children respond differently to such sentences, treating the first noun-phrase as the subject; semantic constraints are over-ridden, and there is a tendency to interpret 'The man was bitten by the dog' as meaning 'The man bit the dog'. Finally, children interpret the sentence correctly again, but for a different reason. It would appear that they now understand passives in general, since at this stage they can also interpret semantically neutral and even reverse-biased sentences (such as 'The dog was bitten by the man') correctly.

## The questions

The phenomena reviewed above raise basic questions about cognitive development. Three of these questions are:

1. Are these different phenomena simply unrelated facts about development in different domains?
2. Are there principles that all of these phenomena exemplify?
3. If there are principles, are they domain specific, or are they general principles about development?

Different kinds of developmental theorists have answered such questions in very different ways. To Piaget, each failure of compensation or conservation reflected a single common developmental stage; the phenomena were intrinsically related by the characteristics of the stage, and these characteristics provided the basis for explanation.

Others have taken a very different approach. Keil (1979), following Chomsky's analogous argument for language, argues for *domain specific principles* of development. His view is that each cognitive domain has its own laws that provide constraints on what can be learned. These constraints limit the hypotheses that the child can entertain, thereby making it dramatically easier for the child to acquire adult abilities in the face of the impoverished information that is provided by experience with the world.

The main thrust of the remainder of this chapter is to argue that recent developments in connectionist learning procedures suggest a dramatic alternative to these kinds of views. The alternative is simply the hypothesis that these diverse developmental phenomena all reflect the operation of a single basic learning principle, operating in different tasks and different parts of the cognitive system.

## The learning principle

The principle can be stated in fairly abstract terms as follows:

*Adjust the parameters of the mind in proportion to the extent to which their adjustment can produce a reduction in the discrepancy between expected and observed events.*

This principle is not new. It might well be seen as capturing the residue of Piaget's accommodation process, in that accommodation involves an adjustment of mental structures in response to discrepancies. (See Flavell, 1963, for a discussion of Piaget's theory.) It is also very similar to the principle that governs learning in the Rescorla–Wagner model of classical conditioning (Rescorla and Wagner 1972). What is new is that there exists a learning procedure for multilayer connectionist networks that implements this principle. Here, the parameters of the mind are the connections among the units in the network, and the procedure is the back-propagation procedure of Rumelhart, Hinton, and Williams (1986; see Hinton, this volume).

The learning principle lies at the heart of a number of connectionist models that learn how to do various different kinds of information processing tasks, and that have applications to phenomena in cognitive and/or language development. Perhaps the simplest such model is the past-tense model of Rumelhart and McClelland (1986). The development of that model pre-dated the discovery of the back-propagation learning procedure, thereby forcing certain simplifications for the sake of developing an illustration of the basic point that lawful behaviour might emerge from the application of a simple principle of learning to a connectionist network. Subsequent models have used back-propagation to overcome some of these limitations. Included in this class are NETtalk (Sejnowski and Rosenberg 1987) and a more recent model of word reading (Seidenberg, Patterson, and McClelland, this volume). The present effort grew out of two observations of similarities between the developmental courses seen in models embodying this principle, and the courses of development seen in children: First, the course of learning in a recent model of concept learning by Rumelhart (in preparation) is similar to aspects of the progressive differentiation of concepts reflected in Keil's (1979) studies of predictability. Second, the course of learning in a recent model of sentence comprehension by St John and McClelland (1988) mirrors aspects of the progression from reliance on semantic constraints, to reliance on word order, to, finally, reliance on complex syntactic patterning such as the passive voice. I do not mean to claim that the models in question are fully adequate models of the developmental progression in either case; I only claim that they seemed suggestive: they raised the possibility that part of the explanation of these and other developmental phenomena might be found in the operation of the learning principle as it adjusts connection strengths in a network subjected to patterns arising in its environment.

The remainder of this chapter presents an experiment assessing the applicability of this conjecture to another developmental phenomenon, namely the acquisition of the ability to take both weight and distance into account in the balance beam task described above. The task has been studied extensively by Siegler and his colleagues (Siegler 1976, 1981; Siegler and Klahr 1982), and quite a bit is known about it. I will first review the developmental findings. Then I will describe a connectionist model that captures these phenomena by applying the learning principle stated above.

**Development of judgements of balance**

In an important monograph, Siegler (1981) studied children's performance in the balance beam task and three other tasks in which two cues had to be taken into account for correct performance. In all cases, as in the balance beam task, the correct procedure requires multiplication. For example, in the balance beam task, to determine which side will go down, one must multiply the amount of weight on a given side of the beam by the distance of that weight from the fulcrum. The side with the greater product will go down; when the products are the same, the beam will balance.

Siegler studied children in several age groups, as well as young adults. Each child was asked to judge 24 balance problems. In each case, the beam was immobilized so that there was no feedback. The 24 problems could be divided into four of each of six types:

1. *Balance*. In this class of problem, the weight is the same on both sides of the beam and the weight is the same distance from the fulcrum on both sides.
2. *Weight*. In these problems, the weights differ but distance from the fulcrum is the same on both sides.
3. *Distance*. Here the weight is the same on both sides, but the distance from the fulcrum differs.
4. *Conflict*. Here both weight and distance differ and are in conflict, in that the weight is greater on one side but the distance from the fulcrum is greater on the other. There are three types of conflict problems:
   (a) conflict-weight. In these cases, the side with the greater weight has the greater torque (i.e. the greater value of the product of weight times distance).
   (b) conflict-distance. In these cases, the side with the greater distance has the greater torque.
   (c) conflict-balance. Here the torques are the same on both sides.

Siegler's analysis of children's performance assumed that children use rule-governed procedures. Four such procedures or *rules* as Siegler called them are shown in Fig. 2.6. Each of these rules corresponds to a distinct pattern of performance over the six problem types. For example, children using Rule 1 should say the side with the greater weight will go down in weight problems and in all three types of conflict problems. They should think the beam will balance on balance problems and distance problems. In general, the mapping from the rules to expected performance is extemely straightforward. The only point that needs explication is the instruction *muddle through* when weight and distance conflict in Rule 3. In practice it is assumed to mean 'guess randomly among the alternatives', so that $\frac{1}{3}$ of the responses would be left-side-down; $\frac{1}{3}$ right-side-down, and $\frac{1}{3}$ balance.

Siegler compared the performance of each child tested with each rule, and counted discrepancies from predicted performance based on the rule. Children who scored less than four discrepancies from a given rule were scored as using that rule.

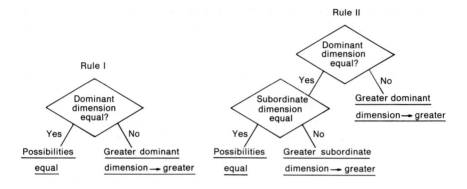
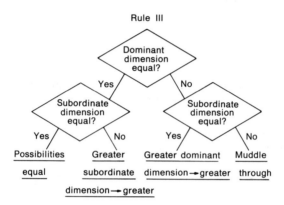
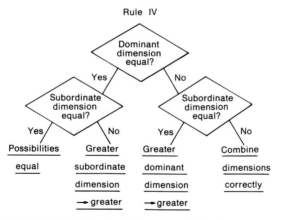

**Fig. 2.6**  Siegler's (1976, 1981) four 'rules' for answering balance beam problems. Each rule is in fact a full procedure, rather than a single rule. (Reprinted with permission from Siegler (1981), Fig. 1.)

For our purposes, there are four basic findings that emerge from Siegler's analysis:

1. *Lawful behaviour*. In general, performance of children over the age of 5 years is extremely regular in the balance beam task. Overall, about 90 per cent of children tested conform to one of the four rules.

2. *Developmental progression*. As children get older, they appear to progress through the use of the different rules. The progression from Rule 1 to Rule 3 can be thought of as a progression in which at first the weight cue is relied on exclusively, while at the end distance and weight are both taken into account. In between (Rule 2), distance is taken into account only if it does not conflict with the weight cue. Children aged 5–7 years typically use Rule 1, and college students typically use Rules 3 or 4. Many college students do not have explicit knowledge of the torque principle. Children younger than age 5 years tend not to be scorable strictly in terms of one of the rules; however, they appear to show an increasing tendency to behave in accordance with Rule 1.

3. *Generality*. The same four rules appear to be adequate to characterize performance in all three of the domains that Siegler studied. Though the developmental progression was not identical across cases, there was in all cases a trend from simpler to more complex rules with development.

4. *Lack of correlation between domains*. Even though children seem to progress through the same rules in different domains, they do not do so in lock-step; the correlation across domains is low, particularly in terms of the higher-numbered rules, so that children who are showing Rule 3 behaviour in one task may be showing Rule 1 behaviour in another and Rule 4 in a third.

**The simulation model**

The model I have developed to capture Siegler's findings is sketched in Fig. 2.7.[5] Of course, the model is a drastic oversimplification of the human mind and of the task; but as we shall see it allows us to capture the essence of Siegler's findings, and to see them emerge from the operation of the learning principle described above.

The model consists of a set of input units, to which balance problems can be presented as patterns of inputs; a set of output units, over which the answer to each problem can be represented; and a set of hidden units, between the input and the output. Connections run from input units to hidden units and from hidden units to output units.

The input units can be divided into two groups of 10. One group is used to

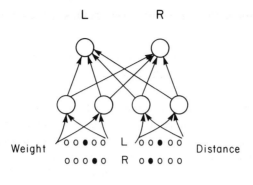

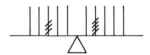

**Fig. 2.7**    The network used in the simulation of the development of performance in the balance beam task.

represent information about weight and the other is used to represent information about distance. In each case I have chosen to use an input representation that imposes as little structure as possible on the input patterns. Each possible value of weight or distance from the fulcrum is assigned a separate unit. The ordering of values from low to high is not given in this representation; the network will have to learn this ordering. For the convenience of the reader, the units are arranged in rows according to which side of the beam they are from, and within each row they are arranged from left to right in order of increasing weight or distance from the fulcrum; but this ordering is unknown to the model before it is trained, as we shall see.

Though the two dimensions are not intrinsically structured for the model, the design of the network does impose a separate analysis of each dimension. This separation turns out to be critical; I will consider the implications of this architectural simplification below. The separation is implemented as follows: there are separate pairs of hidden units for each dimension. Two hidden units receive input from the weight input units and two receive input from the distance input units.

Each of the four hidden units projects to each of the two output units. The left output unit can be thought of as a 'left-side-down' unit, and the right one as a 'right-side-down unit'. Thus a correct network for the task would turn on the output unit corresponding to the side with the greater torque, and would turn off the unit for the other side. For balance problems, I assume that the network should turn both units on half-way. Note that this coding of the output patterns does tell the network that balance is between left-side-down and right-side-down.

*Processing*
Balance problems of the kind studied by Siegler can be processed by the network by simply turning on (i.e. setting to 1) the input units corresponding to a particular problem and turning off (i.e. setting to 0) all other input units. The input from the problem illustrated in Fig. 2.7 is shown by using black to indicate those input units whose activations are 1.0, and white for the units whose activations are 0.

The inputs are propagated forward to the hidden units. Each hidden unit simply computes a net input:

$$net_i = \sum_j w_{ij}a_j + bias_i.$$

Here $j$ ranges over the input units. Each hidden unit then sets its activation according to the logistic function:

$$a_i = \frac{1}{1+e^{-net_i}}$$

In these equations, $w_{ij}$ is the strength of the connection to hidden unit $i$ from input unit $j$, $a_j$ is the activation of input unit $j$, and $bias_i$ is the modifiable bias of hidden unit $i$. This bias is equivalent to a weight to unit $i$ from a special unit that is always on.

Once activations of the hidden units are determined, the activations of the output units are determined by the same procedure. That is, the net input to each output unit is determined based on the activations of the hidden units, the weights from the hidden units to the output units, and the biases of the output units. Then the activations of the output units are determined using the logistic function.

*Responses*
The activations of the output units are real numbers between 0 and 1; to relate the model's performance to the balance beam task, these real-valued outputs must be translated into discrete responses. I used the following simple translation: if the activation of one output unit exceeded the activation of the other by 0.333, I took the answer to be 'more active side down'. Otherwise, the answer was assumed to be 'both sides equal'.

*Learning*
Before training begins, the strengths of these connections from input to hidden units and from hidden to output units are initialized to random values uniformly distributed between $+0.5$ and $-0.5$. In this state, inputs lead to

random patterns of activity over both the hidden and output units. The activations of the output units fluctuate approximately randomly between about 0.4 and 0.6 for different input patterns. The network comes to respond correctly only as a result of training. Conceptually, training is thought of as occurring as a result of a series of experiences in which the network is shown a balance problem as input; computes activations of output patterns based on its existing connection weights; and is then shown the correct answer. The signal that drives learning is the difference between the obtained activation of each output unit and the correct or target activation for that unit. The back-propagation procedure of Rumelhart, Hinton, and Williams (1986) is then used to determine how each connection strength in the network should be adjusted to reduce these differences. The procedure is described in Hinton's chapter in this volume, and it would be redundant to describe it here. Suffice it to say that it exactly implements the learning principle stated above, and restated here in network terminology:

*Adjust each weight in the network in proportion to the extent to which its adjustment can produce a reduction in the discrepancy between the expected event and the observed event, in the present context.*

Here the 'expected event' is the pattern of activation over the output units that is computed by the network; the observed event is the pattern of activation that the environment indicates these units have; and the present context is the pattern of activation over the input units.Note that the direction of change to a connection (positive or negative) is simply the direction that tends to reduce the discrepancy between computed output and the correct or target output.

*Environment*

As I pointed out at the beginning of this chapter, the environment in which a network learns plays a very strong role in determining what it learns, and particularly the developmental course of learning. The simulations reported here were based on the assumption that the environment for learning about balance problems consists of experiences that vary more frequently on the weight dimension than they do on the distance dimension. Of course, I do not mean to suggest that all the learning that children do and that is relevant to their understanding of balance takes the form of explicit balance problems of the kind my network sees. Rather, my assumption that the experience on balance problems is dominated by problems in which there is no variability in weight is meant as a proxy for the more general assumption that children generally have more experience with weight than with distance as a factor in determining the relative heaviness of something.[6] The specific assumptions about the sequence of learning experiences were as follows. The environment consisted of a list of training examples containing the full set of 625 possible problems involving 25 combinations of possible weights (1–5 on the left crossed with 1–5 on the right) crossed with 25 combinations of possible distances (1–5 steps from the fulcrum on the left crossed with 1–5 steps from the fulcrum on the right). Two corpuses were set up. Problems in which the distance from the fulcrum was the same on both sides were listed five times each in one corpus, and 10 times each in the other corpus. Other problems were listed only once in each corpus.

*Training and testing regime*
Four simulation runs were carried out, two with each of the two corpora just described. In each run, training consisted of a series of epochs. In each epoch, 100 patterns were chosen randomly from the full list of patterns in the corpus. In each epoch, weight increments were accumulated over the 100 training trials and then added into the weights at the end of the epoch, according to the momentum method described in Rumelhart, Hinton, and Williams (1986, p. 330); parameters were $\eta = 0.075$, $\alpha = 0.9$).

After weight updating at the end of each epoch, the network was given a 24-item test, containing four problems of each of the six types described above, taken from an experiment of Siegler's. (A few of the examples had to be modified since Siegler's experiment had used up to six pegs.)

*A comment on the simulation model*

The model described above obviously simplifies the task that the learner faces and structures it for him to some degree. In particular, it embodies two principal assumptions which are crucial to the successful simulations we will consider below:

1. *Environment assumption.* The model assumes that the environment is biased, so that one dimension—in this case weight—is more frequently available as a basis for predicting outcome than the other.
2. *Architecture assumption.* The model assumes that the weight and distance dimensions are analysed separately, before information about the two dimensions is combined.

Both these assumptions are crucial to the success of the model. In an unbiased environment, both cues would be learned equally rapidly. Effects of combining the cues from the start, as prescribed by the architecture assumption, are more complex, but suffice it to say for now that the apparent stagelike character of performance is much less clear unless this assumption is adopted.

An important topic for further research will be to examine what variants of these assumptions might still allow the model to be successful. For example, regarding the environment, differences in salience (i.e. strength of input activations) and structuredness of the dimensions might also produce similar results.

The issue of structuredness of the dimensions is a key point that needs to be considered as it relates to the present simulation. For both dimensions, the input representations encode different weights and distances from the fulcrum using distinct units. This means that different values are distinguishable by the model, but they are not structured for it; for example, the input itself provides no indication that a distance or weight of 3 is between 2 and 4. The network must learn to represent the weights and distances in structured ways in order to solve the balance problem. Below we will see that it does so.

*Results*

In general, performance of the model conformed to one of the four rules described by Siegler. Over the four runs, the model fit the criteria of one of Siegler's four rules on 85 per cent of the occasions, not counting an initial, pre-Rule 1 period discussed below (in Siegler, 1981, the conformity figure is about 90 per cent). Of course, the model was not consulting these rules or following the step-by-step procedures indicated in them; rather its behaviour was simply scorable by Siegler's criteria as consistent with the succession of rules. Excluding the initial period, failures to fit the rules were of three types: (1) cases in which a rule fit except for a position bias that gave difficulty on balance problems; (2) cases in which performance was borderline between Rules 1 and 2; and (3) combinations of these two problems. (Siegler (personal communication) does find some borderline cases between Rule 1 and Rule 2, but the position bias cases are not typical of children's performance.)

*Overall development trends*
Epoch by epoch performance in each of the four runs is shown in Figs 2.8 and 2.9. One generally observes the expected developmental progression. Each simulation run is slightly different, due to differences in the random starting weights and the sequence of actual training experiences, but there are clear common trends. Over the first 10 epochs or so, the output of the model was close to 0.5 on all test patterns; by our scoring criteria, all these outputs count as 'balance' responses, but of course they really represent a stage in which neither weight nor distance governs performance. The next few epochs represent a transition to Rule 1, in that in this phase the model is showing some tendency to activate the output unit on the side with the greater weight, but this tendency is variable across patterns and the discrepancy between the activations of the output units is not reliably greater than 0.33 when the weights differ.

After this brief transition, performance of the model had generally reached the point where it was responding consistently to the weight cue while

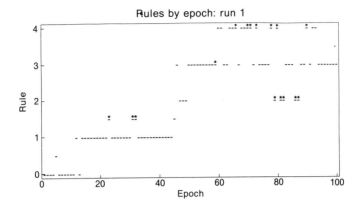

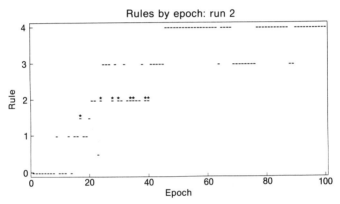

**Fig. 2.8**   Epoch-by-epoch performance of the simulation model in the two runs with a 5 to 1 bias favouring problems in which distance did not vary. Performance is scored by rule. Cases marked by ∗ missed a rule due to position bias. Rule 0 corresponds to always saying 'balance', and occurs at the beginning of training. Rule 1.5 corresponds to performance on the borderline between Rules 1 and 2.

systematically ignoring the distance dimension. This pattern continued for several more epochs. There was a brief transitional period, in which the model behaved inconsistently on the *distance* problems crucial to distinguishing between Rule 1 and Rule 2 behaviour. After several epochs in this phase, use of the distance cue reached the point where performance on all types of conflict problems become variable. The model generally continued in this phase indefinitely, sometimes reaching the point where its performance was generally scorable as fitting Rule 4 and sometimes not.

The variability in the model's performance from epoch to epoch is actually

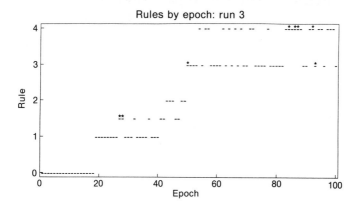

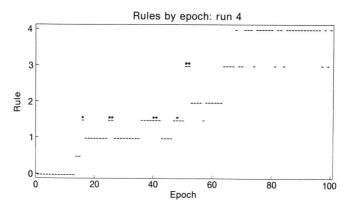

**Fig. 2.9**  Epoch-by-epoch performance of the simulation model in the two runs with a 10 to 1 bias favouring problems in which distance did not vary. Performance is scored by rule, as in Fig. 2.8.

quite consistent with test–re-test data reported in Siegler (1981). Rule 2 behaviour is highly unstable, and there is some instability of behaviour in other rules as well.

*Performance in each phase*
Seigler's criteria for conformity to his rules allow for some deviations from perfect conformity; in fact only 83 per cent of test problems must be scorable as consistent with the rule. Given this, it is interesting to see whether the discrepancies from the rules that are exhibited by the model are consistent with human subects' performances. In general, they seem to be quite consistent, as

Fig. 2.10 indicates. Each panel shows percentage correct performance by the model averaged over the tests on which the model scored in accordance with one of the four rules. Also shown are data from two groups of human subjects as well as the pattern of performance that would be expected from a perfect rule user.

For Rule 1, the model differs very little from human data. For Rule 2, again the correspondence to human data is very close. Both the model and the humans show some slight tendency to get *conflict-distance* problems correct, and to occasionally miss *distance* and *balance* problems. For both Rule 1 and Rule 2, the tendency to miss *balance* problems is slightly greater in the model than in the children's data. For Rule 3, the model exaggerates a tendency seen in the human data to be correct on *conflict-weight* problems more often than on *conflict-distance* problems. The major discrepancy in the data is that the model is too accurate on *conflict-balance* problems. For Rule 4, the model again exaggerates a tendency seen in the human data to have residual difficulties with conflict problems.

With the exception of the *conflict-balance* problems in Rule 3, the human data seem to fall about half-way between the model and perfect correspondence to the rules. It is tempting to speculate that some human subjects—particularly Rule 4 subjects—may in fact use explicit rules such as the torque rule some of the time. It is, indeed, easy for the adult subjects who contribute to the Rule 4 results to follow the torque rule if instructed specifically in this rule. However, it is evident that the subjects who fall under the Rule 4 scoring criteria do not in fact adhere exactly to the rule. Perhaps this group includes some individuals performing on the basis of implicit knowledge of the trade-off of weight and distance as well as some who explicitly use the torque rule, and perhaps some individuals use a mixture of the two strategies.

*Further correspondences between the model and child development*
So far we have seen that the balance beam model captures the pattern of development seen in the studies of Siegler (1976, 1981). There are two further aspects of the developmental data which are consistent with the gradual buildup of strength on the distance dimension that we see in the model:

1. Wilkening and Anderson (in press) present subjects with one side of a balance beam, and allow them to adjust the weight on the other side at a fixed distance from the fulcrum to make the beam balance. Over the age range of 9–20 years, in which children are generally progressing from late Rule 1 or Rule 2 to Rule 3 or Rule 4, according to Siegler's methods, they find an increasing sensitivity to the distance cue. Unfortunately, it is difficult to be sure whether this reflects different numbers of subjects relying on the distance cue, or (as we see in the model) differences in degree of reliance among those who show some sensitivity to the distance cue.

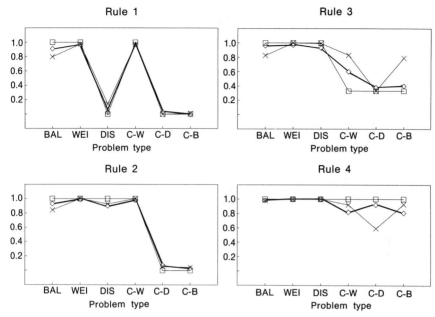

**Fig. 2.10**   Children's performance by problem type on the balance beam task, together with the performance of the simulation model and expected performance based on each rule. The heavy line with diamonds indicates children's performance. The model's performance is given by the light line with × s, while performance predicted from the rule is given by the light line with squares. For each child and each test of the simulation, performance was pre-categorized according to the best-fitting rule. Then, percentage correct responses by problem type were calculated averaging over children or simulation tests falling into each rule.

2.  For children who exhibit Rule 3 on Siegler's 24-item test, careful assessment with a larger number of conflict problems indicates the use of cue compensation strategies, rather than random guessing (Ferretti *et al.* 1985). Thus children are not simply totally confused about conflict problems during this stage but have some sensitivity of relative magnitudes of cues, as does the model. The exact degree of correspondence of the model's performance and human performance on these larger tests remains to be explored.

*The mechanism for developmental change*
Given the generally close correspondence between model and data, it is important to understand just how the model performs, and how its performance changes. To do this, it is helpful to examine the connections in the network at several different points in the learning process: Figure 2.11 displays

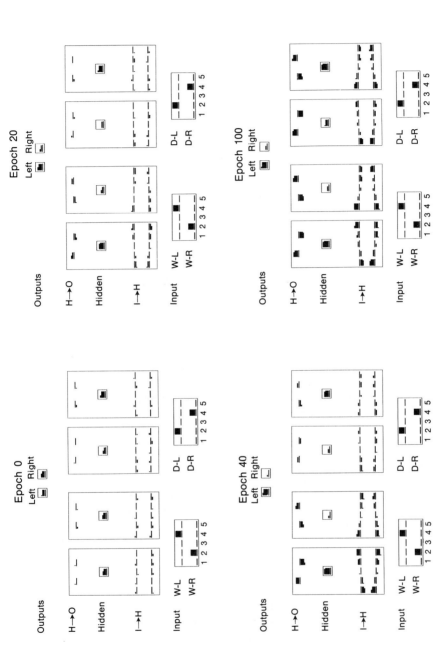

**Fig. 2.11** Connection strengths into $(I \rightarrow H)$ and out of $(H \rightarrow O)$ each of the hidden units, at each of four different points during training. Activations of input, hidden, and output units are also shown, for a conflict balance problem, in which there are two weights on peg 4 on the left and four weights on peg 2 on the right. Magnitude of each connection is given by the size of the blackened area. Sign is indicated by whether the blackened area extends above or below the horizontal baseline. Note that activations are all positive, and range from 0 to 1. The connection strengths range between +6 and −6. See text for further explanation.

the connections from the run that produced the results shown in the top panel of Fig. 2.9, at four different points during learning. At epoch 0, before any learning; at epoch 20, early in the Rule 1 phase; at epoch 40, at the end of the Rule 1 phase; and at epoch 100, when the simulation was terminated. Each of the four subrectangles in each panel shows the weights coming into and out of one of the four hidden units. The two on the left receive input from the weight dimension, and the two on the right receive input from the distance dimension.

In the first panel, before learning begins, all the connection strengths have small random values. In this situation, the output of the hidden units is not systematically related to magnitudes of the weights or distances, and is therefore of no use in predicting the correct output. At this point, the hidden units are not encoding either relative weight or relative distance, and are therefore providing no useful information for predicting whether the left or right side should go down.

The first phase of learning consists of the gradual organization of the connections that process the amount of weight on each side of the balance beam. Recall that the network receives problems in which the distance cue varies much less frequently than problems in which the weight cue varies. Learning to rely on the weight cue proceeds more quickly than learning to rely on the distance cue as a simple result of this fact. The rate of learning with respect to each type of cue is relatively gradual at first, but then speeds up, for reasons that we will explore below. The relatively rapid transition from virtually unresponsive output to fairly strong reliance on the weight cue represents the brief transition to Rule 1 responding. The result of this phase, in the second panel of the diagram, is a set of connections that allow the hidden units on the left to reflect the relative amount of weight on the left v. the right side of the balance beam. The leftmost hidden unit is most strongly excited by large weights on the left and small weights on the right, and most strongly inhibited by large weights on the right and small weights on the left. The activation of this unit, then, ranges from near 0 to near 1 as the relative magnitude of weight ranges from much more on the right to much more on the left. Correspondingly, this unit has an excitatory connection to the left-side-down output unit, and an inhibitory connection to the right-side-down output unit. The second hidden unit mirrors these relationships in reverse. At this point, then, the hidden units can be said to have learned to represent something they were not representing before, namely the relative magnitude of the inputs. Note that this information is not explicitly contained in the inputs, which simply distinguish but do not order the different possible values of weight on the two sides of the balance beam.

At this point, the connection strengths in the distance part of the network remain virtually unchanged; thus, at the hidden unit level, the network has not yet learned to encode the distance dimension.

Over the next 20 epochs, connections get much stronger on the weight dimension, and we begin to see some organization of the distance dimension. While this is going on, the overt behaviour of the network remains Rule 1 behaviour. The network is getting ready for the relatively rapid transition to Rule 2 and then to Rule 3 which occurs over the next several epochs of training (as shown in the top panel of Fig. 2.9), but at epoch 40, the end of the Rule 1 phase, the distance connections are still not quite strong enough to push activations of the output units out of the balance range. With further learning, the distance cue becomes stronger and stronger; this first causes the distance cue to govern performance when the weights are in balance, giving rise to Rule 2 behaviour. Further strengthening causes the distance cue to win out in some conflict problems, giving rise to behaviour consistent with Rules 3 and 4. At epoch 100 of this particular run, the weight dimension maintains a slight ascendancy, so that with the *conflict-balance* problem illustrated, the model activates the left-side-down unit most, corresponding to the side with the greater weight.

A couple of aspects of the developmental progression deserve comment. Learning is slow at first and then accelerates, as shown in Fig. 2.12. As the diagram illustrates, the connection strengths are largely insensitive to differences early on, then go through a fairly rapid transition in sensitivity, and then level off again. The acceleration seen in learning is a result of an inherent characteristic of the gradient descent learning procedure coupled with the architecture of the network. The procedure adjusts each connection in proportion to the magnitude of the effect that adjusting it will have on the discrepancy between correct and actual output. But the effect of a given connection depends on the strengths of other connections. Consider the connection coming into a hidden unit from one of the input units. An adjustment of the strength of this input connection will have a small effect on the output if the connections from the hidden unit to the output units are weak. In this case, the input connection will only receive a small adjustment. If, however, the connections from the hidden units to the output units are strong, an adjustment of the strength of the input connection will have a much larger effect; consequently the learning procedure makes a much larger adjustment in this case. A slightly different story applies to the connections from the hidden units to the output units. When the connections from the input to the hidden units are weak and random, the activations of the hidden units are only weakly related to the correct output. Under these circumstances, the adjustments made to the output weights tend to cancel each other out, and learning progress is very slow. It is only after the input weights become organized that learning can proceed efficiently on the output side of the hidden units.

The story I am telling would be a very sad one, were it not for the fact that it is not all or none. It is not that there is *no* learning at all at first; if there were, there would be no gradual change to the point where learning becomes more rapid. Rather, it is simply that initially learning is *very* gradual; so gradual that

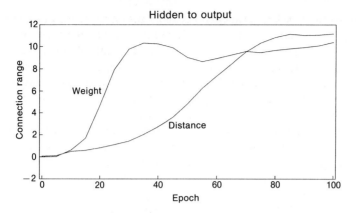

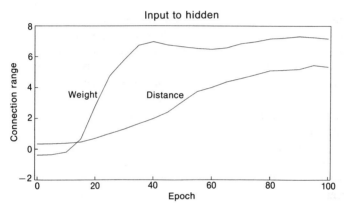

**Fig. 2.12**   Relative magnitude of connection strengths encoding weight and distance, as a function of training. Magnitude is given by the range of connection strengths (most positive minus most negative) coming into one weight or distance hidden unit (lower panel) and coming out of a weight or distance unit (upper panel).

it does not show up in overt behaviour. Gradually, though, this initially slowly learning accelerates, producing an increasing readiness to learn.

This differential readiness to learn allows the model to account for the results of an experiment described in Siegler and Klahr (1982), on the effects of training for young v. old Rule 1 children. They showed 5- and 8-year-old Rule 1 children a series of conflict problems. The children were allowed to try to predict which side would go down, and were then shown what actually happens. The results were striking. The older Rule 1 children were very likely to exhibit Rule 2 behaviour on a post-test. The younger children either continued to behave in accordance with Rule 1 or became inconsistent in their responses. In further experiments on early Rule 1 children, Siegler and Klahr reported that these children do not represent the distance dimension correctly: when asked to reproduce a balance beam configuration, they could usually get the number of weights correct, but could rarely place them on the correct pegs. These findings are in complete conformity with the model: as we have seen, the model does not represent distance information early in Rule 1. Further simulations reported in McClelland and Jenkins (in preparation) show that the model can profit from conflict training of the sort used by Siegler and Klahr at the end of the Rule 1 phase but not at the beginning.

*Shortcomings of the model*

The model exhibits a striking correspondence with many aspects of the developmental facts, but does have a few shortcomings. Three failures to fit aspects of Siegler's data must be acknowledged. First, the model can never actually master Rule 4, though some subjects clearly do. Second, its behaviour during Rule 3 is slightly different from that of humans (though it should be noted that the 'human' Rule 3 pattern is actually a mixture of different strategies according to Klahr and Siegler 1978). Third, it can exhibit position biases which are uncharacteristic of humans, who seem (at least, from the age of 5 years on) to 'know' that there is no reason to prefer left over right.

There are other shortcomings as well. Perhaps the most serious is in the input representations, that use distinct units to represent different amounts of weight and distance. This representation was chosen because it does not inherently encode the structure of each dimension, thereby forcing the network to discover the ordering of each dimension. But it has the drawback that it prevents the network from extrapolating or even interpolating beyond the range of the discrete values that it has experienced.

Finally, Siegler has reported protocol data that indicate that subjects are often able to describe what they are doing verbally in ways that correspond fairly well to their actual performance. It is not true that all subject's verbalizations correctly characterize the rule they are using, but it is true, for example, that subjects who are sensitive to the distance cue mention that they are using this cue and those who are not tend not to mention it. The model is of course completely mute.

What are we to make of these shortcomings in the light of the overall success of the model? Obviously, we cannot take it as the final word on development of ability to perform the balance scale task. I would suggest that the model's shortcomings may lie in two places: first, in details of the encoding of inputs and of the network architecture; and second, in the fact that the model only deals with acquisition of implicit knowledge.

Regarding the first point, it would be reasonable to allow the input to encode similarity on each dimension by using input representations in which each unit responded to a range of similar values so that neighbouring weights and distances produced overlapping input representations; furthermore, the inputs could well make use of a relative code of magnitude to keep values within a fixed range. This would probably overcome the interpolation and extrapolation problems (I have no stand on whether such codings are learned or pre-wired).

These kinds of fixes would not allow the model to truly master Rule 4. This is as it should be, since I believe Rule 4 (unlike the other rules) can only be adhered to strictly as an explicit (arithmetic) rule. Indeed, it must be acknowledged that there is a conscious, verbally accessible component to the problem-solving activity that children and adults engage in when they confront a problem like the balance beam problem. The model does not address this activity itself. However, it is tempting to imagine that the model captures the gradual acquisition mechanisms which establish the possible contents of these conscious processes. One can view the model as making available representations of differing salience as a function of experience; these representations might serve as the raw material used by the more explicit reasoning processes that appear to play a role. This is of course sheer speculation at this point. It will be an important part of the business of my ongoing exploration of cognitive development to make these speculations explicit and testable.

## Implications of the balance simulation

The model captures several of the more intriguing aspects of cognitive development. It captures a stage-like character, while at the same time exhibiting an underlying continuity which accounts for gradual change in readiness to move on to the next stage. It captures that fact that behaviour can often seem very much to be under the control of very simple and narrow rules (e.g. Rule 1), yet to exhibit symptoms of gradedness and continuity when tested in different ways. It captures the fact that development, in a large number of different domains, progresses from an initial over-focusing on the most salient dimension of a task or problem—to the point where other dimensions are not even encoded—followed by a sequence of further steps in which the reliance on the initially unattended dimension gradually increases.

As mentioned previously, the model can be seen as implementing the accommodation process that lies at the heart of Piaget's theory of developmental change. Accommodation essentially amounts to adjusting mental structures to reduce the discrepancy between observed events and expectations derived from the existing mental structures. According to Flavell (1963), Piaget stressed the continuity of the accommodation process, in spite of the overtly stage-like character of development, though he never gave a particularly clear account of how stages arise from continuous learning (see Flavell 1963, pp. 244–9 for a description of one attempt). The model provides such a description: it shows clearly how a continuous accommodation-like process can lead to a stage-like progression in development.

*Changes in representation and attention through the course of development*
When a balance beam problem is presented to the model, it sees it in different ways, depending on its developmental state. At all times, information is in some sense present in the input for determining what is the correct response. However, at first this information produces no real impression; weak, random activations occur at the hidden level and these make weak, random impressions at the output level. At the beginning of the Rule 1 behavioural phase, the model has learned to represent the relative amount of weight. The pattern of activation over the hidden units captures relative weight, since one unit will be more activated if there is more weight to the right, and the other will be more activated if there is more weight to the left; both units take on intermediate activations when the weights balance. At this point, we can see the model as encoding weight, but not distance, information. Indeed, as we have seen at this point the network could be said to be ignoring the distance cue; it makes little impact on activation, and learning about distance is very slow at this point. At the end of the Rule 1 phase, in spite of its lack of impact on overt behaviour, the network has learned to represent relative distances; at this point it is extremely sensitive to feedback about distance; it is ready to slip over the fairly sharp boundary in performance between Rule 1 and Rule 2. Thus, we can see the Rule 1 stage as one in which overt behaviour fails to mirror a gradual developmental progression that carries the model from extreme unreadiness to learn about distance at the beginning of this phase to a high degree of readiness at the end.

This developmental progression seems to resolve the apparent paradoxical relation between observed stage-like behavioural development and assumed continuity of learning. To me this is the most impressive achievement of the model: it provides a simple, explicit alternative to maturational accounts of stage-like progression in development.

It must be noted, however, that the success of the model depends crucially on its structure. In fact the results are less compelling if either of the following changes are made: (1) if balance is treated as a separate category, rather than being treated as the intermediate case between left-side-down and right-side-down; and (2) if the connections from input to hidden units are not restricted as they are here so that weight is processed separately from distance before the two are combined.

More generally, it is becoming clear that architectural restrictions on connectionist networks are crucial if they are to discover the regularities we humans discover from a limited range of experiences (Denker *et al.* 1987;

Rumelhart, in preparation). This observation underscores that fact that the learning principle, in itself, is not the only principle that needs to be taken into account. There probably are additional principles that are exploited by the brain to facilitate learning and generalization. Just what these additional principles are and the extent to which they are domain-specific remains to be understood in more detail.

Extending this observation a step further, we can see the connectionist framework as a new paradigm in which to explore basic questions about the relations of nature and nurture. We may find that successful simulation of developmental processes depends on building in domain-specific constraints in considerable detail; if so this would support a more nativist view of the basis of domain-specific skills. On the other hand, it may turn out that a few other general principles in addition to the learning principle are sufficient to allow us to capture a wide range of developmental phenomena. In this case we would be led toward a much more experience-based description of development. In either case, it seems very likely that connectionist models will help us take a new look at these important basic questions.

## Conclusions

The exploration of connectionist models of human cognition and development is still at an early stage. Yet, already, these models have begun to capture a new way of thinking about processing, about learning and, I hope the present paper shows, about development. Several further challenges lie ahead. One of these is to build stronger bridges between what might be called cognitive-level models and our evolving understanding of the details of neuronal computation. Another will be to develop more fully the application of congitive models to higher-level aspects of cognition. The hope is that the attempt to meet these and other challenges will continue to lead to new discoveries about the mechanisms of human thought and the principles that govern their operation and adaptation to experience.

## Notes

1. The author would like to thank Eric Jenkins for showing the way toward a connectionist model of learning to perform the balance beam task. Thanks are due as well to Robert Siegler and Dave Klahr for useful discussions. This research was supported by ONR contracts N00014-86-K-0167 and N00014-86-K-0678, as well as NIMH Career Development Award MH00385.
2. In a slightly more general formulation, the net input may be the sum of *products* of the activations of groups of contributing units. In this formulation there is a weight

associated with each product, rather than each individual contributing activation. These product terms have no special computational significance, since the effects of multiplicative interactions among inputs can be accomplished by extra layers of units; see Williams (1986).

3. Some variants of connectionist models (e.g. Grossberg 1978) treat the excitatory and inhibitory inputs as separate forces, rather than aggregating them together in a single term.

4. The Hebb rule is about the simplest connectionist learning rule, and it is limited in what it can do, so it has recently been somewhat less popular than other learning rules (but see Linsker 1986a, b, and c). Three learning rules frequently used in current connectionist models are the *competitive learning rule*, the *delta rule* or *least-mean-squared procedure*, and the *generalized delta rule* or *back-propagation procedure* (see Hinton 1987, for details).

5. This model builds on an earlier model of stage transitions in the balance beam task by Jenkins (1986). I am indebted to Eric for indicating the applicability of connectionist models to cognitive development.

6. An alternative assumption which might account for the developmental data just as well is the assumption that the weight dimension is pre-structured before the child comes to consider balance problems, while the distance dimension is not. The assumption that distance varies less frequently than weight but that neither dimension is initially structured allows us to observe the structuring process for both dimensions.

### References

Anderson, J. A. (1977). Neural models with cognitive implications. In *Basic processes in reading perception and comprehension* (eds. D. LaBerge and S. J. Samuels), pp. 27–90. Erlbaum, Hillsdale, NJ.

Bever, T. G. (1970). The cognitive basis for linguistic structures. In *Cognition and the development of language* (ed. J. R. Hayes), pp. 279–362. Wiley & Sons, New York.

Denker, J., Schwartz, D., Wittner, B., Solla, S., Hopfield, J., Howard, R., and Jackel, L. (1987). *Automatic learning, rule extraction, and generalization* (AT&T Bell Labs Technical Report). AT&T Bell Labs., Holmdel, NJ.

Feldman, J. A. (1981). A connectionist model of visual memory. In *Parallel models of associative memory* (eds. G. E. Hinton and J. A. Anderson), pp. 49–81. Erlbaum, Hillsdale, NJ.

Feldman, J. A. (1988). Connectionist representation of concepts. In *Connectionist models and their implications: readings from cognitive science* (eds. D. Waltz and J. A. Feldman), pp. 341–63. Ablex Publishing Corporation, Norwood, NJ.

Feldman, J. A. and Ballard, D. H. (1982). Connectionist models and their properties. *Cognitive Science*, **6**, 205–54.

Ferretti, R. P., Butterfield, E. C., Cahn, A., and Kerkman, D. (1985). The classification of children's knowledge: Development on the balance scale and included plane tasks. *Journal of Experimental Child Psychology*, **39**, 131–60.

Flavell, J. H. (1963). *The developmental psychology of Jean Piaget*. D. Van Nostrand Company, Inc., Princeton, NJ.

Grossberg, S. (1978). A theory of visual coding, memory, and development. In *Formal theories of visual perception* (eds. E. L. J. Leeuwenberg and H. F. J. M. Buffart). Wiley, NY.

Hinton, G. E. this volume.

Hinton, G. E. (in press). Connectionist learning procedures. *Artificial Intelligence.*

Hinton, G. E., McClelland, J. L., and Rumelhart, D. E. (1986). Distributed representations. In *Parallel distributed processing: explorations in the microstructure of cognition. Volume I* (eds. D. E. Rumelhart, J. L. McClelland, and the PDP research group). Bradford Books, Cambridge, Mass.

Inhelder, B. and Piaget, J. (1958). *The growth of logical thinking from childhood to adolescence.* Basic Books. NY.

Jenkins, E. A., Jr (1986). Readiness and learning: a parallel distributed processing model of child performance. Pittsburgh, PA: Carnegie-Mellon University, Psychology Department, 15213.

Jordan, M. I. (1986). Attractor dynamics and parallelism in a connectionist sequential machine. *Proceedings of the Eighth Annual Conference of the Cognitive Science Society.* Amherst, Mass.

Keil, F. C. (1979). *Semantic and conceptual development: an ontological perspective.* Harvard University Press, Cambridge, Mass.

Klahr, D. and Siegler, R. S. (1978). The representation of children's knowledge. In *Advances in child development and behavior* (eds. H. W. Reese and L. P. Lipsitt), pp. 61–116. Academic Press, NY.

Linsker, R. (1986a). From basic network principles to neural architecture: emergence of spatial opponent cells. *Proceedings of the National Academy of Sciences USA,* **83,** 7508–12.

Linsker, R. (1986b). From basic network principles to neural architecture: emergence of orientation-selective cells. *Proceedings of the National Academy of Sciences USA,* **83,** 8390–4.

Linsker, R. (1986c). From basic network principles to neural architecture: emergence of orientation columns. *Proceedings of the National Academy of Sciences USA,* **83,** 8779–83.

McClelland, J. L. (1985). Putting knowledge in its place: a scheme for programming parallel processing structures on the fly. *Cognitive Science,* **9,** 113–46.

McClelland, J. L., Jenkins, E. A., Jr (in preparation). Emergence of stages from incremental learning mechanisms: a connectionist approach to cognitive development. In *Architectures for Intelligence* (ed. K. van Lehn). Erlbaum, Hillsdale, NJ.

McClelland, J. L. and Rumelhart, D. E. (1981). An interactive activation model of context effects in letter perception: Part 1. An account of basic findings. *Psychological Review,* **88,** 375–407.

McClelland, J. L. and Rumelhart, D. E. (1985). Distributed memory and the representation of general and specific information. *Journal of Experimental Psychology: General,* **114,** 159–88.

McClelland, J. L., Rumelhart, D. E., and the PDP research group. (1986). *Parallel distributed processing: explorations in the microstructure of cognition,* Volume II. Bradford Books, Cambridge, Mass.

Rescorla, R. A. and Wagner, A. R. (1972). A theory of Pavlovian conditioning:

variations in the effectiveness of reinforcement and non-reinforcement. In *Classical conditioning* II: *current research and theory* (eds. A. H. Black and W. F. Prokasy). Appleton-Century-Crofts, NY.

Rumelhart, D. E. (in preparation). *Generalization and the learning of minimal networks by back propagation.*

Rumelhart, D. E. and McClelland, J. L. (1986). On learning the past tenses of English verbs. In *Parallel distributed processing: explorations in the microstructure of cognition*, Volume II (eds. J. L. McClelland, D. E. Rumelhart, and the PDP research group). Bradford Books, Cambridge, Mass.

Rumelhart, D. E. and Norman, D. A. (1982). Simulating a skilled typist: a study of skilled cognitive-motor performance. *Cognitive Science*, **6**, 1–36.

Rumelhart, D. E., Hinton, G. E., and McClelland, J. L. (1986). A framework for parallel distributed processing. In *Parallel distributed processing: explorations in the microstructure of cognition*, Volume I (eds. D. E. Rumelhart, J. L. McClelland, and the PDP research group). Bradford Books, Cambridge, Mass.

Rumelhart, D. E., Hinton, G. E., and Williams, R. J. (1986). Learning internal representations by error propagation. In *Parallel distributed processing: explorations in the microstructure of cognition*, Volume I (eds. D. E. Rumelhart, J. L. McClelland, and the PDP research group). Bradford Books, Cambridge, Mass.

Rumelhart, D. E., McClelland, J. L., and the PDP research group. (1986). *Parallel distributed processing: explorations in the microstructure of cognition*. Volume I. Bradford Books, Cambridge, Mass.

Rumelhart, D. E., Smolensky, P., McClelland, J. L., and Hinton, G. E. (1986). Parallel distributed processing models of schemata and sequential thought processes. In *Parallel distributed processing: explorations in the microstructure of cognition*, Volume II (eds. J. L. McClelland, D. E. Rumelhart, and the PDP research group). Bradford Books, Cambridge, Mass.

St. John, M. F. and McClelland, J. L. (1988). *Learning and applying contextual constraints in sentence comprehension.* (AIP Technical Report). Carnegie Mellon University, Departments of Computer Science and Psychology, and University of Pittsburgh, Learning Research and Development Center, Pittsburgh, PA.

Seidenberg, M. S., Patterson, K. E., and McClelland, J. L. this volume.

Sejnowski, T. J. and Rosenberg, C. R. (1987). Parallel networks that learn to pronounce English text. *Complex Systems*, **1**, 145–68.

Shrager, J., Hogg, T., and Huberman, B. A. (1987, May). Observation of phase transitions in spreading activation networks (behavioral change as topology of spreading activation network). *Science*, **236**, 1092.

Siegler, R. S. (1976). Three aspects of cognitive development. *Cognitive Psychology*, **8**, 481–520.

Siegler, R. S. (1981). Developmental sequences within and between concepts. *Monographs of the Society for Research in Child Development*, **46** (189), 1–74.

Siegler, R. S. and Klahr, D. (1982). When do children learn? The relationship between existing knowledge and the acquisition of new knowledge. In *Advances in instructional psychology*, Volume 2 (ed. R. Glaser), pp. 121–211. Erlbaum, Hillsdale, NJ.

Smolensky, P. (1986). Information processing in dynamical systems: foundations of harmony theory. In *Parallel distributed processing: explorations in the microstructure of cognition*, Volume I (eds. D. E. Rumelhart, J. L. McClelland, and the PDP research group). Bradford Books, Cambridge, Mass.

Wilkening, F. and Anderson N. H. (in press). Representation and diagnosis of knowledge structures. In *Contributions to information integration theory* (ed. N. H. Anderson).

Williams, R. J. (1986). The logic of activation functions. In *Parallel distributed processing: explorations in the microstructure of cognition*, Volume I (eds. D. E. Rumelhart, J. L. McClelland, and the PDP research group). Bradford Books, Cambridge, Mass.

# 3

## Learning distributed representations of concepts
### GEOFFREY E. HINTON

**Two simple theories of neural representation**

There have been many different proposals for how conceptual information may be represented in neural networks. These range from extreme localist theories in which each concept is represented by a single neural unit (Barlow 1972) to extreme distributed theories in which a concept corresponds to a pattern of activity over a large part of the cortex. These two extremes are the natural implementations of two different theories of semantics. In the structuralist approach, concepts are defined by their relationships to other concepts rather than by some internal essence. The natural expression of this approach in a neural net is to make each concept be a single unit with no internal structure and to use the connections between units to encode the relationships between concepts. In the componential approach each concept is simply a set of features and so a neural net can be made to implement a set of concepts by assigning a unit to each feature and setting the strengths of the connections between units so that each concept corresponds to a stable pattern of activity distributed over the whole network (Hopfield 1982; Kohonen 1977; Willshaw, Buneman, and Longuet-Higgins 1969). The network can then perform concept completion (i.e. retrieve the whole concept from a sufficient subset of its features). The problem with componential theories is that they have little to say about how concepts are used for structured reasoning. They are primarily concerned with the similarities between concepts or with pairwise associations. They provide no obvious way of representing articulated structures composed of a number of concepts playing different roles within the structure.

**Role-specific units**

One way of using neural nets to implement articulated structures of the kind shown in the semantic net formalism in Fig. 3.1(a) is to assign a group of neural units to each possible role and to make the pattern of activity of the units in that group represent the concept that fills the role (Hinton 1981). Each unit then represents the conjunction of a role with a feature of the concept filling that role (e.g. a unit might be active *iff* the agent is male). A proposition can then be represented by a stable combination of role fillers as shown in Fig. 3.1(b). This is a fundamentally different method of representation than either of the two more obvious methods described above. It has the interesting property that the very same concept will have quite different representations when it is playing different roles. The use of multiple different representations of the same concept appears to be a serious flaw for two reasons. First, it appears to be uneconomical. Second, it is not clear how we know that John in the representation of 'John hit Mary' has anything to do with the John in the representation of 'Mary divorced John'.

The economic considerations are complex. The 'obvious' way to represent that John is the agent of a certain proposition is to combine a canonical representation of John with a canonical representation of agent. In Lisp, for example, a symbolic expression like (agent john) would be an obvious representation and a whole proposition might be represented by the expression ((agent john) (relation hit) (patient mary)). Alternatively, the roles might be implicitly represented by the position of an element in a list and so the whole proposition could be represented by (hit john mary). Either way, the very same symbol is used for John whatever role he plays in the proposition. In logic and in computer programming, the standard way of representing conjunctions is by composing symbolic expressions out of individual symbols. Given a conventional general purpose computer memory, it is easy to store arbitrary compositions of symbols.

If, however, we want to be able to retrieve a proposition from a partial description of its contents, the advantage of always using the very same representation for John is less clear. If the partial description includes the information that John is the agent, we would like this to pick out just those propositions which have John as agent. This is more specific than the propositions which have an agent and also have John in some role. It is the conjunction of John with agent that forms the retrieval cue, and so in a neural implementation it would make sense to have a specific representation for this conjunction. This conjunctive representation can then cause the effects required for completing the whole pattern of activity that represents the proposition. So, even if there is a representation in which John and agent are represented separately, it may be necessary to form a conjunctive representation for retrieval.

A similar argument can be made in other domains. In representing the graphemic structure of the word 'chip', for example, it would be possible to use a representation such as ((4 p) (2 h) (3 i) (1 c)) but for a task like filling in the blank in 'c-ip' it is inefficient to access all words which contain c and i and p. The identities and roles of the letters need to be conjoined to form more

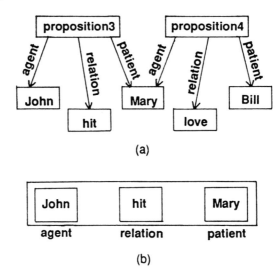

**Fig. 3.1**  (a) Part of a semantic net. (b) Three groups of units which have two *alternative* stable states that represent the two propositions in the semantic net.

specific access cues. This argues that we need quite different neural representations of (1 c) and (4 c). For the purposes of access to the whole word, these representations need have nothing in common.[1] Indeed, parallel network models of reading use separate representations of letters in different positions within the word (McClelland and Rumelhart 1981).

The second problem with role-specific representations is how to recognize the identity of the various different role-specific representations of the same concept. An efficient way to do this is to have a single, canonical representation for each concept and to have a mechanism for translating between role-specific representations and the canonical one. Hinton (1981) shows how this idea can be implemented in a neural net. It will not be discussed further in this paper.

*Choosing the role-specific representations*

From now on, we assume that a concept playing a role within a larger structure is represented by a pattern of activity in a group of role-specific units, and we focus on the issue of how this pattern should be chosen. A simple solution is to use patterns selected at random, perhaps with the additional constraint that no two patterns are too similar. The use of random patterns is quite common in research in this area (Hopfield 1982; Willshaw 1981). It makes analysis easier and it is a sensible default in the absence of any other ideas about representation. However, it entirely eliminates one of the most interesting aspects of distributed representations: the ability to capture the similarity between concepts by the similarity of their representations, and the consequent ability to generalize new information in sensible ways. We illustrate this point in the simple domain of family relationships.

Figure 3.2 shows two family trees. All the information in these trees can be represented in simple propositions of the form (**person1 relationship person2**). These propositions can be stored as the stable states of activity of a neural network which contains a group of units for the role **person1**, a group for the

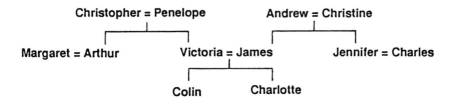

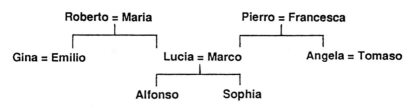

**Fig. 3.2**   Two isomorphic family trees. The symbol '=' means 'married to'.

role **relationship** and a group for the role **person2**. The net may also require further groups of units in order to achieve the correct interactions between the three role-specific groups. Figure 3.3 shows a network in which one further

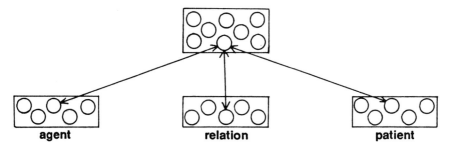

**Fig. 3.3**   An extra group of units can be used to implement higher-order constraints between the role-specific patterns.

group has been introduced for this purpose. Units in this extra group detect combinations of features in the role-specific groups and can be used for causing appropriate completions of partial patterns. Suppose, for example, that one of the extra units becomes active whenever **person1** is old and

**relationship** requires that both people be the same age (e.g. the relationship has-husband in the very conventional domain we use). The extra unit can then activate the unit that represents the feature old within the **person2** group. An extra unit that works in this way will be said to encode a microinference. It uses some of the features of some of the role-fillers to infer some of the features of other role-fillers and it is typically useful in encoding many different propositions rather than just a single one. By dedicating a unit to a microinference that is applicable in many different propositions, the network makes better use of the information carrying capacity of its units than if it dedicated a single extra unit to each proposition. This is an example of the technique of coarse coding described in Hinton, McClelland, and Rumelhart (1986). In describing how a microinference could be implemented, we assumed that there was a single unit within the **person1** group that was active whenever the pattern of activity in that group encoded an old person. This would not be true using random patterns, but it would be true using a componential representation.

Microinferences store propositions by encoding the underlying regularities of a domain. This form of storage has the advantage that it allows sensible generalization. If the network has learned the microinference given above, it will have a natural tendency to make sensible guesses. If, for example, it is told enough about a new person, Jane, to know that Jane is old and it is then asked to complete the proposition (Jane has-husband?) it will expect the filler of the **person2** role to be old. To achieve this kind of generalization of domain-specific regularities, it is necessary to pick a representation for Jane in the **person1** role that has just the right active units so that the existing microinferences can cause the right effects in the other role-specific groups. A randomly chosen pattern will not do.

The real criterion for a good set of role-specific representations is that it makes it easy to express the regularities of the domain. It is sensible to dedicate a unit to a feature like old because useful microinferences can be expressed in terms of this feature. There is another way of stating this point which enables us to avoid awkward questions about whether the network really understands what old means: instead of saying that activity in a unit means that the person is old, we can simply specify the set of people for which the unit is active. Each unit then corresponds to a way of partitioning all the people into two subsets, and good representations are ones for which these partitions are helpful in expressing the regularities. The search for good representations is then a search in the space of possible sets of partitions.[2]

*Giving the network the freedom to choose representations*

The network shown in Fig. 3.3 has the disadvantage that it is impossible to present a proposition to the network without already having decided on the patterns of activity that represent the people and relationships. We would like the network to use its experience of a set of propositions to construct its own internal representations of concepts, and so we must have a way of presenting the propositions which is neutral with respect to the various possible internal representations. Figure 3.4 shows how this can be done. The network

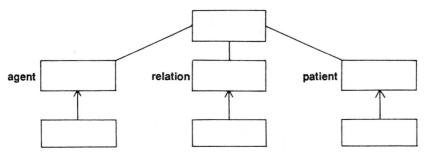

**Fig. 3.4**   The state of each role-specific group can be fixed via a special input group. By varying the weights between the special input groups and the role-specific groups the network can develop its own role-specific representations instead of being forced to use representations that are pre-determined.

translates a neutral input representation in which each person or relationship is represented by a single active unit into its own internal representation before making any associations. In the input representation, all pairs of concepts are equally similar.[3]

## A network that learns distributed representations

In our attempts to show that neural networks can learn sensible distributed representations we have tried several different learning procedures. The most successful of these, so far, is the 'back-propagation' procedure described in Rumelhart, Hinton, and Williams (1986), and the simulation we present uses back-propagation. This learning procedure, which is briefly outlined in the following section, assumes that the units have real-valued outputs between 0 and 1 and which are deterministic functions of their total inputs, where the total input, $x_j$, to unit $j$ is given by

$$x_j = \sum_i y_i w_{ji} \qquad (3.1)$$

A unit has a real-valued output, $y_j$, which is a non-linear function of its total input.

$$y_j = \frac{1}{1+e^{-x_j}} \qquad (3.2)$$

The units are arranged in layers with a layer of input units at the bottom, any number of intermediate layers, and a layer of output units at the top. Connections within a layer or from higher to lower layers are forbidden: all connections go from lower layers to higher ones.

An input vector is presented to the network by setting the states of the input units. Then the states of the units in each layer are determined by applying Equations (3.1) and (3.2) to the connections coming from lower layers. All units within a layer have their states set in parallel, but different layers have their states set sequentially, starting at the bottom and working upwards until the states of the output units are determined.

To use the back-propagation learning procedure we need to express the task of learning about family relationships in a form suitable for a layered network.[4] There are many possible layered networks for this task and so our choice is somewhat arbitrary: we are merely trying to show that there is at least one way of doing it, and we are not claiming that this is the best or only way. The network we used is shown in Fig. 3.5. It has a group of input units for the

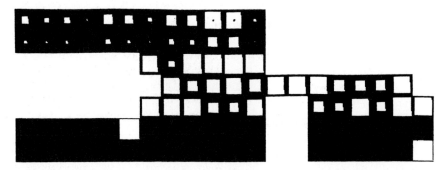

**Fig. 3.5**　The activity levels in a five-layer network after it has learned. The bottom layer has 24 input units on the left for representing **person1** and 12 units on the right for representing the relationship. The white squares inside these two groups show the activity levels of the units. There is one active unit in the first group (representing Colin) and one in the second group (representing has-aunt). Each of the two groups of input units is totally connected to its own group of 6 units in the second layer. These two groups of 6 must learn to encode the input terms as distributed patterns of activity. The second layer is totally connected to the central layer of 12 units, and this layer is connected to the penultimate layer of 6 units. The activity in the penultimate layer must activate the correct output units, each of which stands for a particular **person2**. In this case, there are two correct answers (marked by black dots) because Colin has two aunts. Both the input and output units are laid out spatially with the English people in one row and the isomorphic Italians immediately below.

filler of the **person1** role, and another group for the filler of the **relationship** role. The output units represent the filler of the **person2** role, so the network can only be used to complete propositions when given the first two terms.[5] The states of the units in the input groups are clamped from outside and the network then determines the states of the output units and thus completes the proposition.

For some relationships, such as uncle, there may be several possible fillers for the **person2** role which are compatible with a given filler of the **person1** role. In a stochastic network it would be reasonable to allow the network to chose one of the possibilities at random. In the deterministic network we decided to insist on an output which explicitly represented the whole set of possible fillers. This is easy to do because the neutral representation that we used for the output has a single active unit for each person and so there is an obvious representation for a set of people.

Using the relationships { *father, mother, husband, wife, son, daughter, uncle, aunt, brother, sister, nephew, niece*} there are 104 instances of relationships in the two family trees shown in Fig. 3.2. We trained the network on 100 of these instances. The training involved 1500 sweeps through the 100 examples with the weights being updated after each sweep. The details of the training procedure are given in the following section. After this substantial experience of the domain, the weights were very stable and the network performed correctly on all the training examples: when given a **person1** and a **relationship** as input it always produced activity levels greater than 0.8 for the output units corresponding to correct answers and activity levels of less than 0.2 for all the other output units. A typical example of the activity levels in all layers of the network is shown in Fig. 3.5.

The fact that the network can learn the examples it is shown is not particularly surprising. The interesting questions are: Does it create sensible internal representations for the various people and relationships that make it easy to express regularities of the domain that are only implicit in the examples it is given? Does it generalize correctly to the remaining examples? Does it make use of the isomorphism between the two family trees to allow it to encode them more efficiently and to generalize relationships in one family tree by analogy to relationships in the other?

*The representations*

Figure 3.6 shows the weights on the connections from the 24 units that are used to give a neutral input representation of **person1** to the six units that are used for the network's internal, distributed representation of **person1**. These weights define the 'receptive field' of each of the six units in the space of people. It is clear that at least one unit (unit number 1) is primarily concerned with the distinction between English and Italian and that most of the other units ignore

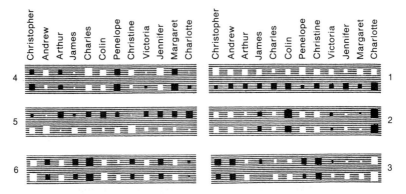

**Fig. 3.6**  The weights from the 24 input units that represent people to the 6 units in the second layer that learn distributed representations of people. White rectangles stand for excitatory weights, black for inhibitory weights, and the area of the rectangle encloses the magnitude of the weight. The weights from the 12 English people are in the top row of each unit. Beneath each of these weights is the weight from the isomorphic Italian.

this distinction. This means that the representation of an English person is very similar to the representation of their Italian equivalent. The network is making use of the isomorphism between the two family trees to allow it to share structure and it will therefore tend to generalize sensibly from one tree to the other.

Unit 2 encodes which generation a person belongs to. Notice that the middle generation is encoded by an intermediate activity level. The network is never explictly told that generation is a useful three-valued feature. It discovers this for itself by searching for features that make it easy to express the regularities of the domain. Unit 6 encodes which branch of the family a person belongs to. Again, this is useful for expressing the regularities but is not at all explicit in the examples.[6]

It is initially surprising that none of the six units encodes sex. This is probably because of the particular set of relationship terms that were used. Each of the 12 relationship terms completely determines the sex of **person2** so the sex of **person1** is redundant. Figure 3.7 shows that one of the six units which encodes the 12 possible relationships is entirely devoted to predicting the sex of **person2**. If we had included relationships like spouse there would have been more pressure to encode the sex of **person1** because this would have been useful in constraining the possible fillers of the **person2** role.

*Microinferences and scientific laws*

There is an interesting analogy between the way in which the network represents propositions and the way in which scientists represent the structure

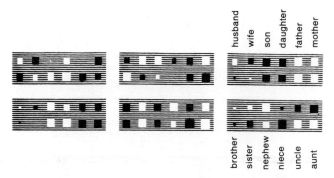

**Fig. 3.7**    The weights from the 12 input units that represent relationships to the 6 units in the second layer that learn distributed representations of the relationships.

of the natural world. In order to express the regularities in the data, a scientist must describe them using appropriate terms. For example, substances with widely different appearances much be grouped together into such categories as 'acid', 'salt', or 'base'. If the appropriate terms are given in advance, the task is much easier than if the terms themselves must be discovered by searching for sets of terms that allow laws to be expressed. The gradient descent procedure used by the network also has its analogue in scientific research. Initial definitions of the descriptive terms can be used to formulate laws and the apparent exceptions can often be used to refine the definitions.

Naturally, there are also many important differences between the way scientists proceed and the way learning occurs in the network. Scientists would not normally be satisfied if their theory consisted of a very large number of statistical 'laws' and they needed a computationally intensive procedure to decide what the laws predicted.

*Generalization*

The network was trained on 100 of the 104 instances of relationships in the two family trees. It was then tested on the remaining four instances. The whole training and testing procedure was repeated twice, starting from different random weights. In one case the network got all four test cases correct and in the other case it got 3 out of 4, where 'correct' means that the output unit corresponding to the right answer had an activity level above 0.5, and all the other output units were below 0.5. In the test cases, the separation between the activity levels of the correct units and the activity levels of the remainder were not as sharp as in the training cases. Figure 3.8 shows the activity levels of all 24 output units for each of the four test cases after training.

Any learning procedure which relied on finding direct correlations between

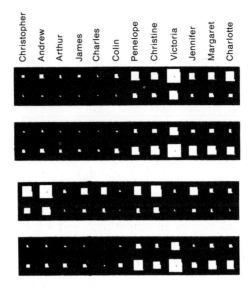

**Fig. 3.8**   The activity levels of the output group in the four test cases that were not shown during training. The dots are on the correct answers. Notice that in every case the network has a slight tendency to activate the isomorphic person in the other family tree.

the input and output vectors would generalize very badly on the family tree task. Consider the correlations between the filler of the **person1** role and the filler of the **person2** role. The filler of **person1** which is used in each of the generalization tests is negatively correlated with the correct output vector because it never occurred with this output vector during training, and it did occur with other output vectors. The structure that must be discovered in order to generalize correctly is not present in the pairwise correlations between input units and output units.

The good generalization exhibited by the network shows that the structure which it has extracted from the training examples agrees with the structure which we attribute to the domain. We would like to be able to say that the training set implicitly contains the information about how to generalize and that the network has correctly extracted this implicit information. But this requires a prescriptive domain-independent theory of how a set of examples should be used for making generalizations. Such a theory would constitute the 'computational level' of understanding for learning research (Marr 1982), and would be a major advance which could guide research at the algorithmic and implementation levels. Unfortunately, we know of no such theory and so we are restricted to showing that the learning procedure produces sensible generalizations in particular domains.

**The back-propagation learning procedure**

The aim of the learning procedure is to find a set of weights which ensure that for each input vector the output vector produced by the network is the same as (or sufficiently close to) the desired output vector. If there is a fixed, finite set of input–output cases, the total error in the performance of the network with a particular set of weights can be computed by comparing the actual and desired output vectors for each case. The error, $E$, is defined as

$$E = \frac{1}{2} \sum_c \sum_j (y_{jc} - d_{jc})^2 \tag{3.3}$$

where $c$ is an index over cases (input–output pairs), $j$ is an index over output units, $y$ is the actual state of an output unit, and $d$ is its desired state. To minimize $E$ by gradient descent it is necessary to compute the partial derivative of $E$ with respect to each weight in the network. This is simply the sum of the partial derivatives for each of the input–output cases. For a given case, the partial derivatives of the error with respect to each weight are computed in two passes. We have already described the forward pass in which the units in each layer have their states determined by the input they receive from units in lower layers using Equations (3.1) and (3.2). The backward pass which propagates derivatives from the top layer back to the bottom one is more complicated.

The backward pass starts by computing $\partial E/\partial y$ for each of the output units. Differentiating Equation (3.3) for a particular case, $c$, and suppressing the index $c$ gives

$$\frac{\partial E}{\partial y_j} = y_j - d_j \tag{3.4}$$

We can then apply the chain rule to compute $\partial E/\partial x_j$:

$$\frac{\partial E}{\partial x_j} = \frac{\partial E}{\partial y_j} \frac{dy_j}{dx_j}$$

Differentiating Equation (3.2) to get the value of $dy_j/dx_j$ gives

$$\frac{\partial E}{\partial x_j} = \frac{\partial E}{\partial y_j} y_j(1 - y_j) \tag{3.5}$$

This means that we know how a change in the total input, $x$, to an output unit will affect the error. But this total input is just a linear function of the states of the lower level units and the weights on the connections, so it is easy to compute how the error will be affected by changing these states and weights. For a weight, $w_{ji}$, from $i$ to $j$ the derivative is

$$\frac{\partial E}{\partial w_{ji}} = \frac{\partial E}{\partial x_j} \frac{\partial x_j}{\partial w_{ji}}$$

$$= \frac{\partial E}{\partial x_j} y_i \tag{3.6}$$

and for the output of the $i$th unit the contribution to $\partial E/\partial y_i$ resulting from the effect of $i$ on $j$ is simply

$$\frac{\partial E}{\partial x_j} \frac{\partial x_j}{\partial y_i} = \frac{\partial E}{\partial x_j} w_{ji}$$

So, taking into account all the connections emanating from unit $i$, we have

$$\frac{\partial E}{\partial y_i} = \sum_j \frac{\partial E}{\partial x_j} w_{ji} \tag{3.7}$$

We have now seen how to compute $\partial E/\partial y$ for any unit in the penultimate layer when given $\partial E/\partial y$ for all units in the last layer. We can therefore repeat this procedure to compute $\partial E/\partial y$ for successively earlier layers, computing $\partial E/\partial w$ for the weights as we go. The amount of computation required for the backward pass is of the same order as the forward pass (it is linear in the number of connections).

One way of using $\partial E/\partial w$ is to change the weights after every input–output case. This has the advantage that no separate memory is required for the derivatives. An alternative scheme, which we used in the research reported here, is to accumulate $\partial E/\partial w$ over all the input–output cases before changing the weights. The simplest version of gradient descent is then to change each weight by an amount proportional to the accumulated $\partial E/\partial w$.

$$\Delta w = -\varepsilon \frac{\partial E}{\partial w} \tag{3.8}$$

This method does not converge as rapidly as methods which make use of the second derivatives, but it is much simpler and can easily be implemented by local computations in parallel hardware. It can be significantly improved, without sacrificing the simplicity and locality, by using an acceleration method in which the current gradient is used to modity the velocity of the point in weight space instead of its position.

$$\Delta w(t) = -\varepsilon \frac{\partial E}{\partial w(t)} + \alpha \Delta w(t-1) \tag{3.9}$$

where $t$ is incremented by 1 for each sweep through the whole set of input–output cases, and $\alpha$ is an exponential decay factor between 0 and 1 that determines the relative contribution of the current gradient and earlier gradients on the weight change. Equation (3.9) can be viewed as describing the behaviour of a ball-bearing rolling down the error-surface when the whole system is immersed in a liquid with viscosity determined by $\alpha$.

The learning procedure is entirely deterministic, so if two units within a layer start off with the same connectivity and the same weights there is nothing to make them ever differ from each other. We therefore break symmetry by starting with small randon weights.

The learning procedure often works better if it is not required to produce outputs as extreme as 1 or 0. To given an output of 1, a unit must receive an infinite total input and so the weights grow without bound. All the examples of back-propagation described in this paper use a more liberal error measure which treats all values above 0.8 as perfectly satisfactory if the output unit should be on and all values below 0.2 as perfectly satisfactory if the output unit should be off. Otherwise, the error is the squared difference from 0.8 or 0.2.

There are many aspects of the learning procedure which make it highly unsuitable as a model of learning in real neural networks. There are ways of removing the prohibition on recurrent connections (Rumelhart, Hinton, and Williams 1986) and it may be possible to overcome the need for an externally supplied desired output vector. But the back-propagation phase is central to the learning procedure and it is quite unlike anything known to occur in the brain. The connections are all used backwards, and the units use a different input–output function. We therefore view this learning procedure as an interesting way of demonstrating what can be achieved by gradient descent, without claiming that this is how gradient descent is actually implemented in the brain. Nevertheless, the success of the learning procedure suggests that it is worth looking for other more plausible ways of doing gradient descent.

*The learning parameters used for the family tree simulation*

We tried several different values for the parameters $\varepsilon$ and $\alpha$ in Equation (3.9). We finally chose to use $\varepsilon = 0.005$ and $\alpha = 0.5$ for the first 20 sweeps through the 100 training examples and $\varepsilon = 0.01$ and $\alpha = 0.9$ for the remaining sweeps. The reasons for varying the parameters during learning and the methods used to choose reasonable parameters are discussed in more detail in Plaut, Nowlan, and Hinton (1986). All the weights were initially chosen at random from a uniform distribution between $-0.3$ and $+0.3$.

To make it easier to interpret the weights, we introduced 'weight-decay'. Immediately after each weight change the magnitude of every weight was reduced by 0.2 percent. After prolonged learning the decay was balanced by $\partial E/\partial w$, so the final magnitude of each weight indicated its usefulness in reducing the error. Weight decay is equivalent to modifying the error function so that, in addition to requiring the error to be small, it requires the sum of the squares of the weights to be small. A side-effect of this modification is that it sometimes causes two units to develop very similar sets of weights with each weight being half as big as it would be if the job was done by a single unit. This is because $(0.5w)^2 + (0.5w)^2 < w^2$.

To achieve negligible error without weight decay required 573 sweeps through the 100 training examples. The weights shown in Fig. 3.6 were obtained by allowing the learning to run for 1500 sweeps with weight-decay.

## Acknowledgements

The research reported here was supported by grants from the System Development Foundation. This paper first appeared in the *Proceedings of the Eighth Annual Conference of the Cognitive Science Society*, Amherst, Massachusetts, 1986 which was published by Lawrence Erlbaum Associates, Hillsdale, New Jersey.

## Notes

1. In a conventional Lisp program, it is easy to separate the representation from the procedures used for retrieval and so it is easy to use a representation that is not in a form that is helpful for retrieval. In a neural net it is probably more important to choose representations that can directly cause the required effects without the intervention of a complex interpreter. This is one of the many differences in representation considerations that follows from the difference between the von Neumann architecture and a massively parallel network.

2. If the units can have intermediate activity levels or can behave stochastically, they do not correspond to clean cut partitions because there will be borderline cases. They are more like fuzzy sets, but the formal apparatus of fuzzy set theory (which is what defines the meaning of 'fuzzy') is of no help here so we refrain from using the term 'fuzzy'. In much of what follows we talk as if units define clearcut sets with no marginal cases. This is just a useful idealization.

3. The words of a natural language seem to work in a very similar way. They stand for concepts while indicating very little about how those concepts should be represented internally. Monomorphemic words with similar meanings do not generally have similar forms. So a pattern of activity based on the form of the word is not a good way of capturing the similarities between meanings. There must be a process that maps word forms into word meanings. This process must be far more complex than the simulations we present here because many word forms, like 'bank', are ambiguous and so the process of going from the input representation to a representation of the word meaning cannot be performed separately for each word. The meaning of whole phrases or sentences must be used for disambiguation (Waltz and Pollack 1985).

4. Rumelhart *et al.* describe another version of the procedure which does not require a layered net. It works for arbitrary recurrent networks, but requires more complex units that remember their history of activity levels. We have not applied this version to the family relationships task.

5. We would have preferred it to perform completion when given *any* two terms. This could have been done by using a bigger network in which there were three input groups and three output groups, but learning would have been slower in the large network and so we opted for the simpler case.

6. In many tasks, features that are useful for expressing regularities between concepts are also observable properties of the individual concepts. For example, the feature male is useful for expressing regularities in the relationships between people and it is also related to sets of observable properties like hairyness and size. We carefully chose the input representation to make the problem difficult by removing all local cues that might have suggested the appropriate features.

# References

Barlow, H. B. (1972). Single units and sensation. A neuron doctrine for perceptual psychology? *Perception*, **1**, 371–94.

Hinton, G. E. (1981). Implementing semantic networks in parallel hardware. In *Parallel models of associative memory* (eds. G. E. Hinton and J. A. Anderson). Erlbaum, Hillsdale, NJ.

Hinton, G. E., McClelland, J. L., and Rumelhart, D. E. (1986). Distributed representations. In *Parallel distributed processing: explorations in the microstructure of cognition* (eds. D. E. Rumelhart, J. L. McClelland, and the PDP research group). Bradford Books, Cambridge, Mass.

Hopfield, J. J. (1982). Neural networks and physical systems with emergent collective computational abilities. *Proceedings of the National Academy of Sciences USA*, April, **79**, 2554–8.

Kohonen, T. (1977). *Associative memory: a system-theoretical approach*. Springer, Berlin.

Marr, D. (1982). *Vision*. Freeman, San Francisco.

McClelland, J. L. and Rumelhart, D. E. (1981). An interactive activation model of context effects in letter perception, part I: an account of basic findings. *Psychological Review*, **88**, 375–407.

Plaut, D. C., Nowlan, S. J., and Hinton, G. E. (1986). *Experiments on back-propagation*. Technical Report CMU-CS-86-126, Carnegie-Mellon University, June.

Rumelhart, D. E., Hinton, G. E., and Williams, R. J. (1986). Learning internal representations by error propagation. In *Parallel distributed processing: explorations in the microstructure of cognition* (eds. D. E. Rumelhart, J. L. McClelland, and the PDP research group). Bradford Books, Cambridge, Mass.

Waltz, D. L. and Pollack, J. B. (1985). Massively parallel parsing: a strongly interactive model of natural language interpretation. *Cognitive Science*, **9**, 51–74.

Willshaw, D. J., Buneman, O. P., and Longuet-Higgins, H. C. (1969). Nonholographic associative memory. *Nature*, **222**, 960–2.

Willshaw, D. (1981). Holography, associative memory, and inductive generalization. In *Parallel models of associative memory* (eds. G. E. Hinton and J. A. Anderson). Erlbaum, Hillsdale, NJ.

# Part II

## Implications for psychology

# 4

## Parallel distributed processing and psychology
### GLYN W. HUMPHREYS

**Introduction**

Connectionist models attempt to carry out complex tasks using highly interconnected networks containing large numbers of computationally simple units. Each unit in the network performs a simple function, such as summing the activity along its input lines and giving an output if the incoming value exceeds some threshold. The levels of activity on the lines connecting the units are a function of two variables: the activity in the preceding 'input' unit and the weight assigned to the connections between the units. Thus the weights on the connections govern the way in which input activity is mapped between units, and ultimately they govern the mapping from a stimulus on to a response. Connection weights can be amended by experience. Various algorithms exist to 'teach' networks to associate particular responses with particular stimuli, by modifying the weights on the connections (see Grossberg 1978; Hinton and Sejnowski 1986; Rumelhart, Hinton, and Williams 1986). By means of such learning algorithms, a network initially assigned random weights on its connections can become tuned to the most frequently occurring aspects of input patterns, so that the system can in a sense 'extract out' subtle correlations between co-occurring aspects of the input. In such systems individual units could be devoted to the representation of particular stimuli, or a given stimulus could activate many units, each of which is involved in the coding of other stimuli. In the latter case, stimuli are identifiable from the pattern of activation distributed across the units in the network. Once such a distributed system has come to learn to associate a particular response to a stimulus, it makes little sense to talk of there being some form of discrete internal representation of the stimulus in the system. Rather, the system re-computes the internal representation in terms of the pattern of activation generated across the network on each repeated presentation. In such systems, processing is both parallel (taking place simultaneously across many units) and distributed, hence the term PDP.

These and other aspects of PDP models have now been rehearsed many times (McClelland and Rumelhart 1986; Rumelhart and McClelland 1986a; Smolensky 1988a,b, and commentaries). We know that PDP models can do many things. They can solve the XOR problem (Rumelhart, Hinton, and Williams 1986); they can learn the past tenses of English verbs (Rumelhart and McClelland 1986b); they can learn to associate spelling patterns with associated distinctive phonemic features (Seidenberg and McClelland, in press), and so on. As computational and learning devices, PDP models are impressive and powerful. But what relevance is this to psychology? Should psychologists be excited by the possibilities such models offer?

As discussed by Longuet-Higgins (this volume), there is a long history of models based on patterns of activity transmitted between computationally simple units, dating back at least as far as the perceptron (Rosenblatt 1962). The more recent models, incorporating layers of 'hidden' units that mediate the mapping between input and output layers in a network, are computationally more powerful than the perceptron. In the initial optimistic flush following the development of such models, advocates made various strong claims about the relevance of PDP models to psychology, some of which I discuss below. Time has now passed. We have been able to see how well these models account for psychological data. Many experimental psychologists have also started to gain hands-on experience with PDP models, and, where this is not the reality already, most will have their own 'toy' networks on their personal computers in the imminent future. It is thus appropriate to begin to evaluate the utility of such models for psychology. The four chapters that follow this introduction begin this process. However, before discussing each chapter further it is useful to highlight what connectionist models may offer to psychology, their possible limitations, and what directions might be taken by future work relating parallel distributed processing and psychology.

**Positive aspects of PDP models**

Whittlesea (this volume) discusses three ways in which computational models (in general) can be useful to psychologists.

First, computational models can lead to the formalization of theories, so that processes are defined explicitly and their implications are fully worked through. This can be illustrated using examples from almost any area of psychology, but I focus here on models of reading. For instance, 'dual-route' models of reading hold that word recognition is accomplished by mapping the printed input on to a word recognition system (a logogen, or whatever) and that non-words are read aloud by a process of grapheme-to-phoneme conversion followed by phoneme blending (see Coltheart 1985; Humphreys and Evett 1985; and commentaries). The trouble here is that such accounts are too imprecise to enable a working computational model to be constructed. We need to define the mapping and blending processes; we need to know what types of representation are involved, how information is transmitted between representations over time, etc. Computational models define these processes explicitly.

Second, computational models provide a means of finding out whether particular assumptions really have the processing implications that the author intends. In dual-route models of reading, it is typically assumed that a 'horse race' operates between a word-specific lexical process and a rule-governed non-lexical process (using grapheme-to-phoneme conversion rules), with the first 'horse' past the post determining performance. However, left alone to complete their race, the result would be that subjects would make naming errors whenever an irregular word is presented and the non-lexical rule-based system completes first (since the rule-based system will 'regularize' such words). Since this is not what is observed, theorists need to posit some way of comparing lexical and non-lexical outputs prior to a response taking place (e.g. Norris and Brown 1985). The point here is that any initial processing assumptions, for example concerning the existence of independent processing routes, have implications that must be fully worked out in terms of the details of particular tasks. As is obvious from the above example, this point is not unique to PDP models, or even to computer simulations in general. Nevertheless, simulation stresses this point since, within a working model, any intitial processing assumptions have an end result.

Whittlesea's third proposal is that PDP models can serve as the source of new theoretical, and perhaps even empirical, insights. Again this attribute is not unique to PDP models, as it can arise from what Marr (1982) termed a 'computational analysis' of the problem at hand. For instance, in vision research, Marr (Marr 1982; Marr and Nishihara 1978) argued that object-centred representations were a necessary precursor to object recognition, because of the computational problems encountered in storing every viewer-centred representation of an object and trying to match such viewer-centred representations to the input in order to enable recognition to occur. The procedures he suggested for deriving object-centred representations were influenced by the computational constraints involved in choosing some fixture of an object to serve as a consistent perceptual reference frame. The procedures he suggested, such as finding the object's major axis of elongation or symmetry, have since led to considerable empirical research and to a refining of Marr's account (e.g. Humphreys 1987; Humphreys and Quinlan 1987; Palmer 1982). Thus the development of an explicit computational account of a process can lead to empirical tests, and in turn to further development of the model.

However, the excitement over PDP models arises because they attempt to do more than this. For instance, they challenge traditional psychological theories that assume the existence of discrete symbolic representations which operate by the application of rules. As Pinker and Prince (this volume) discuss, in symbol-based systems a symbol can correspond to any exemplar from a class of stimuli. Rule-based operations can then be applied to the symbol irrespective of the identity or properties of the stimulus at hand. Any present-tense English verb can be transformed into an identifiable past-tense form by the application of a rule of the form: past tense = present-tense stem + suffix (ed/d). Similarly, any printed word can be assigned a regular pronunciation by the application of grapheme-to-phoneme conversion rules, based on the most frequent phonemes assigned to individual graphemes in English. These rules can be applied irrespective of the particular word concerned—though in a language such as English, which has many irregular past-tense forms and spelling-to-sound correspondences, the rules are not *guaranteed* success. Nevertheless, the rules would allow us to make a passable attempt at producing the past tense or at reading aloud letter strings that we have never seen before.

PDP models do not have explicit rules. They do have learning algorithms that are sensitive to statistical regularities in the input that the network receives, even when the regularities are highly complex and difficult to conceptualize within any single rule set. Such models thus come to exhibit rule-like behaviour by responding on the basis of these internalized regularities. Accordingly, following suitable training with regular and irregular past tenses of English verbs, Rumelhart and McClelland's (1986b) system produced 'regularization' errors, where irregular past-tense verbs were erroneously regularized. Similarly, following training to assign a set of distinctive phonemic features to orthographic input representations, Seidenberg and McClelland's (in press) model of reading finds it more difficult to assign the correct phonological representation to low-frequency irregular words than to low-frequency regular words. In the psychological literature, both results have been reported with humans and have been taken as evidence for rule-based operations (e.g. Berko 1958; Humphreys and Evett 1985; Patterson and Coltheart 1987). At the very least, PDP models provide alternative ways of conceptualizing such findings. More strongly, to the extent that the world contains statistical regularities, and to the extent that humans internalize and act upon them, the models provide detailed and important accounts of human processing.

PDP models hold promise for psychologists in other respects, too. For instance, the models exhibit instance-based learning. Yet, by allowing weights on the connections to decay, the systems can come to respond most efficiently to prototypes, even when the prototype is an unseen member at the centre of a class of stimuli (McClelland and Rumelhart 1985). A system can abstract properties from a set of instances, and so can be sensitive to both abstractions and specific instances in its behaviour. Here is another way in which interesting and non-obvious properties emerge from the operations of the system, which again have a correspondence with the experimental literature (see Whittlesea, this volume).

The final promise of PDP models that I will mention concerns their potential to facilitate interactions between workers in different areas of psychology, and even workers in different disciplines. Rumelhart and McClelland (1986c) speculate that

some of the differences between rats and people lie in the potentiality for forming connections that can subserve the vital functions of language and thought that humans exhibit and other animals do not.

Thus, by means of PDP models, we may be able to develop models of animal and human learning within a common framework. Psychologists working on human experimental psychology and those working on animal learning may consequently address each other using a common language and common concepts. The paper by McLaren, Kaye, and Mackintosh (this volume) illustrates just this point. Similarly, PDP models can be 'lesioned' in a way that symbol-based systems cannot (e.g. weights may be put to zero, or random noise added to the weights). PDP models thus provide a natural way of linking cognitive modelling to neuropsychological studies. Patterson *et al.*'s paper (this volume) is an elegant example of this. Modellers also enjoy the claim that PDP models have neuron-like properties (but see Smolensky 1988a). Although we might quibble about the strength of the analogy with physiology (see Sejnowski 1986), it is nevertheless the case that the models enable physiologists, psychologists and computer scientists to address each other using a common conceptual framework—a development seen in the third section of this book.

## Some problems

However, all is not rosy in the connectionist garden. In the last few years we have seen the emergence of a number of counter-arguments against PDP models and favouring symbol-based systems. For instance, Fodor and Pylyshyn (1988) and Pinker and Prince (this volume) point out that symbol-based systems facilitate the computation of similarity between stimuli formed by the conjunction of two or more attributes, such as AB and BA. This is because symbol-based systems have combinatorial structures so that representations can be built from constituent elements (A and B in the above example). AB and BA are similar because they have the same constituents. In connectionist models in general the means of computing the similarity of conjunction stimuli is often not obvious. In an extreme case, individual units in a connectionist network could be devoted to individual letters and to individual positions in a string (as in McClelland and Rumelhart's, 1981, original interactive activation model of word recognition). In this instance, the units activated by AB and BA are completely different, and similarity cannot be computed on the basis of the common input units activated. The extension of the argument made by these critics is that constituent structure is useful, and facilitates the development of combinatorial syntax and semantics.

We can think of such criticisms as aimed at fundamental principles in the design of PDP models. Such criticisms are clearly important for constraining modelling. For instance, they warn against the proliferation of models in which semantic and syntactic structures are generated from increasingly complex feature-lists, with units in the network corresponding to particular features—simply because of the huge numbers of features needed to cover subject, verb and object relations and their token identifiers in natural language (see Fodor and Pylyshyn, 1988, for a full working through of this point). Perhaps what is needed here is some way of formally computing constituent relations in PDP models, and work is indeed underway to shore-up the models against formal problems like this (Smolensky 1988b).

However, even with the likely further developments in formal aspects of connectionist modelling, psychologists will still have to assess the value of the models as explanatory devices. Given that a model produces an end result that fits (or, perhaps even worse, doesn't fit) the empirical findings, is it a valid psychological model?

In this respect, a second line of attack on PDP models is apparent. This attack is directed at specific models. Two examples are presented in this volume. Pinker and Prince's arguments about the validity of distinctive phonemic features (Wickelphones) as representative of phonological representations in humans are of this sort. Pinker and Prince make a number of telling arguments against the psychological reality of Wickelphones (e.g. that some languages contain different words that decompose into the *same set* of Wickelphones). This is a criticism relevant to the particular instantiation of past-tense learning in Rumelhart and McClelland's (1986b) PDP model, which represents phonology in terms of patterns of activation distributed across sets of context-sensitive Wickelphones. Note, though, that it is not a knock-down argument against PDP modelling. Some other type of representation could be developed to remedy such problems.

A second example is contained in the attempt by Patterson *et al.* (this volume) to 'lesion' a PDP model of spelling-to-sound translation, and to compare the output from the 'damaged' model with well-studied neuropsychological syndromes, such as surface dyslexia. The model provides a good first approximation to surface dyslexia—for example, it makes more reading errors to irregular than to regular words. However, it gets the details wrong. It does not produce regularization errors to irregular words at any greater frequency than other (non-regularization) errors that differ by a distinctive feature from the target word. In a sense (and *only* a sense, since the model is actually not able to pronounce anything), the model is no more likely to say

/pint/ than /pent/ to PINT when it makes a reading error. This is unlike the behaviours of at least some patients (e.g. Shallice, Warrington, and McCarthy, 1983).

Now note again that this model uses distinctive phonemic features as output representations (indeed, they are a 'graft-on' from the past-tense learning model). Thus the choice of representation—an implementational detail—could again be held responsible for the discrepancy between the human data and the model. Also, 'naming' is based on the goodness of fit between: (1) the output given to the word by the model; and (2) each of a number of possible outputs (e.g. the 'correct' output or a regularized output for an irregular word). Outputs are derived from the pattern of activation distributed across the phonemic features, but they are not influenced by past learning about the plausible phonological representations in English—there is no process of autoassociation to enable cross-correlations between phonological segments to be learned. The problem in reproducing the regularization errors could arise for various reasons, but among them it could be that the wrong representations have been adopted or that the system is not sensitized to regular phonological patterns (via autoassociation). Options such as choosing the input or output representations, or choosing whether to employ autoassociation, are implementational. Criticisms addressed to such implementational points ought not to demand rejection of the whole approach, only a particular version of a model. Of course when models fail to give a good fit we can still learn from them. The tendency the model of Patterson *et al.* to be influenced by the number of distinctive features separating target words and error responses has led to interesting re-analyses of the reading errors of surface dyslexic patients. The failure of the model to make a preponderance of regularization errors has led to tests of normal reading under deadline conditions (the assumption being that the insult might produce effects analogous to precipitate responding). Both these points are taken up in the chapter by Patterson *et al.* Our understanding of human behaviour can be advanced even by modelling failures.

From the above analysis it seems important to separate *formal* from *implementational* critiques of PDP models, because they essentially serve different purposes. In a sense, the critiques address different levels of theoretical description (cf. Marr 1982). Formal critiques are concerned with whether connectionist architectures are capable of performing certain computations. Implementational critiques are concerned with whether the algorithms adopted in PDP models match those found in humans. Yet other types of critique may concern how well the models match relevant physiological data. In the longer term, formal critiques may help constrain the topic areas that PDP models are applied to—PDP models might be inappropriate for natural language or certain types of problem solving, but appropriate for vision. Implementational critiques should lead to the development of models that are more psychologically plausible. Psychological evidence is relevant for both types of critique. Most especially, there is a good deal of work concerning the nature of internal representation in humans. It would be useful to draw on this work when deciding upon the nature of the input and output representations within a network. In the *ultimate* PDP model input units may link to sensory inputs and output units to motor systems, perhaps by-passing the need for the programmer to 'label' intermediary representations (all intermediary representations being tuned through experience; see Lakoff 1988). For how, however, such labelling is required. Whenever it is, it should be guided by the available psychological data.

## To the future

It is often easy to confuse formal and implementational critiques of PDP models. Partly, this is because it is not made clear that the models can address different levels of theoretical description (and perhaps are not necessarily perched at a single level of theory, contra Smolensky 1988*a*). Partly, it is because the modellers themselves have not distinguished formal aspects of modelling from simulation. Some PDP models can be conceptualized as theorem proofs—showing that PDP models can perform certain tasks or act in certain ways. I take attempts to solve the XOR problem (Rumelhart *et al.* 1986), to show prototype formation (McClelland and Rumelhart 1985) or to show discrete transitions during learning (McClelland, this volume) as (essentially) attempts at theorem proving. Other PDP models attempt to capture data in a more serious way (e.g. Seidenberg and McClelland's, in press, model of reading), and can be thought of more accurately as simulations. Implementational critiques are most appropriate to simulations.

Leading on from the last point, one way forward is to develop connectionist simulations in areas where there are rich bodies of psychological data. Further, the model should preferably be one that can be applied to several tasks—so reducing the danger of models being developed to account for single phenomena, where solutions can nearly always be found but need not generalize. Seidenberg and McClelland's (in press) model is again a good example, since it can be applied to a rich body of lexical decision and naming task results. In vision we might look to models that account for the body of visual search and pattern segmentation data, and so forth. Models that apply across a range of tasks may be more usefully constrained and more psychologically plausible than those accounting for single phenomena.

This work will also be facilitated by the development of better formal modelling techniques. It is useful here to distinguish what I will term Mark 1 and Mark 2 PDP models. Mark 1 models typically operate by mapping activation values continuously between pre-labelled layers in a network (e.g. between letter and word representations in McClelland and Rumelhart's, 1981, interactive activation model). Mark 2 models use learned weights and sets of hidden units that mediate between pre-labelled input and output layers in a network. Once the weights are set, processing takes place in a single step. Mark 2 models are interesting because of their learning capabilities, but they do lose the ability to reproduce the time course of information processing (and so to model effects that are a function of this time course). The development of models that learn and are sensitive to time-course constraints will be welcome. So, too, would be improved techniques for analysing when a given problem must be solved by a number of networks, where processing within each network is essentially modular—perhaps something akin to Marr's (1982) modularity principle would be useful, and provide one way of formally breaking up networks which may in turn make them more psychologically plausible. We also need better techniques for analysing hidden units and their role in behaviour once learning has taken place. Understanding the role of these units is clearly important for any attempts to parallel psychological data. Unless analysis techniques are refined there is a danger that any working models will mimic, but not *explain*, behaviour: what, apart from theorem proving, do we learn from building a connectionist model of a given behaviour if we do not understand how the system performs the task?

**The book**

I have tried to cover some of the characteristics and some of the aspirations of current PDP models—highlighting the importance of mutual interplay between the models and empirical tests, if the models are to be relevant to psychology. The following chapters take up these points in more detail.

Whittlesea's chapter deals with how parallel distributed processing systems can, like humans, be sensitive to task demands, bringing flexible coding into the model via the operation of an attentional-gating mechanism. The issue of how control can be exerted within PDP networks is important and Whittlesea's work provides a step in this direction. It also illustrates how simple networks can be usefully developed on small machines when the task and encoding demands are highly constrained.

The chapter by McLaren *et al.* shows how connectionist models can be used to link human and animal work. The chapter is concerned with how two contrasting results in the animal learning literature (on how previous conditioning can retard the learning of new associations to a stimulus, while also facilitating perceptual discrimination) can be reconciled—and naturally so—in a PDP system. Thus such models can be used to link findings within, as well as across, areas.

I have already discussed the chapters by Patterson *et al.* and Pinker and Prince extensively. At the very least, both chapters have important implications for the implementation of PDP models, and I believe that both will serve as landmarks in the future development of such models. These developments should further clarify the relevance of parallel distributed processing to psychology.

## Acknowledgements

The arguments made in this chapter have arisen from a number of discussions with other workers in the field. In particular, from talks and discussions that took place during the Venice meeting on cognitive neuropsychology in October 1988, and from discussions with a number of individuals including Jane Riddoch, Andrew Mayes, and Paul Smolensky. Without them this chapter would not be what it is, but the individuals concerned bear no responsibilities for any misrepresentation of an argument on my part. The work was supported by grants from the ECRS, the MRC, and the SERC of Great Britain.

## References

Berko, J. (1958). The child's learning of English morphology. *Word*, **14**, 150–77.

Coltheart, M. (1985). The cognitive neuropsychology of reading. In *Attention and performance XI* (eds. M. I. Posner and O. S. M. Marin). Erlbaum, Hillsdale, NJ.

Fodor, J. A. and Pylyshyn, Z. W. (1988). Connectionism and cognitive architecture: a critical analysis. *Cognition*, **28**, 3–71.

Grossberg, S. (1978). A theory of human memory: self-organization and performance of sensory-motor codes, maps, and plans. In *Progress in theoretical biology*, Volume 5 (eds. R. Rosen and F. Snell). Academic Press, NY.

Hinton, G. E. and Sejnowski, T. J. (1986). Learning and relearning in Boltzmann Machines. In *Parallel distributed processing: explorations in the microstructure of cognition*, Volume 1 (eds. D. E. Rumelhart and J. L. McClelland). MIT Press, Cambridge, Mass.

Humphreys, G. W. (1987). Objects, words, brains and computers: framing the correspondence problem in object and word recognition. *Bulletin of the British Psychological Society*, **40**, 207–10.

Humphreys, G. W. and Evett, L. J. (1985). Are there independent lexical and nonlexical routes in word processing? An evaluation of the dual-route theory of reading. *The Behavioral and Brain Sciences*, **8**, 689–740.

Humphreys, G. W. and Quinlan, P. T. (1987). Normal and pathological processes in visual object constancy. In *Visual object processing: a cognitive neurospychological approach* (eds. G. W. Humphreys and M. J. Riddoch). Erlbaum, London.

Lakoff, G. (1988). Connectionism and semantics. *The Behavioral and Brain Sciences*, **11**, 39–40.

Marr, D. (1982). *Vision*. W. H. Freeman, SF.

Marr, D. and Nishihara, K. (1978). Representation and recognition of the spatial organisation of three-dimensional objects. *Proceedings of the Royal Society, London, Series B*, **200**, 269–94.

McClelland, J. L. and Rumelhart, D. E. (1981). An interactive activation model of context effects in letter perception: part 1, an account of basic findings. *Psychological Review*, **88**, 375–407.

McClelland, J. L. and Rumelhart, D. E. (1985). Distributed memory and the representation of general and specific information. *Journal of Experimental Psychology: General*, **114**, 159–88.

McClelland, J. L. and Rumelhart, D. E. (1986) (eds.). *Parallel distributed processing: explorations in the microstructure of cognition*, Volume 2. MIT Press, Cambridge, Mass.

Norris, D. and Brown, G. (1985). Race models and analogy theories: A dead heat? A reply to Seidenberg. *Cognition*, **20**, 155–68.

Palmer, S. E. (1982). Symmetry, transformation and the structure of the perceptual system. In *Organization and representation in perception* (ed. J. Beck). Erlbaum, Hillsdale, NJ.

Patterson, K. E. and Coltheart, V. (1987). Phonological processes in reading: a tutorial review. In *Attention and Performance XII* (ed. M. Coltheart). Erlbaum, London.

Rosenblatt, F. (1962). *Principles of neurodynamics*. Spartan, NY.

Rumelhart, D. E. and McClelland, J. L. (1986a) (eds). *Parallel distributed processing: explorations in the microstructure of cognition*, Volume 1. MIT Press, Cambridge, Mass.

Rumelhart, D. E. and McClelland, J. L. (1986b). On learning the part tenses of English verbs. In *Parallel distributed processing: explorations in the microstructure of cognition*, Volume 2 (eds. J. L. McClelland and D. E. Rumelhart). MIT Press, Cambridge, Mass.

Rumelhart, D. E. and McClelland, J. L. (1986c) PDP models and general issues in cognitive science. In *Parallel distributed processing: explorations in the microstructure of cognition*, Volume 1 (eds. D. E. Rumelhart and J. L. McClelland). MIT Press, Cambridge, Mass.

Rumelhart, D. E., Hinton, G. E., and Williams, R. J. (1986). Learning internal representations by error propagation. In *Parallel distributed processing: explorations in the microstructure of cognition*, Volume 1 (eds. D. E. Rumelhart and J. L. McClelland). MIT Press, Cambridge, Mass.

Seidenberg, M. S. and McClelland, J. L. (in press). A distributed developmental model of word recognition and naming. *Psychological Review*.

Sejnowski, T. J. (1986). Open questions about computations in cerebral cortex. In *Parallel distributed processing: explorations in the microstructure of cognition*, Volume 2, (eds. J. L. McClelland and D. E. Rumelhart). MIT Press, Cambridge, Mass.

Shallice, T., Warrington, E. K., and McCarthy, R. (1983). Reading without semantics. *Quarterly Journal of Experimental Psychology*, **35A**, 111–38.

Smolensky, P. (1988a) On the proper treatment of connectionism. *The Behavioral and Brain Sciences*, **11**, 1–74.

Smolensky, P. (1988b) Distributed representation of structured data. Paper presented at Neuro-Image 88, University of Bordeaux II, October.

# 5

## Selective attention, variable processing, and distributed representation: preserving particular experiences of general structures
### BRUCE W. A. WHITTLESEA

**Introduction**

The ease with which humans perform many activities, including making summary judgements about ourselves and others, reading unfamiliar texts, and behaving discriminatively towards objects belonging to different categories, demonstrates that we are sensitive to the general structure of classes of events. Such sensitivity is puzzling, because we do not directly experience classes of events, but only the events themselves. This has led many investigators to conclude that we must chronically abstract general properties out of the raw data of particular experiences, and retain this summary knowledge in the form of stereotypes, linguistic rules and schemata. However, recent evidence suggests that this conclusion overestimates our reliance on general information, and that memory may retain only our experiences of particular events.

Because parallel distributed processing (PDP) models superimpose information about successive events in a composite matrix, they are usually assumed to work by abstracting the common or regular aspects of the events, and their success in simulating human performance is taken as support for a similar function in humans. However, it will be argued that this description of PDP is misleading. This chapter demonstrates a PDP model, variable integration and selective attention (VISA) that simulates a variety of the phenomena of human sensitivity to general structure, and succeeds precisely because it preserves particular experiences rather than abstracting general properties. Its use of this form of knowledge also permits it to respond flexibly to changes in attentional demands, and suggests a means of understanding attention, remembering, perception and classification, not as separate mental functions, but as alternative perspectives on the interactions of memory with the world.

## Parallel distributed processing and the integration issue

### Unconfounding the general and the particular

The basic distinction between models of chronic abstraction and models of particular experiences is that the former assume canonical representation of events, while the latter assume that different experiences of the same event may result in representations that differ in important ways. One variable which may cause such differences between experiences is processing integration, or the degree to which the components of an event are processed as a unit or as separate parts. The next two sections present evidence that variations in processing integration do result in different representations of the same event, and argue that such a function is fundamental to the success of PDP models in simulating human data. To introduce those issues, this section provides some background on how memory might interact with general and specific properties of experience.

The evidence that humans chronically abstract general properties begins with dissociations observed between reflective tasks that explicitly require the use of memory, such as recognition, and unreflective tasks in which the use of memory is incidental, such as perception and word completion (e.g. Jacoby and Dallas 1981; Tulving, Schacter, and Stark 1982), suggesting that the tasks depend on independent forms of memory (Tulving 1983). Because recognition clearly requires memory for particular events, the second form of memory is thought to retain general knowledge of events, a conclusion supported by observations that performance in unreflective tasks is frequently correlated with general properties of experience. Taking classification as an example, typical category members are usually judged faster, more accurately and more confidently than less typical members (e.g. Rosch 1977). This is usually interpreted to mean that people learn what is typically true about members of a category, and use this summary, or prototype, to classify other members. This summary is thought to be abstracted automatically, because the correlation occurs even with stimuli learned when no classification test was expected (e.g. Homa, Sterling, and Trepel 1981).

However, this evidence is also consistent with the conclusion that memory only preserves information about particular events. Dissociations between such tasks as classification and recognition would be expected because they provide different retrieval cues, and thus are likely to activate different sets of representations (Jacoby and Witherspoon 1982). The correlation of typicality and performance would also be expected, because the typicality of an item is also generally correlated with its similarity to familiar instances (Brooks 1978; Medin and Shaffer 1978).

In fact, when general and specific properties of experience are uncon-founded, performance in conceptual and perceptual tasks also appears to be determined by memory for particular events. As an example, I constructed a stimulus domain of letter-string stimuli in which the similarity of test items to the prototype could be manipulated independently of their similarity to particular training instances (Whittlesea 1987). Subjects were required to copy selected training stimuli, and then to identify briefly presented test items. The accuracy of identification was found to be correlated with the similarity of probes to the set of training items, but not systematically related to the typicality of the probes. This denies the conclusion that regular or typical stimulus properties automatically have a special status in memory, and suggests that performance in unreflective tasks such as perception of category members may also rely on idiosyncratic information about particular events.

### Integration and memory for particular events

The conclusion that both reflective and unreflective tasks rely on memory for particular events rather than on memory for the common components of those events may seem to imply that humans invariably encode events as configural wholes, never attending to the individual components. However, the claim is that *humans do not chronically or automatically process individual components or summarize commonalities.* Instead, processing is expected to vary with circumstances, so that on different occasions the subject may encode a particular stimulus either as a whole or as a collection of parts, or even attend to one component exclusively, and may compare or not compare the components of the present stimulus with past stimuli. The major thrust of this account is that current processing depends on the demands of the task in conjunction with whatever memory traces are made available by current contextual and stimulus cues, that memory preserves whatever experience one has of the stimulus, whether of the whole or the parts, and that future performance depends on preserved representation of the particular properties of that experience.

This chapter focuses on how different demands cause us to process a stimulus as a whole unit or as a collection of independent parts. This is the issue of processing integration, or the degree to which processing one component of a stimulus involves processing others. Some tasks require analytic processing, focusing attention on each stimulus aspect individually, resulting in independent encoding and representation of each component. In contrast, processing each component in a non-analytic task involves processing others to some degree, and the representation of each involves information about the others, so that following highly integral tasks, memory effectively retains configural information about whole items. This account assumes that analytic and non-analytic processing differ only in the degree of integration of stimulus components, so that the resulting representations differ only in the extent and organization of the encoded detail, and do not constitute different forms of memory.[1]

This description of the characteristics of analytic and non-analytic tasks provides a loose operational definition, permitting us to select tasks which we expect to be at least relatively analytic or non-analytic. However, we also employ a rigorous manipulation check, defining the degree of processing integration required by a task in terms of its consequences for later performance. If a stimulus is presented in a perceptual test after exposure in an analytic task, the probability of identifying one element should be independent of the probability of identifying any other elements, because representations of each should be independently available to assist perception. By contrast, following non-analytic encoding, the identification of each component will depend to some degree on the identification of the others. The degree of this interdependence in identification will vary with the degree to which the components were integrated in the earlier task, and the measurement of the interdependence of identification serves as an index of the integration demands of the earlier task.

Applying this principle to the concept experiment mentioned above, suppose that a subject had copied the item FURIT in a training session, and was later required to identify both FURIT and FURIK in a tachistoscopic test. If the subject had originally encoded FURIT as five independent elements, then each encoded element should facilitate later identification of itself in any item, and should do so independent of the identities of other elements of the test stimulus. In consequence, the first four letters would be perceived with identical success in both familiar and novel items, although the subject would be more likely to identify the T of FURIT than the K of FURIK. In contrast, if the subject had encoded FURIT as a single event, integrating its components within the representation, then later perception of each component would depend on activation of the representation of all components, and in turn that activation would depend on the proportion of the encoded item reinstated by the probe. In this case, subjects should make more errors on all letters of the novel item. The experimental data gave exactly this result and, in general, the probability of identifying any letter was found to depend on the degree to which other letters of the original item were reinstated. This interdependence suggested that rather than abstracting typical features from successive items either automatically or deliberately, subjects had encoded the training stimuli as relatively integral units, and that in this case perception depended on memory for particular items.

*Parallel distributed representation of particular events*

Perhaps the most obvious way in which memory might preserve information about particular events is to retain each as a separate trace. This assumption is basic to a number of models of memory, including the Medin and Shaffer

(1978) context model, Hintzman's (1983) multiple-trace model and my own (1983, 1987) episode model. These models assume that traces are recruited in parallel by cues provided by current processing, and that cues succeed in activating traces to the extent that they share information. In consequence, although it is assumed that all events one has experienced are retained in memory, the ability to retrieve an event independent of others may be lost because other events are too similar. Because the representations of past experience are represented separately and interact only when recruited by a new stimulus, these models are referred to as 'post-computational'. In such models, concepts are distributed over traces of events, but the traces remain distinct.

McClelland and Rumelhart's (1985) model carried distribution a step further, assuming that the traces themselves are distributed across the storage medium. This assumption is definitional to the class of models which has come to be known as parallel distributed processing. With this step, the unique identities of particular events are lost. At first glance, this loss appears to conflict with the conclusion of the last section, that perception in that experiment depended on the preservation of information about individual events. I was thus surprised when McClelland and Rumelhart demonstrated that their model could simulate the patterns of perception on which that conclusion was based. However, closer examination of McClelland and Rumelhart's model revealed that it succeeds precisely because it preserves information about stimuli as integrated units, because learning, in a PDP model, consists of the development of interdependence among the processing units which represent stimulus components. In fact, the model preserves complete information about the configurations of components within particular events, but distributes this information across a matrix representation so that the unique identities of the events are not preserved explicitly. It thus maintains precisely the same detail of information as a post-computational model, but in a kind of pre-computed form. However, it differs in important ways from other pre-computed models, such as prototypes, which involve actual loss of information about atypical components and the configurations of components within items.

To explain in greater detail, PDP models consist of a system of interconnected processing units (see McClelland, this volume). Initially, these units are inactive, and the system contains no information. Under the impetus of a signal pattern from the external world, the processing units become active, and begin to modify each others' activity. They also modify the strength of the interconnections that permit them to affect each other. After some period of time, changes in the activities of units and in the strengths of their interconnections stabilize. The activities of the units are transient, decaying back to resting levels when the stimulus is removed. The only permanent impact of a stimulus is that the pattern of interconnectivity is altered. This change alters the way the system will respond to another stimulus, and thus constitutes learning within the system.

Although the pattern of interconnectivity is the internal representation of the stimulus, no particular part of that pattern can be identified with any particular feature of the external signal. This is because processing of each stimulus element is distributed across the entire network of units: even if one unit has direct input from one particular stimulus aspect, it will receive and pass activity from and to units responding to other aspects, so that the response of any unit to a particular stimulus aspect depends upon its interconnections with every other unit and the activities of those units, which in turn depends upon the response of those units to other stimulus aspects. Thus the model constructs a representation in which knowledge of every stimulus component depends on knowledge of the others.

Successive learning trials modify the pattern of interconnectivity, so that the final pattern is not isomorphic with that resulting from any one experience. For this reason, it is tempting to think of the resultant pattern as a form of abstract representation that retains some idiosyncracies of specific events. However, critically, the process of modifying the connectivity pattern does not cause loss of any information: unlike a prototype or semantic memory it does not automatically result in a summary of typical or regular properties of the events. Just as a Fourier sum of sine waves can always be decomposed into the separate frequencies on which it is based, so the connectivity matrix implicitly maintains information about all the specific patterns of which it is composed. The system may lose the ability to retrieve a particular event independent of similar events, but the influence of that event remains, however difficult to discern among the simultaneous influences of other events.

This point becomes particularly important in understanding data on human performance, indicating that the indiosyncratic characteristics of unusual events are clearly influential, even after long periods (e.g. Jacoby 1983; Kolers 1976). Moreover, it demonstrates the essential commonality between PDP models and other distributed models, such as those discussed at the beginning of this section. Parallel distributed processing models retain the same information, but represent it in a network form that grants computational ease, permits close investigation of the development of representations of successive events and the effects of these representations on performance, and makes a start toward co-ordinating cognitive processes with their neurophysiological substrate.

*Variable processes and particular experiences*

Thus the McClelland and Rumelhart model succeeded in simulating the human data because the model is inherently integral, and in that experiment humans encoded items integrally. Since the publication of that model, however, some of us (e.g. Whittlesea 1987; Whittlesea and Brooks 1988; Whittlesea and Cantwell 1987) have explored tasks that cause humans to vary the integration of encoding and representation.

We assume that each encounter with a stimulus occurs for a purpose, which dictates the allocation of attention to various parts of the stimulus, and thus determines the way the stimulus is processed. This suggests that task variation should entail variation in the organization of stimulus components in memory, and consequently in performance on subsequent tasks. This is clearly not a novel idea: effects of processing manipulations on tasks such as recognition and recall are well documented (e.g. Craik and Lockhart's, 1972, 'levels of processing' paradigm). The novelty of our approach was to investigate such episodic effects in the context of tasks that do not explicitly require the use of memory, such as perception and classification, which were generally thought to depend on memory for information abstracted across episodes. We have observed that encounters with the same stimulus for different purposes cause varying degrees of perceptual interdependence among the stimulus components, and interpret these findings as indications that different encoding tasks invoke differing degrees of processing integration. We concluded that perception depends upon highly specific memories, preserving not only the properties of particular stimuli, such as their components, but also the properties of particular experiences of stimuli, such as the organization imposed on the stimulus components by the demanded processing.

Evidence of variable integration is a challenge to PDP models, because the basic learning mechanism, the development of interconnections between processing units, constitutes a built-in, inflexible tendency to code stimulus components integrally. The following two sections present evidence of such variable integration, and describe a novel mechanism whereby PDP models can accommodate such findings.

## Evidence of variable processing integration

The word superiority effect (Reicher 1969; Wheeler 1970) has long been taken to be an illustration of how perception depends on memory. It consists of the observation that a letter is generally easier to perceive when presented in a word than when presented either alone or in a pseudoword. Because the perceptibility of letters is correlated with the orthographic (Baron and Thurston 1973) or phonological (Gibson, Shurcliff, and Yonas 1970) regularity of stimuli, the effect has been thought to demonstrate that word perception depends on memory for regular aspects of experience.

The problem in interpreting this evidence is similar to that described above regarding the correlation of typicality and performance measures, namely that the regularity of a stimulus is, to a great extent, confounded with the number of particular experiences the subject is likely to have had with that stimulus. In order to determine whether perception depends on specific familiarity *per se*, we (Whittlesea and Brooks 1988) adopted the strategy of manipulating familiarity independent of regularity prior to a perceptual test. Specifically, we showed subjects a number of pronounceable pseudowords (e.g. FURIG, NOBAL) in one of several training conditions, and then measured the relative perceptibility of letters presented alone or in the context of pseudowords. If perception depends primarily on memory for general lexical properties, we would expect that letters presented in pseudowords would show a stable superiority over letters presented alone, no matter what the training condition in which the items had been pre-exposed. In contrast, if the particular characteristics of the training experience are preserved in memory and influence perception, we would expect that the relative perceptibility of letters alone and in pseudowords would depend on the nature of the pre-exposure.

In a first (baseline) condition, subjects identified letters alone and in pseudowords without specific prior experience. (Precise details of the method are given in Whittlesea and Brooks 1988.) Briefly, trials consisted of a 30 ms presentation of a CVCVC pseudoword or a single letter, and were terminated by a display of pattern masks in the five positions in which a letter could occur. Single letters were displayed in the same screen position they would occupy in a pseudoword, the remaining positions being filled with the same symbols used to create the mask. Co-incident with the presentation of the mask, a caret was displayed beneath a position in which a letter had just occurred, cuing the subject to give a free report of the letter's identity. In this baseline condition, we observed no difference in subjects' accuracy in identifying letters presented alone or in pseudowords (see Fig. 5.1). This was an ideal starting point, suggesting that perception of letters in pseudowords received no more assistance than perception of letters alone, whether from knowledge of orthographic regularity, particular experiences of words, familiar units, phonological codes, or any other source.

In the second condition, we began investigating the perceptual consequences of particular experiences by introducing a training phase in which subjects were required to copy pseudowords that would be presented later in the identification test. On the basis of earlier studies of word and pseudoword repetition (e.g. Kolers 1975; Salasoo, Shiffrin, and Faustal 1985), we expected this pre-training to facilitate later perception of pseudoword stimuli. The novel question was the degree to which the experience of copying items would facilitate identification of their constituent letters when presented alone. If the repetition benefit is due only to learning about the components of items, then perception of letters presented alone should be facilitated as much as perception of letters presented in pseudowords. However, if subjects additionally learned something about the organization of letters within

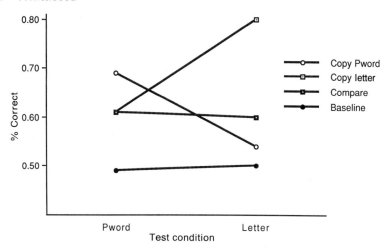

**Fig. 5.1** Accuracy of identification of human subjects in pseudoword and single-letter test conditions, following training in Conditions 1 (baseline), 2 (copy pseudowords), 3 (compare pseudowords), and 4 (copy single letters).

specific pseudowords, we should observe a greater benefit for letters presented in pseudowords.

As shown in Fig. 5.1, the copying experience facilitated perception of letters in pseudowords considerably, but had little or no effect on perception of single letters, although the same letters also occurred in the pseudowords, and in the same position. We interpreted this to mean that perception of each component depended on the reinstatement of context in which it had been processed earlier, and concluded that subjects had learned something about the interrelationships of components within items, rather than simply learning about individual components. We also speculated that the requirement of the training task, to copy whole stimuli, had caused subjects to encode stimuli relatively integrally, and that this organization could be modified by other encoding tasks.

To test this possibility, in Condition 3 we replicated the entire methodology of Condition 2, with the exception that whereas subjects in Condition 2 copied stimuli in the pre-training phase, subjects in Condition 3 performed a letter-comparison task. Each training stimulus had to be matched with a comparison item, copying matching letters in one location of a response sheet and non-matching letters in another, which might encourage learning about the individual stimulus components rather than their organization within items. Any differences in the patterns of identification accuracy between Conditions 2 and 3 could be attributed to the difference in experience of the stimuli, because all other aspects of the two conditions, including the stimulus displays, were identical.

As shown in Fig. 5.1, identification in both conditions was facilitated relative to the baseline condition, indicating that subjects had learned something from the training experience. Moreover, letters were identified with equal accuracy alone and in pseudowords, meaning that the identification of each component was independent of the presence or absence of others. We interpreted this context-free perception as an indication that under the task demand to compare items, subjects had encoded each component analytically, without reference to other components of the stimulus, so that each could be accessed as a resource for perception independent of the others.

It is clear that the change in task requirements from Condition 2 had an effect on performance: letters alone were better perceived, and letters in pseudowords worse, than in Condition 2. We interpreted these differences to mean that the integration of components within large units grants an advantage to perception if the integrated context is reinstated. However, integration also has a cost, in that perception fails if the context of a component is not reinstated. Analytic coding does not support perception as well as integral coding, but is more robust across conditions of test.

Because Conditions 2 and 3 were identical in all regards except the purpose for which stimuli were encountered, we concluded that memory preserves, and perception depends on, the specific characteristics of particular experiences. If this is true, then we should be able to produce a perceptual advantage for letters presented alone. We tested this hypothesis in Condition 4, showing subjects single target letters in the same display (other string positions filled with masks) that would be used in the perceptual test. Following this training condition, the identification of letters presented in pseudowords should be at a relative disadvantage, because the perceptual context provided by a pseudoword at test does not match the context in which target letters were seen in training.

As seen in Fig. 5.1, single letters in this condition are perceived more easily than letters presented in pseudowords. This is a striking result, because the information available in training about the identity and location of letters is equally useful in both cases. The difference cannot be attributed to confusions among letters in the pseudoword case, because letters in pseudowords were perceived equally well in the baseline condition. The only information available in the training displays that is differential between pseudoword and single-letter tests is the presence of the non-letter contextual elements. Superior performance in single-letter tests thus suggests that under the demand to copy the letters, subjects had encoded the earlier single-letter displays as integrated wholes that included the non-letter contextual elements. We concluded that single-letter presentations earned a benefit from maintaining this non-linguistic context, whereas pseudoword presentations, which failed to reinstate that context, did not receive this benefit. (In a later study, we found that blank contexts caused similar effects.)

Together, these four conditions suggest to us that when specific familiarity is unconfounded from general lexical properties, perception depends on memory for particular experiences. In order to increase the generality of this conclusion, we have induced integration and analysis through a variety of tasks, and have conducted similar experiments over a 24-hour span (Whittlesea and Cantwell 1987), and with comparisons and natural words v. single letters, and phrases v. words (Whittlesea and Brooks 1988), and natural objects (Brooks and Whittlesea 1988); we have found similar results in each case. We conclude that optimal perception occurs when the original context of an element is reinstated, but that context is given at least in part by the processing conducted on the element in the original encounter, and that the kind of processing to which a stimulus is subjected depends on the purpose for which the encounter took place. Thus we conclude that particular experiences exercise a dominant and enduring influence in perception.

### Simulating variable context dependence

The four conditions outlined above present extreme examples of the ways in which performance on a perceptual task can be made to vary by changing the context and processing demands of earlier experiences of the target. A model capable of simulating these results would seem to require the ability to process stimuli non-analytically, encoding stimuli as relatively integral wholes, in order to account for the results of Condition 2. It must also be able to process stimuli analytically, encoding stimulus aspects independently, in order to account for Condition 3, and it must make the switch from one style of processing to the other under instructional control, rather than as a reaction to stimulus structure. Lastly, it should be capable of sensitivity to 'nothing' as an effective context, in order to simulate the superiority of single-letter over pseudoword presentation in Condition 4. This section describes an example of a PDP model incorporating such variable processing, called VISA (for variable integration and selective attention).

To avoid all suspense, the results of simulating the four conditions are shown in Fig. 5.2. Clearly, the model is capable of approximating human performance in these tasks. What is important is the mechanisms that enabled the model to achieve this success, and whether these mechanisms give us any insight into more general problems of memory.

### Overview of the model

The chief novel feature of VISA is a selective attention mechanism. This mechanism determines which aspects of a stimulus receive extensive processing, and whether stimulus components are processed integrally or

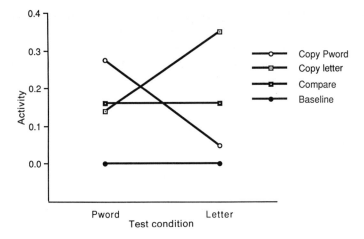

**Fig. 5.2**   Activity of model's response units in simulation of test and training conditions shown in Fig. 5.1.

analytically. To understand how this mechanism controls processing, it is useful to know a little about the model's gross architecture and function.

*External demands*
The external world can present three kinds of input to VISA. The first is a nominal stimulus, to be processed for some purpose. It may consist of letter strings, compounds of letters and blanks, or other patterns. The second input is a demanded response, which may be the name of the stimulus or of some part of it, or the name of a paired associate. This demanded response is also a stimulus, and the model must learn to perceive it in the same way it learns to perceive the nominal stimulus. On training trials, the demanded response forms part of the purpose for processing the nominal stimulus. It is omitted on test trials to determine the model's unguided response to the stimulus. The third input to the model consists of attentional demands, and will be described shortly.

*Internal structure*
VISA consists of two processing subsystems, differing only in the external sources from which they receive input. One responds primarily to cues about the nominal stimulus, the other to cues about the demanded response. Each subsystem consists of two layers of units. The first is a communication layer, which receives energy from the appropriate external sources and passes it to the second layer. Besides this communication function, the communication layer receives input from attention cues, and also enhances the contrast between units responding to letters and units responding to blanks.

The second, or association layer, receives energy from the communication layer and from selective attention cues, but also receives and passes energy from and to the association layer in the other subsystem. On training trials, the activity of these units converges on the activity of the communication units, but the development and maintenance of their activity becomes dependent on the activity of units in the association layer of the other subsystem. The model thus builds up a combined representation of the nominal stimulus and demanded response, consisting of mutual stimulation of the association units of the two subsystems. This representation is enduring, and determines the response of the system in subsequent test trials.

The response of the entire system to the nominal stimulus and/or demanded response consists of the pattern of activity on the association units of the response subsystem. On training trials, these units come to reflect the activity of their respective communication units. On test trials, those communication units are inactive, because no demanded response is presented. However, presentation of the nominal stimulus activates the association units of the stimulus subsystem, and these units activate the response units through the interconnections built up in training. Thus the response of the system in test trials depends on what the system learned about the nominal stimulus and demanded response on preceding trials.

*Selective and non-selective attention*
The model distinguishes among three conditions of attention: pre-cued selective attention, in which the subject knows in advance which stimulus aspect to attend; post-cued selective attention, in which the basis of the selection is not established until the stimulus has been presented and removed; and uncued, or non-selective attention, in which case the subject is to attend and report the entire stimulus. Intuitively, these conditions present a subject with different problems. In the case of non-selective attention, the subject is likely to process and encode the stimulus as a whole. This is particularly true if the subject has previously integrated those components in similar stimuli, as demonstrated by Condition 2 of the experiment discussed above. If, instead, a stimulus is pre-cued, it may be possible for the subject to orient processing toward a particular physical location, passively ignoring the remainder of the stimulus. Ignored contextual elements would have no impact on current processing, and would not be encoded with the representation of the target aspect. (Actively ignored elements might have different effects, as discussed below in the section covering the implications of the model.)

In contrast, if the cue occurs after stimulus offset, the subject has little choice but to encode the entire stimulus, and suppress the unwanted portions in report. If the stimulus presentation is brief and immediately followed by the cue, the perceptual processing of the stimulus is likely to interact with the suppressing effects of the cue. For example, if the subject has already coded the same stimulus integrally, perception of the target element will depend in part on perception of the context. A selection cue suppressing processing of context elements may thus actually interfere with the identification of the element it indicates.

VISA is sensitive to all three conditions of attention, and responds in much the way described. If attention is demanded without selection, the model permits all aspects of the stimulus and demanded response to enter and receive extensive processing. In consequence, it constructs a representation integrating all aspects of the nominal stimulus and demanded response. On subsequent test trials, which omit presentation of the demanded response, the system can regenerate some portion of its earlier response through the interconnections of the stimulus and response association units. The interconnected assembly of association units responds optimally to re-presentation of the stimulus components to which it was originally tuned. If the stimulus is altered between training and test by the substitution of novel elements for old ones, the assembly responds less well, not only to the novel features, but also to the reinstated elements, because the activity of each unit depends on feedback through all the others. Thus the ability of the system to identify a particular component in test depends on reinstatement of the context in which the component was originally encoded.

In the experiment to be simulated, pre-cuing is conducted only in training trials. It causes the model to function in an 'early selection' mode (e.g. Broadbent 1958); however, as discussed below, the 'filter' is not a separate mechanism, but simply a response to the cue, learned in the same way that responses to other stimuli are learned. In VISA, pre-cued selection operates on the stimulus subsystem, preventing non-target parts of the stimulus from entering the processing system. Both communication and association units of the stimulus subsystem are held at their resting levels, except for those units corresponding to the position from which a feature is to be reported. At the same time, the demanded response consists of a single element, the name of the stimulus feature in the position to be reported, so that most of the association units of the response subsystem are also quiescent. The event is represented by the development of interconnections between the few active response units and the selected stimulus units, while the dormant units are unaffected. Successive pre-cuing trials on other components of the same stimulus involve different sets of stimulus and response units, so that earlier representations are unaffected by the development of later ones. When a stimulus component is re-presented at test, the system is capable of regenerating its earlier response to some extent. Alteration of non-target (contextual) elements of the nominal stimulus between training and test does not affect its ability to regenerate the response to the target feature, because the representation formed in the training trial between that feature and its response is independent of representations of contextual elements.

Post-cuing is generally reserved for test trials. To simulate the fact that the stimulus has already been presented before the cue is given, the model is allowed to process all features of the nominal stimulus, while selection is applied to the demanded response. In consequence, information about the entire nominal stimulus enters the system, but processing is suppressed on all of the units of the response subsystem, except those representing the target location. In this case, the system is operating in a 'late selection' mode (e.g. Deutsch and Deutsch 1963), in which a learned response to the selection cue interacts with, rather than prevents, processing of the stimulus elements. The effect of this interaction depends on the type of representation the system constructed in the training trial. If earlier processing was non-selective, then the activity of each stimulus unit depends on every other stimulus unit, but the dependence is mediated through the response units. Suppression of some of the response units means that all stimulus processing is degraded, leading to poorer performance on the demanded response position. However, if earlier processing was analytic, the stimulus and response units corresponding to each position of the stimulus are interconnected separately from those corresponding to other positions, and thus the target stimulus units do not depend on feedback from other stimulus units through the suppressed response units. In consequence, earlier analytic encoding makes the system relatively immune to the effects of post-cuing.

*Simulation conditions*

These three demands on attention permit VISA to duplicate the variations in processing integration that human subjects displayed in the perception experiment above. In the training phase of that experiment, subjects were exposed to no stimulus (Condition 1), a pseudoword (Conditions 2 and 3) or a single letter in a context of masks (Condition 4), in a task designed to foster integral encoding of the components (Conditions 2 and 4) or relatively analytic encoding (Condition 3). The test phase of all conditions required the subject to report a target letter presented alone (surrounded by masks) or in a pseudoword, one of these displays reinstating the physical context of the target letter.

To simulate Condition 1, VISA was given only test trials, consisting of a nominal stimulus (a letter compound or a letter presented with blanks) and a post-cue specifying a target position to report. Because the model had built up no stimulus–response representation, the activation of the stimulus subsystem had no effect on the response subsystem in either test condition (see Fig. 5.2). In the training trials of Condition 2, the model was given a letter compound as both nominal stimulus and demanded response, and non-selective attention was demanded. In consequence, it developed an integral representation of the components of the stimulus and response. The test was identical to Condition 1. Because presenting the compound maintained the encoding context, stimulus processing was successful in regenerating the response, despite the limitations imposed by the post-cue. In contrast, the single-letter test provided too little stimulus information to regenerate the response.

In the training trials of Condition 3, the model was given the same stimulus compound, but with a pre-cue specifying one of the stimulus positions, and a demanded response consisting of the name of the cued feature, also presented in the cued position. Learning trials were repeated until each stimulus position has been cued. The analytic processing caused by pre-cuing caused each stimulus aspect to be coded with its name independent of other stimulus–response representations, so that the system was able to generate the response with equal ease whether the test stimulus was a single letter or compound. However, its response was not as great in this condition as in the pseudoword test of Condition 2 (see Fig. 5.2). In Condition 4, the model was given a single letter surrounded by blanks as both nominal stimulus and demanded response, and non-selective attention was demanded. Owing to a contrast enhancement mechanism (described in greater detail in the following section), the model responded to blanks as actual information, and formed an integral representation of the configuration of letters and blanks. Reinstatement of this pattern at test resulted in superior ability to regenerate the response, whereas the substitution of letters for blanks forced the system to rely on information about the one familiar component, thus reducing its ability respond. The difference between the patterns of performance of Conditions 2 and 4 (see Fig. 5.2), which both require integral stimulus processing, results from the fact that the contrast enhancement mechanism acts by increasing the activity of units representing letters and decreasing the activity of units representing blanks, thus giving special prominence to the single letter.

## Detailed assumptions of the model

### External world

As indicated above, the external world can make three kinds of demands on VISA, consisting of a nominal stimulus, a demanded response and various kinds of attention cues. In order to reduce the complexity of front-end computation, demands presented by the world are recoded as standardized input patterns. (This simplification ignores the problem of mapping the same physical pattern occurring in different locations in the world onto the same set of processing units—but see McClelland 1985). Each feature was recoded as a pattern of four elements, permitting different patterns to represent different features. The choice of four units is arbitrary, but sufficiently large that increases in the number of units do not significantly affect the performance of the model.

The elements of these patterns take values from zero, indicating that no input is occurring at that point, to unity, indicating that some aspect of a stimulus or cue is acting on the organism. In the present simulation, the nominal stimuli 'AA' and 'A–' were used to represent the pseudoword and single-letter conditions described above. The letter 'A' is represented as '1111', the compound 'AA' as '11111111', the compound 'A–blank' as '11110000'. Attention instructions are similarly encoded, the command 'Report the letter in the left position' being represented as '11110000'. In effect, the code '1' means 'attend to this information', and '0' means 'ignore this information'. A complete command to the system in a training trial might consist of the pattern '111111111111000011110000011111111', translating as a presentation of the stimulus AA coupled with a pre-cue instruction to attend only to the left letter, a demand to report A–blank, and an instruction to attend the entire demanded response.

*The cycle of processing*

As indicated earlier, VISA consists of two subsystems, one primarily concerned with the nominal stimulus and one with the demanded response, and each subsystem consists of two layers of units, a communication and an association layer. Conceptually, there are no differences between units in the two subsystems, and the distinction between subsystems arises not because of hardwired circuitry, but because particular units and not others happen to respond to a particular stimulus, and become committed to responding to that stimulus in future. In order to simulate parallel processing on a serial computer (an Apple IIe), the model cycles repetitively through its subsystems, layers and components computing tiny adjustments in each until it reaches stable activity.

*Communication layer*
The processing cycle begins with the units of the communication layer. The communication layer of each subsystem consists of eight units, each receiving input from one of the units in the external energy pattern of a stimulus or demanded response. This input is constant, for as long as the stimulus is present. Additionally, each unit is connected to all the other units in the communication layer of the same subsystem. These connections are responsible for contrast enhancement, and become active only if the external signal pattern is non-uniform, causing differences in the activity of units within a layer. Moreover, the activity of these units may be modified by attention demands.

The units can take values between 1 and $-1$, but are initially at rest, with activity of zero. A unit receiving input from the outside world or from another unit within the system responds by altering its activity in the direction of the sign of the input. The input from an external source to a unit, $u$, is written as $e_u$, and the internal input from a paired unit $p$ to a unit $u$ is written as $i_{up}$. The inputs from internal and external sources are summed to form a net input, $n_u$. The unit responds to this net input by altering its current activity, $a_u$, by an amount proportional to the net input it receives, $En_u$, where $E$ is a proportional constant, usually set at 0.2. (The actual values of this and other proportional constants given below matter very little, except that the system becomes unstable if they are set high.) It is also assumed that units become increasingly resistant to altering their activity as it approaches ceiling (1) or floor ($-1$) levels, and so the change in activity is proportional to the difference between the current activity level and the maximum level, written as $1 + (Va_u)$, where $V$ takes the value of $-1$ if the activity is greater than zero, and 1 otherwise. Further, it is assumed that unit values tend to decay toward their resting state at a rate proportional to their current activity, the amount of decay being $Da_u$, where $D$ is a second proportional constant, usually set at 0.1. Thus, the change in activation of a unit resulting from all inputs in one cycle, $\Delta a_u$, is $\Delta a_u = En_u(1 + (Va_u)) - Da_u$. (This rule is borrowed from McClelland and Rumelhart 1985.)

If one unit becomes more active than another as a result of differences in the energy pattern presented by the external source, the units begin to provide inputs to each other. The internal input, $i_{up}$, that a unit, $u$, receives from each paired unit, $p$, depends on the activity of the paired unit, $a_p$, and the gain or weight of the connection from the second unit to the first, $w_{up}$, so that $i_{up} = a_p w_{up}$. Initially, the gain of the connections between units is zero, but as units become differentially active, the gain may take on values between 1 and $-1$. The gain is proportional to the difference in the activities of the units, so that $w_{up} = S(a_s - a_l)$, where $a_s$ is the smaller of the activities of the target and paired units, and $a_l$ is the larger, and $S$ is a (final) proportional constant, usually set at 0.2. In consequence, if the activity of one unit rises above zero and that of a second unit remains at zero, the first will present negative inputs to the second, and as the activity of the second becomes negative it will provide positive inputs to the first. One effect of this rule is that any differences between the activities of units within a communication layer become magnified, so that contrasts in the presented display are enhanced. A second and vital effect of this mechanism is that blanks in the presented display are encoded integrally with other aspects of the display. Without such a positive feedback mechanism, the activity of a unit corresponding to a stimulus aspect with zero energy would remain at zero, and it would therefore develop no interconnections with other units. The effect of this mechanism is seen most clearly in the simulation of Condition 4, above.

The response of processing units to stimulation from the outside world or from other units is modulated by attentional demands. As a first approximation of how attention might affect perception, I have given VISA a set of attention units, each of which is responsible for receiving the attentional demand for a particular external input, and is linked to the communication and association units for that input through a gated negative feedback loop.

Each communication unit is connected to a gate unit which in turn is connected back to the communication unit. The gain of the connection from a communication unit, $c$, to a gate unit, $g$, is unity, so that as the activity of the communication unit increases, its input to the gate unit is $i_{gc} = a_c$. In consequence, the activity of the gate unit corresponds to the activity of the communication unit. The gain from the gate to the communication unit is $-1$, and its input to the communication unit is $i_{cg} = -a_g$, so that the gate unit exactly cancels the current activity of the communication unit. The effect of this loop is to keep the activity of the communication units at zero, no matter what inputs they receive from the external world.

Thus the system is insensitive to stimuli in the world, and remains so until an attentional demand is made. Attention units respond to these cues, using the same rule that governs the activity of communication units. Each attention unit $a$ is connected unidirectionally to a gate unit $g$. The gain of this connection is $w_{gc} = (0 - a_g)a_a$, and the input to the gate unit is $i_{gc} = a_a w_{gc}$. If an attention demand is made, the activity of the attention unit rises to a maximum, and in consequence it drives the gate unit toward its resting level of zero. When the gate unit's activity is at zero, it has no effect upon the communication unit to which it is connected. Thus negative feedback to the communication unit is cancelled, and the communication unit is free to respond to its external stimulus or to lateral input from other communication units. If no attention is demanded, the attention unit remains at resting level, the gate unit is free to respond to the communication unit, and the consequent negative feedback prevents the communication unit from becoming active. (As a computational shortcut, the effects of the attention circuit may be approximated by multiplying the activity of each communication unit by the value of the stimulus cue on each cycle of the model.) As discussed above, attention cues can operate on either the stimulus or response subsystem, but their effects are quite different in the two cases.

This is by no means an ideal circuit for incorporating variable attention, but does permit the model to demonstrate the importance of including an attentional mechanism in simulations of memory. Conceptually, the effect of the attention codes is learned in the same way that all patterns are learned, through presentation of the cue patterns and modification of the interconnectivity matrix, and exercises its influence through interactions of communication units responding to different stimuli in the world.

*Association Layer*

The association layer of each subsystem also consists of eight units. These units each receive input from one unit in the communication layer of the same subsystem, and from all units of the association layer in the other subsystem, but not from any units in the association layer of the same subsystem. The activity of these units converges on the activity of the single communication unit to which each is connected, because the inputs from the other association units are modified under that restriction. Specifically, the gain of the connection from a communication unit to an association unit is always unity, so that the input to the association unit equals the activity of the communication unit. Between association units, the change in the gain of the connection from any pair unit, $p$, and any target unit, $u$, is proportional to the product of the activity of the pair unit, $a_p$, and the difference between the input to that unit from the communication layer, written as $c_u$, and the current activity of that unit, $a_u$, so that $\Delta w_{up} = (c_u - a_u)a_p S$, where $S$ is a proportional constant mentioned above. (This rule is a modification of McClelland and Rumelhart's, 1985, delta rule.) The current gain of the connection is equal to the gain on the preceding cycle plus the change in gain computed in the present cycle. Computing the current gain in this way prevents it from falling to zero as the activity of the association unit converges on that of its paired communication unit. This is important because the pattern of interconnectivity of the association units forms the enduring representation of the system's experience, and determines how the model performs on subsequent trials.

The input from each paired unit to each target unit is computed as it was for communication units, as the product of the activity of the paired unit, $a_p$, and the gain, $w_{up}$, although the gain is defined differently in the two cases. The net input to each association unit is computed as the sum of the inputs from each pair unit plus the input from the relevant communication unit, and the current activity of the unit is computed according to the general rules given above. Attention cues are also applied to units in this layer, according to the rules given above.

*Termination of processing and response*

This completes one processing cycle of the model. Cycling continues until the system achieves stability, which I define as no change in the second decimal place of the activation of any unit for 25 cycles. At that time, the activity of response-side association units constitutes the final response of the model under the demands of a particular run. These units could be connected to some motor output units to make the model produce an overt response.

Because of the way they are defined, the pattern of interconnectivity in the association level is permanent, whereas the weights of the connections among communication layer units are transient. Thus when the system is faced with a second stimulus to learn, the only enduring effect of the first stimulus is in the interconnectivity matrix of the association layer. For test trials, this matrix is frozen, so that the response to a test stimulus depends on what the system learned in the training trial.

**Implications of the model**

Psychological models can be useful adjuncts to theory construction and empirical observation in a number of ways. They serve as a means of formalizing a theory, providing objective and rigorous definitions of theoretical constructs and their interactions. They provide a means of testing whether a complex package of assumptions actually contains the implications that its author intends. Frequently, they serve as the source of new insights, as heuristic devices for developing fresh ideas about the nature of the problem.

VISA has served me in all of these ways. First, it allowed me to verify that variable processing integration was a reasonable explanation of the variable context dependence I had observed in studies of concept formation and word perception, and that objectively defined changes in processing integration do cause differences in performance, such as the ones observed in humans. Second, although the idea of processing integration was originally conceived to explain variations in concept application, I found that in order to cause the model to process the same stimulus in different ways, I had to consider how task instructions modify processing. Phrased in this way, it was clear that selective attention was an important aspect of the story. As the model developed, it became apparent that the issues of selective and non-selective attention could be considered identical with the issues of analytic and non-analytic processing, and that both could be thought of simply as aspects of the operation of memory. Further, the attentional concepts of early and late selection could be tied to the experimental operations of pre-cuing and post-cuing, and both could be incorporated within a larger framework of interactions of current task demands and representations of past experiences.

Third, because the model consists of fundamental processes stated in objective and neutral language, rather than in the abstract and loaded terms frequently used to state psychological theories, I hoped that it could transcend the artificial barriers between areas of study in psychology, and help to provide a common account of basic perceptual and memorial processes. The model has been a good beginning in this endeavour, being capable not only of simulating data from studies of perception, such as those demonstrated above, but also data from studies of concept learning, such as analytic and non-analytic generalization of performance to novel and degraded stimuli, data from memory studies such as the general superiority of recognition over recall and dissociations between reflective and non-reflective tasks, and data from the social literature on stereotype and attitude formation. Moreover, the model can simulate a number of the phenomena of animal learning, such as Pavlovian conditioning, extinction and fast recovery, and blocking and overshadowing. The latter simulations were particularly exciting to me, because I have long been frustrated by the elusive parallels between animal learning issues and the study of human cognition, such as the relationship between occasion-setting and context specificity, conditioning and expectation, motivation and cuing, or reinforcement and attention. The neutral language of PDP assumptions has enabled me to begin explorations of these issues with colleagues studying conditioning (see McLaren, Kaye, and Mackintosh this volume).

As a final example of the heuristic utility of PDP models incorporating attention, I wish to present some current work on what happens when people actively ignore one stimulus while attending to another, resulting in the 'negative priming' phenomenon (e.g. Tipper 1985). The paradigm consists of presenting a display of two familiar stimuli, one of which is to be reported and the other ignored. Following this training, the subject is required to identify each of the stimuli, as well as novel stimuli, in brief displays. For a short time after the training experience, the previously reported stimulus is more easily identified than the novel stimulus, and the novel stimulus more easily than the previously ignored stimulus.

This phenomenon has invited speculation that the representation of the ignored stimulus is inhibited during the selection trial. The background assumption of this speculation is that familiar stimuli have a pre-formed, abstract and unitary representation whose activation threshold can undergo temporary modification either downward, resulting in priming, or upward, resulting in negative priming. This assumption conflicts with evidence about memory such as that presented in the first sections of this chapter, which suggests that memory preserves each experience of a stimulus, and that performance is determined by the similarity of current and prior processing episodes.

VISA produces results similar to the human data, and does so far a reason which may assist understanding of the interaction between memory and selective ignoring. The simulation consists of two learning trials followed by a selection trial, with test trials interspersed. On the first learning trial, the model is presented the stimulus *A–blank* and on the second the stimulus *blank–B*. In both cases, the model is instructed to attend and respond to the letter only, thus becoming familiar with each letter in isolation. In consequence, it develops independent stimulus–response representations of each letter. In the first set of tests, conducted by freezing the connectivity matrix and presenting the training stimuli without a demanded response, the model responds (generates activity on the response-side association units) with equal strength to both stimuli.

To simulate the selection trial, the model is presented the compound $AB$ and required to output the response $A$. No selective cues are imposed, so that the system processes the entire stimulus–response compound of $AB$–$A$. Thus the system is actually selectively responding during the trial rather than attending selectively. In consequence, the model learns to use perceptual cues about the ignored stimulus as part of the stimulus–response representation leading to report of the attended stimulus.

When the same pair of test trials is conducted following the selection trial, the system is less able to identify the $B$ stimulus than before, although its ability to identify the $A$ stimulus is unimpaired. However, the degraded performance on the previously ignored stimulus does not result from inhibition or unlearning of a representation. The $B$ stimulus is actively processed in interaction with the composite stimulus–response representation formed under the training and selection trials, but that representation is less appropriate for producing a $B$ response given a $B$ stimulus than an $A$ response given an $A$ stimulus.

The focus of human studies of negative priming has been on the fate of the ignored item. VISA's simulation suggests that the subject's ability to perform on the attended item after the event is at least as important in discovering the processes leading to the phenomenon. Following the selection trial, the model can identify both $A$ and $B$ better if the compound $AB$ is presented than if either is presented alone (although it still identifies $A$ more readily). This indicates that its ability to identify the attended stimulus is dependent on the representation formed during the selection experience, in the same way as its ability to identify the ignored stimulus. Systematic human data are not available for comparison, but anecdotal evidence suggests that humans show the same effect. This is important, because if true it suggests that attended and ignored stimuli are not processed independently, as suggested by the inhibition account, but rather that humans, like the model, form a representation of the total selection experience that results in strong performance under some specific conditions of test and degraded performance under others. In this case the effects of ignoring a stimulus can be understood through the same means used to account for the effects of attending.

Thus the simulation raises the intriguing possibility that the negative priming phenomenon depends on standard learning procedures rather than on a special inhibitory mechanism. However, human subjects recover quickly from the experience, which appears to contradict the learning hypothesis. A possible resolution is that the purpose of the encounter (to identify or select a stimulus) forms part of the representation of the event, and on a later occasion serves as an additional cue or stimulus context interacting with the representation, resulting in performance specific to the current demands. The transience of the phenomenon may reflect a shift of effective processing context from selection to identification as time since the selection trial passes. (If the demands of trials are included as context in the model, the effect is extremely transient: the system immediately responds with facilitation for both ignored and attended stimuli.) We are currently investigating this issue through experiments with humans, varying the familiarity of stimuli and the purposes for which stimuli have been encountered, and also determining whether the experience of selecting are enduring and specific to the configural properties of the compound selection display. In parallel, we are continuing simulation studies, examining the effects of different kinds of context changes on later perceptual success and attempting to model the time course of negative priming.

## Conclusion

Although VISA is very crude in some respects, it illustrates the utility of PDP models in studying fundamental processes of memory and their interactions. The model achieves its success by preserving specific organizations of stimuli imposed by the purpose of encountering the stimuli. Its sensitivity to the demands of the task is due to flexible attention and processing integration, and its ability to retain the separate influence of multiple experiences is due to its parallel processing and distributed representation. Because it incorporates these functions, the model is able to simulate human sensitivity to the general structure of the world and to the specific circumstances of particular experiences.

## Acknowledgements

The author is indebted to Lee Brooks and Larry Jacoby for their theoretical leadership, to Alisa Cantwell for her empirical contributions and to Henry James for his constructive criticism. Preparation of this article was supported by Grant No. A0573 from the National Science and Engineering Research Council of Canada. Requests for reprints should be sent to the author, c/o The Department of Psychology, Mt Allison University, Sackville, NB, Canada E0A 3C0.

## Note

1. A related processing difference is the completeness of encoding, varying from processing the whole stimulus to processing a single element. A particular task may focus attention only on typical stimulus aspects and thus effectively cause abstraction

of general properties. However, such processing is assumed to occur only under the demands of particular tasks rather than chronically, and creates a representation which is the same in kind as traces resulting from other tasks, although different in detail.

## References

Baron, J. and Thurston, I. (1973). An analysis of the word superiority effect. *Cognitive Psychology*, **4**, 207–88.

Broadbent, D. E. (1958). *Perception and communication*. Pergamon Press, London.

Brooks, L. R. (1978). Non-analytic concept formation and memory for instances. In *Cognition and Categorization* (eds. E. Rosch and B. B. Lloyd). Erlbaum, Hillsdale, NJ.

Brooks, L. R. and Whittlesea, B. W. A. (1988). Critical influence of particular experiences in the identification of objects. Unpublished manuscript.

Craik, F. I. M. and Lockhart, R. S. (1972). Levels of processing: a framework for memory research. *Journal of Verbal Learning and Verbal Behavior*, **11**, 671–84.

Deutsch, J. A. and Deutsch, D. (1963). Attention: some theoretical considerations. *Psychological Review*, **70**, 80–90.

Gibson, E. J., Shurcliff, A., and Yonas, A. (1970). Utilization of spelling patterns by deaf and hearing subjects. In *Basic studies in reading* (eds. H. Levin and J. P. Williams). Basic Books, NY.

Hastie, R. (1981). Schematic principles in human memory. In *Social cognition: the Ontario Symposium* (eds. E. T. Higgins, C. P. Hermand, and M. P. Zanna). Erlbaum, Hillsdale, NJ.

Hintzman, D. (1983). Schema abstraction in a multiple-trace memory model. Paper presented at conference on 'The priority of the specific'. Elora, Ontario.

Homa, D., Sterling, S., and Trepel, L. (1981). Limitations of exemplar-based generalization and the abstraction of categorical information. *Journal of Experimental Psychology: Human Learning and Memory*, **7**, 418–39.

Jacoby, L. L. (1983). Perceptual enhancement: persistent effects of an experience. *Journal of Experimental Psychology: Learning, Memory and Cognition*, **9**, 21–38.

Jacoby, L. L. and Brooks, L. R. (1984). Non-analytic cognition: memory, perception and concept formation. In *The psychology of learning and motivation*, Volume 18 (ed. G. H. Bower). Academic Press, NY.

Jacoby, L. L. and Dallas, M. (1981). On the relationship between autobiographical memory and percpetual learning. *Journal of Experimental Psychology: General*, **3**, 306–40.

Jacoby, L. L. and Witherspoon, D. E. (1982). Remembering without awareness. *Canadian Journal of Psychology*, **36**, 300–24.

Kolers, P. A. (1975). Memorial consequences of automatized encoding. *Journal of Experimental Psychology: Human Learning and Memory*, **1**, 689–701.

Kolers, P. A. (1976). Reading a year later. *Memory & Cognition*, **8**, 322–8.

McClelland, J. L. (1985). Putting knowledge in its place: a scheme for programming parallel processing structures on the fly. *Cognitive Science*, **9**, 113–46.

McClelland, J. L. and Rumelhart, D. E. (1985). Distributed memory and the representation of general and specific information. *Journal of Experimental Psychology: General*, **114**, 159–88.

Medin, D. L. and Shaffer, M. M. (1978). Context theory of classification learning. *Psychological Review*, **85**, 207–38.

Reicher, G. M. (1969). Perceptual recognition as a function of meaningfulness of stimulus material. *Journal of Experimental Psychology*, **81**, 274–80.

Rosch, E. (1977). Principles of categorization. In *Cognition and categorization* (eds. E. Rosch and B. B. Lloyd). Erlbaum, Hillsdale, NJ.

Salasoo, A., Shiffrin, R. M., and Faustal, T. C. (1985). Building permanent memory codes: codification and repetition effects in word identification. *Journal of Experimental Psychology: General*, **114**, 50–77.

Tipper, S. (1985). The negative priming effect: inhibitory priming by ignored objects. *Quarterly Journal of Experimental Psychology*, **37**, 571–90.

Tulving, E. (1983). Elements of episodic memory. Oxford University Press, London.

Tulving, E., Schacter, D. L., and Stark, H. A. (1982). Priming effects in word-fragment completion are independent of recognition memory. *Journal of Experimental Psychology: Learning, Memory and Cognition*, **8**, 336–42.

Wheeler, D. D. (1970). Processes in word recognition. *Cognitive Psychology*, **1**, 59–85.

Whittlesea, B. W. A. (1983). The representation of concepts: an evaluation of the abstractive and episodic perspectives. Unpublished doctoral dissertation, McMaster University, Hamilton.

Whittlesea, B. W. A. (1987). Preservation of specific experiences in the representation of general knowledge. *Journal of Experimental Psychology: Learning, Memory and Cognition*, **13**, 3–17.

Whittlesea, B. W. A. and Brooks, L. R. (1988). Critical influence of particular experiences in the perception of letters, words, and phrases. *Memory & Cognition*, **5**, 387–99.

Whittlesea, B. W. A. and Cantwell, A. L. (1987). Enduring influence of the purpose of experiences: encoding-retrieval interactions in word and pseudoword perception. *Memory & Cognition*, **6**, 465–72.

# 6

## An associative theory of the representation of stimuli: applications to perceptual learning and latent inhibition[1]

I. P. L. McLAREN, H. KAYE, and
N. J. MACKINTOSH

### Introduction

Connectionist theories of parallel distributed processing (PDP) models postulate a system containing a large number of elements which become associated in accordance with certain rules. Associationist theories have a long history in psychology—indeed, they long antedate modern experimental psychology. But within experimental psychology today, the best worked-out theories of association are those developed to account for simple Pavlovian conditioning in animals. It would be surprising, therefore, if there were no parallels to be found between connectionist theories and theories of Pavlovian conditioning, and equally surprising if insights from one area of research cannot shed light on the problems of the other. Pavlovian conditioning in animals may provide unusual opportunities for studying fundamental associative processes uncluttered by the complexity of optional control processes. Equally, however, we shall argue that some connectionist ideas prove to have powerful implications for the understanding of a hitherto rather intractable set of problems for theories of Pavlovian conditioning.

As has been widely recognized, connectionist and Pavlovian conditioning theories have developed rather similar learning rules (Sutton and Barto 1981). Classical associationism made do with a small handful of simple rules to account for the establishment of associations between events or ideas, the standard ones being temporal and spatial contiguity and constant conjunction. It is now apparent that these laws will produce inefficient and maladaptive learning, which would leave animals at the mercy of chance conjunctions of events. Pavlovian conditioning can be regarded as the process by which animals discover what predicts those events of consequence to themselves which psychologists call reinforcers. It allows them to establish an accurate representation of the causal structure of their environment, and it does so precisely because it is not adequately characterized by the standard laws of classical associationism. Modern conditioning theory has added a new law, that of relative predictive validity. Repeated paired presentations of a conditioned stimulus (CS) and reinforcer are not sufficient to guarantee their association: the CS must provide information about the occurrence of the reinforcer not otherwise available; it must be a more valid predictor of the reinforcer than any other event. The idea was first expressed informally by Kamin some 20 years ago (Kamin 1968), and given its first formal statement by Rescorla and Wagner in 1972. Alternative versions of the rule have been proposed (Mackintosh 1975; Pearce and Hall 1980), but in one form or another it seems as securely established today as it was 20 years ago (Durlach 1988).

The implications of this insight are not confined to the production of better models of salivary conditioning in dogs. Modern conditioning theory describes an effective system for detecting correlations or contingencies between events, and as such can be applied to people as well as inarticulate animals. There is, of course, nothing novel in suggesting that some of our emotional attitudes and irrational phobias are the product of a primitive conditioning process. It is more interesting to suggest that the associative principles of conditioning theory provide a surprisingly satisfactory account of the way university students attempt to judge which of several events is the cause of a particular effect, or to diagnose which of several possible diseases is indicated by a particular constellation of symptoms (Dickinson and Shanks 1985; Gluck and Bower 1986).

Sutton and Barto (1981) were the first to notice the striking similarity between the Rescorla–Wagner equation and the Widrow–Hoff or delta rule frequently used to determine the formation of connections in a PDP system (e.g. McClelland and Rumelhart 1985; Rumelhart, Hinton, and McClelland 1986). According to the Rescorla–Wagner model, the association between a CS and reinforcer will change on a given conditioning trial only if there is a discrepancy between the obtained and expected reinforcer on that trial. According to the delta rule, connections between elements are changed only in so far as is necessary to bring them into line with the external input to those elements. The power of Pavlovian conditioning paradigms is that they permit one to observe the operation of this rule very much more directly than in most PDP studies. Kamin's blocking experiment provides the simplest illustration. Kamin (1968) showed that if animals received a series of conditioning trials on which two CSs, say a light and a tone, occurred simultaneously followed by a reinforcer, the conditioning that would normally have accrued to the tone was prevented or blocked if the light had already been established as a signal for the reinforcer. According to the Rescorla–Wagner model, as a consequence of this prior conditioning to the light the reinforcer was already fully expected when the tone was added, and conditioning to the tone was prevented because there was no discrepancy between the obtained and predicted reinforcer in its presence.

This parallel between the Rescorla–Wagner and delta rules is probably sufficiently familiar to require little further comment from us. In what follows we take it for granted, and the modified delta rule incorporated into the model that we propose allows us to explain such phenomena as blocking in much the same way as did Rescorla and Wagner. As far as we are aware, however, a second parallel has been entirely ignored, probably because the conditioning theory in question has fallen out of favour. Most contemporary theories of conditioning take as their point of departure the naïve assumption that the stimuli used as CSs, tones, buzzers, flashing lights, etc., may be conceptualized as simple, unitary events, given direct to the animal, and standing in need of no further analysis. Occasional lip service acknowledges that this is a naïve oversimplification, but little serious attention has been paid to developing a more adequate account of the perception and representation of stimuli in conditioning experiments. According to stimulus sampling theory, however, even a simple CS should be regarded as a set of elements, only a randomly selected and partial subset of which is sampled on each trial (Estes 1950; Neimark and Estes 1967). And only sampled elements control performance and enter into new associations on each conditioning trial.

The assumptions of stimulus-sampling theory hardly constitute a radical departure from those of other conditioning theories, but already they provide plausible explanations of a number of phenomena. The gradual increase in performance over a series of conditioning trials, superimposed on substantial variability from one trial to the next, is explained by supposing that although sampled elements are conditioned in an all-or-none manner, only a random subset is sampled on each trial, so that on early trials the sample will contain relatively few conditioned elements. The learning-rate parameter of other conditioning theories finds a natural interpretation in terms of the proportion of all elements sampled on each trial. Variability of performance is a consequence of chance variation in the proportion of conditioned elements sampled from one trial to the next, and forgetting (and spontaneous recovery following extinction) is explained by appeal to the fluctuation of elements with the passage of time. The explanation of generalization provided by stimulus-sampling theory has seemed so persuasive that it has been widely borrowed by other theorist (e.g. Blough 1975; Pearce 1987): after a response has been conditioned to one stimulus, it will be elicited by another, similar, stimulus to the extent that the two stimuli share elements in common.

So far, so good. But not very far. Stimulus-sampling theory assumes that associations are formed only between different events, a CS and a response or a reinforcer. A connectionist perspective suggests that we should allow associations to be formed not only between the elements of different events, but also between the various elements comprising a single event, such as the CS itself. Every time a set of elements is activated together, connections will be formed between them; repeated presentation of a CS should therefore establish associations between the random subset of its elements sampled on each trial, and thus eventually between all its elements. This seemingly innocuous assumption has far-reaching consequences. In general terms, it provides a mechanism for the establishment of representations of events, allowing an animal to identify a repeatedly seen stimulus better than one seen for the first time, or to re-construct a complete representation of a familiar stimulus from an isolated fragment. More specifically, as we hope to show, it allows us to explain a seemingly paradoxical and hitherto unintegrated set of findings from experiments in which animals are simply exposed to one or more stimuli in the absence of reinforcement.

## Changes in behaviour to a repeatedly presented stimulus

It is certain that animals learn something when a stimulus is repeatedly presented to them, even without reinforcement, for such treatment has enduring effects on their behaviour: apart from causing a decline in their initial responses to the stimulus—the phenomenon of habituation—it has two further, contrasting effects. First, and more commonly, it slows down the rate at which conditioning occurs to the stimulus when it is subsequently paired with a reinforcer. This is latent inhibition (Lubow 1973), a phenomenon of wide generality, observed in essentially all standard conditioning preparations: while a novel stimulus conditions rapidly, a familiar one, which the animal has come across before with no further consequence, conditions slowly. The results of a typical experiment are shown in Fig. 6.1(a).

The second effect is less common: occasionally, exposure to two stimuli, far from retarding subsequent conditioning, enhances the rate of subsequent discrimination learning between them. The classic demonstration of this perceptual learning effect (Gibson and Walk 1956) involved rearing rats with metal circles and triangles hanging on the walls of their cages, and showing that, when adult, they learned to discriminate between them more rapidly than control animals reared under comparable conditions, but without these shapes present (see Fig. 6.1(b)). Subsequent research, however, has established that the effect occurs with a rather wider array of stimuli, does not require such extensive exposure as that provided by Gibson and Walk, and certainly does not depend on exposure in infancy (Hall 1980; Honey and Hall 1988).

We shall argue that both latent inhibition and perceptual learning are a consequence of the elaboration of representations of stimuli with their

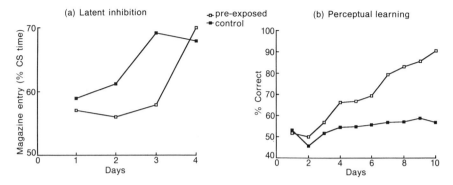

**Fig. 6.1** Demonstrations of latent inhibition and perceptual learning. (a) Rate of conditioning to a CS (tone) signalling the delivery of water, in animals pre-exposed to the tone and in controls for whom the tone was novel. (From Kaye *et al.* 1987, Experiment 1.) (b) Rate of learning whom animals are required to discriminate between a circle and a triangle which have either been pre-exposed in their home cages or which, for the control group, are novel. (From Gibson and Walk 1956.)

repeated presentation. The procedures employed in these experiments are as simple as can be: one or more stimuli are repeatedly presented with no further consequence. But we do not believe that there exists a fully satisfactory account of either phenomenon, let alone one which might encompass both. The problem is lack of adequate theory, rather than inconsistency of experimental outcome. Latent inhibition and perceptual learning are, on the face of it, diametrically opposite effects, but the experimental operations responsible for this apparent difference in outcome seem reasonably clear. The first important variable is whether conditioning or discrimination learning takes place in the same context as that in which the stimuli were initially exposed (Lubow, Rifkin, and Alek 1976; Channell and Hall 1981). When it does, the almost invariable outcome is slower learning (latent inhibition). Exposed to a pair of stimuli in the apparatus in which they are subsequently required to discriminate them, rats will learn this discrimination more slowly than control animals given no prior exposure to the stimuli (Channell and Hall 1981; see Fig. 6.2). Conversely, if animals are exposed to a CS in one context and subsequently conditioned to that CS in a different context, latent inhibition is normally attenuated, and sometimes abolished (Lovibond, Preston, and Mackintosh 1984; Kaye *et al.* 1987). But significant facilitation of learning (i.e. a perceptual learning effect) requires more than a change of context. Typical perceptual learning experiments employ stimuli, such as circles and triangles, or horizontal and vertical striations, which are presumably rather more complex than the tones and buzzers used in simple conditioning experiments, and an experiment by Oswalt (1972) suggests that

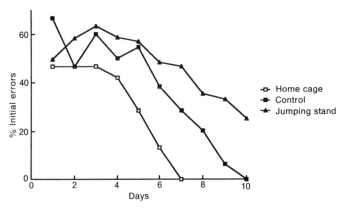

**Fig. 6.2**   The effect of context on latent inhibition and perceptual learning. By comparison with a control group for whom the stimuli are novel, pre-exposure to the stimuli in the jumping stand (the test apparatus) retards subsequent discrimination learning—a latent inhibition effect, while pre-exposure to the stimuli in the home cage facilitates subsequent discrimination—a perceptual learning effect. (From Channell and Hall, 1981.)

perceptual learning is more likely to be found with more difficult discriminations. More important, perceptual learning is measured not in terms of the rate of conditioning to one stimulus, but in terms of the discrimination between two. An experiment reported by Hall and Honey (1988) suggests that prior exposure to a stimulus may simultaneously retard conditioning to that stimulus and enhance its discrimination from another, similar, stimulus. They first exposed rats to horizontal and vertical striations, then trained them to respond to one of these stimuli, and finally measured the extent to which responding generalized to the other. Prior exposure both retarded the rate of conditioning in the second phase of the experiment and decreased generalization in the final phase. A decrease in generalization is, of course, equivalent to an increase in discrimination. Thus the same animals showed both latent inhibition (retarded conditioning) and perceptual learning (improved discrimination).

The implications of these observations seem rather clear. As Hall and Honey (1988) have argued, we need to distinguish between a change in the *associability* of a stimulus and a change in its *discriminability*. Prior exposure to a stimulus will tend to reduce the readiness of that stimulus to enter into new associations (its associability). Such exposure typically, therefore, retards subsequent conditioning, although this effect is somehow attenuated by a change of context. But at the same time exposure to a stimulus may make it easier to discriminate that stimulus from another, similar, stimulus. Experiments on simple conditioning make minimal demands on discrimination (the animal is required only to discriminate the presence of the CS from its absence), and are therefore unlikely to show a perceptual learning effect. But even where animals are required to discriminate between two similar stimuli, any increase in their discriminability may be more than offset by a decrease in their associability. An increase in the speed of discrimination learning is normally observed only where a change of context has disrupted latent inhibition. The implication is that the processes underlying any increase in discriminability (or at least some of these processes) survive a change of context better than do those underlying the decline of associability.

The main problem remains, however, that of proposing a theoretical framework which might, even in principle, explain both experimental outcomes, let alone the circumstances which pre-dispose towards one or the other. There is no shortage of theories of latent inhibition (see Mackintosh 1983), and we do not propose to review them all here. Our own account will assume that latent inhibition reflects a decline in the associability of a repeatedly presented stimulus, which occurs as a consequence of the associations formed between stimulus elements during these presentations.[2] It is thus related to the accounts provided by Wagner (1981) and by Pearce and Hall (1980). According to Pearce and Hall, the associability of a stimulus depends on the extent to which it predicts its consequences. Animals are said to attend to a novel stimulus with unknown consequences, but as its consequences become expected (i.e. associated with it), so its associability declines. An interesting feature of the theory has been the attempt to use an animal's orienting responses to a stimulus as an overt index of attention or associability, and the theory is nicely supported by the demonstration that such orienting responses habituate during the course of repeated, unreinforced presentations of a stimulus, recover when the stimulus is paired with a reinforcer on a series of conditioning trials, but once again habituate as conditioning proceeds and the reinforcer becomes well predicted (Kaye and Pearce 1984, 1987).

As originally formulated, however, the Pearce–Hall theory has no means of predicting that latent inhibition is disrupted by a change of context between exposure and conditioning trials. But the gap is filled by Wagner's account which directly predicts this effect. According to Wagner, latent inhibition occurs because a representation of a repeatedly presented stimulus is associated with the context in which it occurred, and is retrieved whenever the animal is replaced in that context. But only unexpected stimuli are well processed: if a stimulus is already 'primed' in memory, this will be sufficient to reduce processing of that stimulus, and therefore its associability with any other event, when it is actually presented. From this it follows that if animals are exposed to a CS in one context and subsequently conditioned to it in another, latent inhibition will be abolished. While this accounts nicely for the basic observation, there are additional effects of contextual variables on latent inhibition which are much harder to explain in terms of Wagner's account. We shall return to some of these below.[3]

## A connectionist theory of perceptual learning

The associative accounts of latent inhibition provided by Wagner (1981) and Pearce and Hall (1980) have much to commend them. We believe that it is possible to subsume aspects of both into a more general theory, which then handles, without great difficulty, some of the findings which created problems for the original theories. But the major problem for both is how to account for perceptual learning. We believe that the solution to this is to take seriously the implications of the idea that stimuli (even simple stimuli like tones and flashing lights) should be conceptualized as sets of elements. Both Wagner (1981) and Pearce (1987) have indeed acknowledged that stimuli may be regarded as sets of elements, and Pearce in particular has used this idea in an analysis of generalization and generalization decrement. But neither has worked out some of the implications that follow from the basic idea, let alone those that follow from the further idea that associations can be established between these elements.

We assume a PDP system containing a large number of elements. An input to the system (a stimulus such as a tone) causes a pattern of activation over many of the elements of the system. The advantages of such a distributed system, in terms of resistance to noise or degradation of the input, and its ability to explain generalization, do not need to be rehearsed further. We also assume that only a subset of the elements potentially activated by a stimulus will be sampled on any given trial. And finally, we assume that associations are formed between all elements activated at the same time. According to the modified delta rule which we shall use, connections are formed between elements in such a way as to minimize the discrepancy between their external inputs (activation from the presentation of stimuli) and internal, associative inputs from other elements within the system. (A more detailed and formal exposition of the model is provided in the appendix to this chapter.)

We follow stimulus sampling theory in assuming that only a subset of the elements of a stimulus is sampled on any one trial, but we depart from the theory in assuming that the sampling process is not random, but depends on the nature of the stimulus and of the animal's interaction with it. For the 'simple' stimuli typically used as CSs, tones, coloured lights, etc., there will be little variability in input from one occasion to the next; in other words, a relatively large proportion of the elements of the stimulus will therefore be sampled on each trial. For more 'complex' stimuli, such as circles, triangles, horizontal or vertical striations, the position may be different. There is potentially much greater variability in input and hence in the elements sampled from one trial to the next: the defining characteristics of such stimuli are multiple and distributed (in these instances in space), and animals can sample from only a limited region of space at any given moment. They will therefore sample only a small subset of the elements of such stimuli on each trial.

Successive presentations of the same stimulus, therefore, will not necessarily activate exactly the same set of elements on each trial, and this variability will be related to the complexity of the stimulus. Even in the most variable case, however, the application of the learning rule will ensure that a particular set, corresponding to the 'central tendency' of the stimulus, will eventually be activated together. Elements common to successive presentations of the stimulus will become connected and thus activate each other, while elements only occasionally activated, i.e. noise, will acquire only weak connections with this central tendency. The process is exactly the same as that proposed by McClelland and Rumelhart (1985) to account for the learning of concepts: as they note, since 'the delta rule can be used to extract the structure from an ensemble of inputs, and throw away random variability . . . the distributed model acts as a sort of signal averager, finding the central tendency of a set of related patterns' (pp. 167–8).

There are more general parallels with earlier views on perceptual learning. Following Hebb (1949), we are appealing to the development of associations between the elements of a stimulus to account for the elaboration of a representation of that stimulus. But this associative process will have effects similar to those postulated by other accounts. If the initial presentation of a complex stimulus directly activates only a small subset of its elements, including (as we shall argue below) a disproportionate number of the elements that do not differentiate it from other, similar, stimuli, this is tantamount to saying that its initial representation will be vague and imprecise. As more elements of the stimulus are sampled on succeeding trials and become associated with one another, then whatever elements are sampled on any one trial they will retrieve other elements, and a complete and accurate representation of the stimulus, which includes all its defining features, will be activated. The mechanism underlying this change in representation is simply the formation of associations between elements; but the consequences seem to correspond to the development of Sokolov's 'neuronal model' or Konorski's 'gnostic unit' (Sokolov 1963; Konorski 1967), and even appear to capture the essentials of the Gibsons's account of perceptual differentiation where 'percepts change over time by progressive elaboration of qualities, features, and dimensions of variation . . . and the world gets more and more properties as the objects in it get more distinctive' (Gibson and Gibson, 1955 p. 34).

As a consequence of this process of 'unitization', novel and familiar stimuli will have different effects on the system. Presentation of a novel stimulus will activate a random subset of its elements; even if those elements are associated with a reinforcing consequence on that trial, there is no guarantee that a sufficient number of them will be directly activated by the next presentation of the 'same' stimulus to generate the required response. The importance of this process of unitization will depend on the 'complexity' of the stimulus. With stimuli of sufficient complexity, unitization will lead to more reliable conditioning, with less variability in responding from trial to trial. Other things being equal (which, as we shall see, they are not), this would mean more rapid conditioning.

Perceptual learning, however, is a matter of enhanced discrimination, i.e. reduced generalization, between two similar stimuli, and to understand it we need to understand why generalization occurs in the first place. According to stimulus-sampling theory, generalization will occur from one stimulus to another to the extent that they share elements in common. Consider a pair of stimuli, A and B, each consisting of a set of unique elements, *a* and *b* respectively, and a set of elements, *x*, common to both (see Fig. 6.3). Exposure

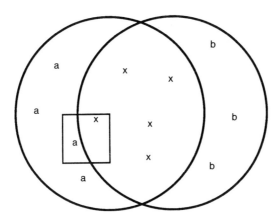

**Fig. 6.3**   A schematic representation of two stimuli, each composed of a large number of elements, some of which they share in common. The similarity of the two stimuli is represented by the proportion of common elements. On any one trial, only a subset of the elements of a stimulus is directly sampled—the sample being represented in the diagram by the small square box.

to these two stimuli will have a number of effects. First, to the extent that such exposure produces latent inhibition (the mechanism for which we shall discuss below), it will be more marked for the common elements, *x*, which occur twice as often as the unique elements, *a* and *b*. In the case of the stimuli typically used in perceptual learning studies, moreover, the unique elements may well be sampled more variably than the common elements. The features common to a circle and a triangle are that they are both, for example, solid black shapes, and these attributes will presumably be sampled regardless of how the animal fixates them. The unique features, straight or curved lines in various orientations, corners, etc., permit of greater variability of input, and, unless the animal always fixates exactly the same part of the stimulus, any one element is less likely to be sampled on a given trial. This will provide an additional reason why the unique elements might be less subject to latent inhibition than the common elements. As a consequence, if stimulus $A$ is subsequently paired with reinforcement, conditioning will occur more strongly to the unique $a$ elements than to the common $x$ elements, and generalization to $B$ will be reduced.

A second consequence of exposure to $A$ and $B$ will be the establishment of a number of interconnections between their various elements. The $a$ elements will be connected with one another, as will the $b$, and the $x$ elements will become connected to both $a$ and $b$ elements (and vice-versa). The formation of these associations will have a number of consequences. We have already suggested that in the case of stimuli such as a circle (A) and a triangle (B) there is a higher probability of sampling the elements they share in common than any particular set of unique elements. A naïve animal learning to discriminate between them, therefore, will initially associate $x$ elements with both reinforcement and non-reinforcement, a rather variable set of $a$ elements with reinforcement, and a similar variable set of $b$ elements with non-reinforcement. The probability of correct choice will increase only slowly. But the establishment of associations between the $a$ elements will mean that the presence of one or two $a$ elements in a sample will retrieve others and thus increase both the probability of correct choice on that trial and the rate of excitatory conditioning to $a$ elements. The process of unitization should enhance the rate of discrimination learning.

But the formation of other associations between the elements of A and B may initially act to increase *generalization* between them. As a result of associations between common and unique elements, the occurrence of A will now activate not only $a$ and $x$, but also, by association, $b$ elements, and reinforcement of A will therefore increase the association between $b$ and reinforcement. A final process, however, will cancel this effect: *inhibitory* connections will be established between the $a$ and $b$ elements. This follows from the application of the delta rule, since there will be a negative correlation between the activation of the two types of element (if A and B are distinct stimuli, they will not be perceived exactly simultaneously). Conditioning theorists may find the derivation from the Rescorla–Wagner model easier to follow: the presence of $x$ elements is associated with, and hence predicts, the presence of both $a$ and $b$ elements, but the presence of $a$ signals the absence of the otherwise predicted $b$ (and vice-versa). The consequence of these inhibitory connections will be to prevent the generalization that would otherwise arise as positive associations are formed between the common and unique elements. Since these positive associations will be formed during the course of discrimination training when the stimuli are novel, and more rapidly than the inhibitory associations between the unique elements, the net effect of pre-exposure will be to facilitate the discrimination between the two stimuli.

Perceptual learning will thus occur for at least three rather distinct reasons. First, when two stimuli are pre-exposed, the elements common to both, which are responsible for generalization between them, will be subject to a stronger latent inhibition effect that those unique to each. We have seen that perceptual learning is more likely to be found after a change of context has attenuated latent inhibition, but our own account of latent inhibition allows for some transfer of the effect across a change of contexts. Second, the process of unitization will ensure that the presentation of a complex stimulus activates elements belonging to the central representation of that stimulus, rather than a small, variable subset of its elements, dominated by those it shares in common with other, similar, stimuli. Finally, there will be some tendency to generalization between two stimuli caused by the formation of interconnections between their common and unique elements during the course of discrimination training, but this will be cancelled in pre-exposed animals by the establishment of additional, inhibitory connections between their unique elements.

We believe that this represents the first analytic attempt to come to terms with perceptual differentiation, and one which has the added virtue both of explaining the detailed results of a number of published experiments, and of making novel, testable predictions. Differential latent inhibition, for example, seems to provide a compelling explanation for results such as those of Forgus (1958a,b), where perceptual learning has been more evident with a slight change in the stimuli between pre-exposure and discriminative training. Rats learned a circle–triangle discrimination especially rapidly following exposure to a triangle lacking its three corners: latent inhibition will have reduced the associability of many of the elements of the triangle which it shares in common with a circle, but will have left intact the associability of those features, the angles, which most effectively differentiate it from a circle.

The suggestion that the formation of inhibitory connections between unique elements provides one mechanism of perceptual learning seems to capture the essential part of the idea, advanced by Bateson and Chantrey (1972), that the beneficial effects of pre-exposure depend on animals learning to classify the stimuli apart rather than together, and provides a ready explanation for the finding that perceptual learning is enhanced by an increase in the temporal separation between stimuli during pre-exposure (Chantrey 1974).

One of the most obvious predictions derivable from our account is that perceptual learning should depend on the proportion of elements common to the two pre-exposed stimuli. We have some initial evidence to support this idea. In a study of perceptual learning and latent inhibition in a maze discrimination, Chamizo and Mackintosh (1989) found that an increase in the number of features common to the intramaze cues which differentiated positive and negative arms turned a significant latent inhibition effect (pre-exposure retarded subsequent discrimination learning) into a marginal perceptual learning effect. In some preliminary experiments on flavour aversion conditioning, we have shown that when an aversion is conditioned to a compound flavour of saline plus lemon, generalization to a sucrose–lemon compound is reduced by prior exposure to the two compounds, but generalization to sucrose alone from saline alone is unaffected by exposure to these two elements. In the former case, moreover, the discrimination between saline–lemon and sucrose–lemon compounds is more effectively enhanced by exposure to the two compounds than by exposure to the various elements in isolation.

### A connectionist theory of latent inhibition

The establishment of interconnections between elements in a network may thus provide an explanation of perceptual learning with exposure to a pair of discriminative stimuli. But the more common effect of pre-exposure is latent inhibition. In order to accommodate latent inhibition, we must introduce a further assumption to the model in the form of a modulator (see Fig. 6.4),

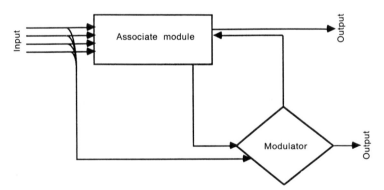

**Fig. 6.4**   A representation of the system architecture. External input activates nodes in the associative module, corresponding to stimulus elements, and also feeds directly into a modulator. The modulator also receives input directly from nodes in the associative module and can thus compare the external and internal input to each node. The modulator feeds back to the associative module to regulate the activation of each node.

which detects the discrepancy between external and internal inputs to an element, enhancing the activation of those elements where the mismatch is large. Elements with high activation form new associations rapidly. The delta rule itself, of course, ensures that the change in connectivity between the elements of a CS and a reinforcer will be proportional to the discrepancy between external and internal inputs to the elements of the reinforcer. The effect of the modulator is to ensure that the change is also proportional to the discrepancy between external and internal inputs to the elements of the CS. A novel CS, which has no internal inputs and thus a large discrepancy between external and internal inputs, will therefore enter into association with other elements more rapidly than a familiar CS.

We may distinguish two possible sources of internal input to a stimulus element and, hence, two possible sources of latent inhibition. First, repeated presentation of a stimulus establishes a representation of that stimulus consisting of a network of connections between elements corresponding to the central tendency of the stimulus. This process of unitization will itself cause a decline in the associability of the elements of the stimulus with any new consequence. As we noted above, all else being equal, unitization will also reduce variability and may increase discriminability. But all else is not equal: connections between the elements that constitute a stimulus will tend to reduce their associability. The second source of latent inhibition arises when a stimulus is repeatedly presented in the same, unchanging, context. Here the entire set of elements comprising the stimulus will form connections with the entire set of elements comprising that context, and when the stimulus is again presented in that context, the match between external and internal inputs to each element of the stimulus will ensure their low associability. Moreover, since these connections go in both directions, the presentation of a stimulus associated with a particular context will lower the associability of those contextual stimuli, so that the entire set of elements comprising the stimulus plus context, which must be associated with the reinforcer during conditioning, will have lower activation.

We are now in a position to explain the major facts of latent inhibition. Repeated presentation of a simple, salient CS, such as a bright light, will tend to retard conditioning to that CS when it is subsequently paired with a reinforcer. Since there will be little variability in the elements sampled from one trial to the next, the representation of the stimulus will be established rapidly; and since animals are not required to discriminate it from any other stimulus during the course of conditioning, the process of unitization will have little beneficial, and considerable adverse, effect on subsequent conditioning. The repeated presentation of the CS in the same context will establish connections (in both directions) between the CS and contextual stimuli, reducing associability yet further and therefore also retarding subsequent conditioning in that context. But if the CS is presented in a new context for conditioning, the loss of internal input from the elements of the old context will restore the associability of the CS elements and sharply attenuate latent inhibition.

The importance of contextual stimuli in latent inhibition is also affected by animals' experience with them. One prediction derivable from Wagner's (1981) theory is that exposure to the context alone, either before or after exposure to the CS in that context, should attenuate latent inhibition. Prior exposure to the context alone should cause latent inhibition of contextual stimuli themselves and thus retard their association with the subsequently presented CS on which latent inhibition depends. The evidence suggests, however, that such exposure does nothing to diminish latent inhibition (Hall and Channell 1985a). The second problem for Wagner's account is that exposure to the context alone after exposure to the CS in that context, i.e. between latent inhibition and conditioning, should tend to extinguish the association between context and CS on which latent inhibition is assumed to depend. Although there are reports of such an effect (Wagner 1979, pp. 66–67; Baker and Mercier 1982), in the majority of relevant studies no evidence of the extinction of latent inhibition has been found (Baker and Mercier 1982; Hall and Minor 1984).

Neither of these findings is as problematical for our model as they are for Wagner's. The crucial feature of our account is that we postulate additional sources of latent inhibition, which will continue to generate an effect in the absence of any associations between CS and context.[4] Indeed, the model makes some novel predictions. We should expect that the latent inhibition effect still seen when animals are exposed to the context *before* exposure to the CS in that context will generalize to other contexts, whereas any latent inhibition still seen when animals are exposed to the context alone *after* exposure to the CS in that context will fail to generalize. McLaren, in some unpublished experiments, has confirmed the former prediction.

We have spent what some may regard as a disproportionate amount of time discussing the role of context. We make few apologies for this. The contextual specificity of latent inhibition is a striking, and imperfectly understood, phenomenon. It is striking, since it is unusual for a change of context to have similarly dramatic effects on other forms of learning. Although there have been claims to the contrary (e.g. Bouton and Bolles 1979; Balaz et al. 1981), the results of several properly controlled experiments have suggested that conditioning can transfer perfectly from one context to another (Lovibond, Preston, and Mackintosh 1984; Kaye et al. 1987; Kaye, Swietalski, and Mackintosh, unpublished observations; but for contrary results, see Honey and Hall 1989): when steps are taken to ensure that animals have equivalent experience with two contexts, the responses conditioned to a CS in one may transfer without loss when the CS is presented in the other. Similarly, when orienting or startle responses habituate to a stimulus repeatedly presented in one context, they may remain completely habituated when the stimulus is presented in another (Hall and Channell 1985*b*; Churchill, Remington, and Siddle 1987; Mackintosh 1987). In some of these experiments, indeed, explicit comparison has shown that conditioning or habituation will transfer from one context to another when latent inhibition will not (Hall and Channell 1985*b*; Kaye *et al.* 1987). The simplest explanation from our point of view would be to assume that the modulator, which detects a mismatch when a CS is presented in a new context, affects only the associability of that CS, not the responses it generates.[5]

### Conclusions

Sutton and Barto (1981), in their account of an adaptive network system based on the delta rule, acknowledged that their theory 'does not, for example, include the effects of experience on stimulus salience [the prime example of which is the phenomenon of latent inhibition] . . . and does not address stimulus representation problems' (p. 166). The same deficiencies in the Rescorla–Wagner model have always been acknowledged by its authors (e.g. Wagner and Rescorla 1972; Rescorla 1971). We believe that the model which we have sketched in outline here goes some way towards filling this gap. We do not claim any great novelty for the ideas on which it is based. We have borrowed from stimulus sampling theory the idea that stimuli should be conceptualized as sets of elements, only a subset of which is sampled at any one moment, and have merely added the further assumptions that the sampling process depends on the nature of the stimulus and of an animal's interaction with it, and that the elements of a single stimulus become associated with one another, in accordance with a standard learning rule, as they repeatedly occur together. But these further assumptions (particularly the second) turn out to have surprisingly powerful consequences. They provide a mechanism for the establishment of representations of stimuli which will allow familiar and novel stimuli to have quite different effects on the system, and they suggest a variety of ways by which exposure to several similar stimuli should enhance their discriminability. Interestingly enough, our model implies that perceptual learning or differentiation is not a unitary phenomenon: different processes can contribute to the effect, and their relative importance will depend on the nature of the stimuli and the experimental procedures employed. The addition of a further assumption, in the form of a modulator which compares external and internal inputs to an element and enhances the activation of elements where there is a mismatch between these inputs, allows the model to account for latent inhibition (again in a variety of ways). This assumption, too, is hardly novel: it is quite similar to ideas proposed by Wagner (1978; 1981) and by Pearce and Hall (1980).

One point worth emphasizing is that our discussion has been about the development of representations in an associative network: we have appealed to no processes beyond those of association and changes in associability dependent on associations. We have had no recourse to any additional rule or intermediary processes to account for the data. One possible candidate for enhancing the discriminability of repeatedly presented stimuli would be an intermediate learning stage employing a competitive learning algorithm of the type proposed by Rumelhart and Zipser (1986). This stage would learn, over a number of trials, a coding of the stimuli that would allow them to be differentiated, even though they were intially indiscriminable. We conclude that it is not necessary to appeal to such a process to account for the improvement in discrimination seen in studies of perceptual learning (it may, of course, be necessary for other purposes).

Our explanation of latent inhibition states that the activation of a stimulus, and hence its associability with other events, changes with experience of that stimulus. There are no further necessary consequences. But we acknowledge that it would be quite natural to assume that the activation of a stimulus should also affect the responses controlled by that stimulus. This would then imply that the modulator affected not only learning but also performance. As we have seen, there are problems with this assumption: it appears to predict, for example, that a response which has habituated to a repeatedly presented stimulus in one context will be restored when the stimulus is presented in a different context; and it further implies that a response conditioned to a CS over a long series of trials in one context should actually be elicited *more* strongly when the CS is presented in a different context. There is very little published evidence consistent with the former prediction, and none with the latter. For the time being at least, it may be more prudent to assume that the modulator affects only the ease with which a stimulus enters into new associations, rather than determining the vigour of the responses it elicits.

We can place a further restriction on the scope of the model with even greater confidence. By comparing external and internal inputs to a stimulus, the modulator produces a different response to a novel stimulus (which has no internal input) and a familiar one (whose internal input will eventually match its external input). The modulator thus appears to provide a mechanism for discriminating novel from familiar stimuli, and our model might be thought to imply, therefore, that animals must be capable of solving discrimination problems solely on the basis of their relative novelty or familiarity. But it is actually rather difficult to teach animals to perform one arbitrary response to a large set of stimuli on their first presentation and another response when they are presented a second time (Mackintosh 1987). The solution of such a generalized novelty–familiarity discrimination, however, would require that the output from the modulator were itself available for association with other consequences. There is no guarantee that it will be. In our model, the modulator plays a particular role in a single, encapsulated system, that of determining the associability of the element whose external and internal inputs it is comparing. There is no reason why it should be accessible to other systems. As Rozin (1976) has suggested, such inaccessibility is a common feature of many learning mechanisms, and their gradually increasing accessibility may be a feature of the evolution of intelligence.

## Appendix

Here we give formal details of a model that implements variations in associability within an associative network employing a modified delta rule. We take the delta rule (see McClelland and Rumelhart, 1985, for a discussion) as our starting point, but later introduce a number of necessary modifications.

Figure 6.5 shows three elements or nodes interconnected by links or weights. All nodes are interconnected, but the strength of the link between any two nodes may vary. When activation ($\Omega$) tries to pass along a link, i.e. when one node tries to influence another, the link strength or weight ($w$) determines

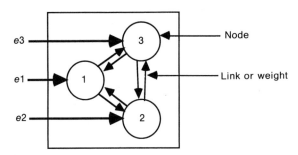

**Fig. 6.5**   A representation of a set of nodes in the associative module, with their external and internal inputs.

how successful this is. The activation of the emitting node is multiplied by the weight for the link from that node to the recipient, hence a weight of zero prevents any activation from passing. Note that links are unidirectional.

The nodes themselves can have an activation of between $+1$ and $-1$. This activation is the result of two types of input, external input ($e1$, $e2$, $e3$) and internal input, the latter simply being the input received by a node from other nodes via the links. The summed external input for a given node will be termed $e$, and the summed internal input $i$.

The latter is given by Equation (I):

$$i_i = \sum w_{ij} \Omega_j \tag{I}$$

where $i_i$ is the summed internal input to the $i$th node, $w_{ij}$ is the weight from node $j$ to node $i$, and $\Omega_j$ is the activation of the $j$th node.

When input is applied to a node, its activation changes, and when the input ends, the level of activation in the node reverts to its original level. The time course of these changes in activation is described by Equation (II):

$$
\left.
\begin{aligned}
d\Omega/dt &= E(e+i)(1-\Omega) - D\Omega \qquad \text{for } \Omega > 0 \\
\delta\Omega/dt &= E(e+i)(1+\Omega) - D\Omega \qquad \text{otherwise}
\end{aligned}
\right\}
\qquad \text{(II)}
$$

where $E$ and $D$ are the (positive) constants for excitation and decay respectively. Broadly speaking, these equations ensure that the level of activation changes until the excitation, $E(e+i)(1-\Omega)$ for $\Omega > 0$, equals the decay, $D\Omega$, at which point the rate of change of activation is zero and the node is in equilibrium. For example, if $e$ and $i$ are positive and $\Omega$ is small, then excitation will prevail over decay and activation will rise, but this decreases the excitation and increases the decay, hence the rate of increase of activation slows and activation settles towards some equilibrium level. If the input to the node is now terminated, then the decay term smoothly reduces the activation to zero.

However, activation is not the only quantity varying over time; the weights change with time as well, in a manner which gives the delta rule its name and reveals it to be of the Widrow–Hoff error-correcting type. While activation is controlled by the sum of $e$ and $i$, the weights vary in a manner controlled by the difference between $e$ and $i$, the rule being given in Equation (III):

$$
dw_{ij}/dt = S(e_i - i_i)\Omega_j \qquad \text{(III)}
$$

where $S$ is a positive constant. The term $(e-i)$ is often referred to as delta ($\Delta$). The effect of this rule is that the weights into a node are changed until $e$ and $i$ are equal, i.e., until the external input is matched by the internal input. In doing this the weights from the more active nodes are changed the most. It is as if a given node checks to see how close $i$ is to $e$, then looks around for links where a change might make a really substantial difference because of a very active node at the end of it, and changes those weights preferentially.

The account of the delta rule given up to this point has been the standard one. Typically, systems employing the rule would be simulated by treating the differential equations given as difference equations, with features such as weight decay and noise treated in a rather *ad-hoc* manner. However, in the model discussed here, the simultaneous differential equations are solved using techniques of numerical integration (fourth order Runge–Kutta). All the processes discussed in this treatment act on-line and continuously: for example there is no waiting for the system to settle before changing the weights. This represents a rather more realistic and efficient state of affairs than the commonly used technique of dividing the learning cycle up into discrete phases.

We add some further assumptions. First, the system is noisy, with the noise having both exogenous and endogenous components. The former component is due to both random variation in the external world and in the peripheral input systems that process the signal before it reaches the system of interest here. Noise endogenous to the system is assumed to be intrinsic to the hardware implementing the system and is not considered further here. Exogenous noise may have more of an all-or-none quality to it: quite simply, some inputs may fail to arrive while others may be produced spuriously. It would be unrealistic to expect the perception of a given stimulus to be completely stable, since there will be variation in accompanying stimuli and the stimulus itself will probably vary. This might be rather crudely modelled by randomly setting a proportion of the es that should be on, off, and a proportion of the es that should be off, on. The effects of noise will be to render the representation of some input pattern initially unreliable. This unreliability will attenuate with repeated presentation of the pattern, and the variability in response to the pattern or a portion of the pattern will decline.

Another addition to the basic rule is to add the notion of weight decay. This can be justified on computational grounds, since if no decay were to occur, then the system would be prone to unnecessary interference between associative representations, and would not be making optimal use of its computational resources. Decay represents a mechanism by which transient relationships can be distinguished from stable ones, and the latter given preferred status. We assume that each increment to a weight decays exponentially until a fixed proportion of that increment remains, at which point no further decay to that increment ever occurs. If this seems rather impenetrable, consider the following example. Some learning episode changes a weight by $+0.32$. If the system were now left entirely to its own devices that increment would decay in a smooth exponential until it had reached some fixed proportion of its original value, say one-twentieth. Hence decay would cease when the increment had been reduced to $+0.016$. The total weight at any given time will be composed of many increments, some of which will be decaying, while others will have reached asymptote. Thus any weight can be divided into a part that is decaying and a part that is not, and any weight left for long enough would settle to an asymptotic value representing the long-term learning for that part of the system. The effect of this is that learning episodes may now show dissociable short- and long-term effects. For example, massed learning will typically lead to a short-term advantage (on some appropriate test) over spaced learning, but vice-versa in the long term. Another important consequence of the decay mechanism is that it can directly limit learning if decay comes to equal the rate of increment of link strength; this will typically occur in mass presentations of input patterns. Finally, only stable relationships between inputs will ever build up a substantial permanent representation in the system: transient relationships will be quickly learnt, and then forgotten, an efficient use of the computational resources available.

The above, of course, is a high-level characterization rather than a definition. For completeness, the equations governing weight change are given in Equation (IV):

$$dw_{ij}/dt = S\,\Delta\Omega_j - Km_{ij}$$

> where $K$ is a constant and $m_{ij}$ is a dummy variable

$$dm_{ij}/dt = S\,\Delta\Omega_j - LM_{ij}$$                                           (IV)

> where $L$ is a constant such that $L > K$ $(L, K > 0)$

Taking the enhanced implementation of the delta rule (delta +) developed in the preceding discussion as a starting point, it is clear that its basic computation is best characterized as a form of association. One problem is that, typically, PDP models of sufficient power to be interesting tend to learn rather slowly. An obvious first step, then, is to devise an architecture that allows rapid, efficient association. An architecture that accomplishes this is the modulator–associator arrangement shown earlier in Fig. 6.4 (see p. 114).

As can be seen, the suggested architecture has an associative module (AM) linked to a modulator. The AM contains many interlinked nodes obeying delta +; for simplicity, complete connectivity is assumed, though this assumption could be relaxed somewhat. The modulator functions on an individual basis for each node in the AM, receiving its external input and activation. Given this input, it is possible to compute the $i$ coming into the node. The modulator then returns to the node an external input proportional to $\Delta$. This boost is treated by the node as another component of external input to be summed with the rest to give $e$. The modulator, however, allows for its output to a node in computing $\Delta$.

The effect of this arrangment is to improve the learning shown by the nodes in the associative module. The boost a node receives will be large when $e - i$ is large, and this is typically when in a novel situation. In these circumstances the effect of the extra $e$ is to increase the node's $\Delta$ and $\Omega$, the former effect having the consequence of speeding the formation of incoming associations (increased associativity), while the latter effect enhances the node's ability to form outgoing associations (increased associability). The boost thus enhances both the associativity and associability of any node it acts on, and it acts quite independently on each node. As learning progresses, $\Delta$ decreases and the modulator's output to each node wanes. But if the modulator is to affect the associability of a node (determined by $\Omega$) as well as its associativity (determined by $\Delta$), the parameters of the system must be set so that as the boost declines the $\Omega$ of that node declines even though its $i$ is increasing.

This architecture is designed to promote rapid association between nodes, given the appropriate circumstances; as it stands, however, it has some unfortunate side-effects. Nodes which are internally rather than externally activated will be swamped by the modulator boost and take activations opposite to those they should have. The summed modulator outputs will tend to cancel, as a number will be negative, and will not be interpretable as a novelty measure. Further amendments to the delta + rule are needed.

A first step is to restrict the range of activation values to $0 \leq \Omega \leq 1$, i.e. to forbid negative activations. Thus Equation (II) becomes:

$$\left. \begin{array}{ll} d\Omega/dt = E(e+i)(1-\Omega) - D\Omega & \text{for } \Omega \geq 0 \\ \delta\Omega/dt = 0 & \text{otherwise} \end{array} \right\} \qquad (V)$$

Another modification consistent with this is to constrain $e$ to be positive, as a negative $e$ would now be in danger of having no visible effect on the node it inputs to. While a negative $e$ would have little utility in representational terms, however, note that it could be used as a means of control.

Now only a small alteration to the modulator is needed to ensure that the problems previously mentioned are obviated. The dependence of the output on $e-i$ remains, with the proviso that if $\Delta$ is negative, then no output occurs. It is as though the difference between $e$ and $i$ controls a gate with the output proportional to $\Delta$ when positive; however, when $i$ exceeds $e$, then the gate is closed and no output can emerge.

These changes have a number of further consequences which are worth listing:

1. It is now impossible for the modulator to have a negative output.
2. Internally activated nodes will never receive any modulator boost, and their activations will be determined entirely by their internal input.
3. A corollary of this is that inhibitory associations will be formed more slowly than excitatory associations, since the formation of an inhibitory association depends on the absence of a predicted consequence, i.e. on the node to which associations are to be made being internally rather than externally activated.
4. Excitatory associations will extinguish relatively slowly as internally activated nodes are involved.
5. Extinction of inhibitory associations will not occur at all. One way to see this is to note that an attempt to evoke a node via inhibitory associations will simply keep that node's activation at zero. Since the $i$ value used in computing $\Delta$ is estimated from knowledge of $e$ and $\Omega$, and since $e$ will be zero (there is no external input to the US node since no US is present) $i$ must also be estimated as zero. Hence $\Delta$ will be zero and no weight change can occur.

The equations governing this system can now be summarized as Equation (VI) (with all constants positive) . . .

$$d\Omega_i/dt = E(e_i + i_i)(1 - \Omega_i) - D\Omega_i \quad \text{for } \Omega_i \geq 0$$

$$d\Omega_i/dt = 0 \qquad\qquad\qquad\qquad \text{otherwise}$$

$$dw_{ij}/dt = S\Delta_i\Omega_j - Km_{ij} \qquad \text{where } S, K \text{ are constants} \\ \text{and } m_{ij} \text{ is a dummy variable}$$

$$dm_{ij}/dt = S\Delta_i\Omega_j - Lm_{ij} \qquad \text{where } L \text{ is a constant such} \\ \text{that } L > K$$

$$\Delta_i = e_i - i_i \qquad\qquad\qquad\qquad i > 0 \qquad\qquad\qquad\qquad (\text{VI})$$

$$\Delta_i = e_i \qquad\qquad\qquad\qquad\qquad \text{otherwise}$$

$$c_i = P\Delta_i \qquad\qquad\qquad\qquad \Delta > 0, P \text{ constant, and} \\ c_i = \text{modulator's output} \\ \text{to } i\text{th node}$$

$$c_i = 0 \qquad\qquad\qquad\qquad\qquad \text{otherwise}$$

$$e_i \geq 0$$

Recall that the modulator's output is treated as a component of $e$ (i.e. $e = e + c$), except in the case of calculating $\Delta$ for $c_i$, when it is omitted.

This is, of course, just one possible implementation of the modulator; there remain many possibilities with little to distinguish one from the other at present. However, the functional description given is sufficient for some modelling of the system to be possible without worrying about the details of modulator function, and a paper giving the results of some simulations using the equations presented here is in preparation.

## Notes

1. The work reported here was supported by the Science and Engineering Research Council, with a research grant to N. J. Mackintosh and a research studentship to I. P. L. McLaren. We are deeply indebted to A. Dickinson and G. Hall for numerous discussions and for their dissection of an earlier draft, to R. G. M. Morris and J. Russell for their helpful comments, and to G. Hall and R. Honey, from whom we have borrowed a number of ideas (although they will certainly not wish to be associated with our use of them).

In order to make what follows even remotely intelligible to those psychologists not intimately familiar with the details of conditioning theory and conditioning experiments, we have confined some of our more tedious discussions of these minutiae to footnotes. We believe that the main text can stand alone without these additions, and apologize to our conditioning colleagues for putting many of the parts which will concern them into such an inconvenient format.

2. Latent inhibition has been explained in numerous other ways. One possibility is that

it can be simply reduced to habituation. According to Hawkins and Kandel (1984; see also chapter 10), for example, habituation occurs because repeated presentation of a stimulus raises the threshold for the transmission of activation from that stimulus to the response it normally elicits. Since their theory of conditioning assumes that the presentation of a US shortly after a CS has the reverse of this effect, augmenting the response normally elicited by the CS (which is then called the conditioned response), they could simply argue that prior habituation of this response inevitably implies that more conditioning trials will be needed to restore it. We do not believe that latent inhibition can be reduced to the habituation of the responses normally elicited by the CS (any more than conditioning can be reduced to their augmentation). For one thing, latent inhibition retards not only excitatory, but also inhibitory, conditioning (Rescorla 1971; Baker and Mackintosh 1977).

An alternative theory is that presentation of a CS alone causes it to be associated with its experienced consequence, namely nothing. This association between the CS and nothing may then pro-actively interfere with the establishment of an association between the CS and either an increase or decrease in the probability of a reinforcer (Testa and Ternes 1977). But latent inhibition should not, in our judgement, be confused with any simple form of associative interference. Associative interference occurs when prior pairing of a CS with one reinforcer (e.g. weak shock) retards subsequent conditioning when that CS is paired with a different reinforcer such as water (Scavio 1974). But such interference may be distinguished from latent inhibition by a change in the context of conditioning. Conditioning established in one context can transfer perfectly to another (Lovibond et al. 1984). Similarly, if a CS is initially paired with weak shock in one context, this will interfere with subsequent conditioning when the CS is paired with water, both in the original context and in a quite different one (Kaye et al. 1987). But latent inhibition, as we have seen, does not survive a change of context (see also Lovibond et al. 1984; Kaye et al. 1987). Prior exposure to a CS alone, which severely retards conditioning when the CS is paired with a reinforcer in the same context, may have no effect on subsequent conditioning when the CS is paired with a reinforcer in a different context.

3. The model we are proposing incorporates only a very limited part of Wagner's (1981) model. An earlier formalization (Wagner 1978) simply proposed that, just as in the Rescorla–Wagner model an already predicted reinforcer would not act to reinforce further conditioning, so an already predicted CS would not enter into new associations. It is this assumption that we are, in effect, borrowing. We do not need the underlying mechanism which Wagner has postulated, which appeals to the priming of stimuli in short-term memory. We neither postulate any distinction between 'self-generated' and 'retrieval-generated' priming (we are concerned only with the latter), nor do we suppose that short-term memory is of strictly limited capacity. The former distinction is said to be supported by the difference between short-term and long-term habituation or latent inhibition, but the data do not seem to us to require such a theoretical distinction (Mackintosh 1987). The latter assumption is supposedly required because both habituation and latent inhibition are disrupted by a 'distractor' presented immediately after the target stimulus (e.g. Green and Parker 1975; Best et al. 1979). These results seem more simply interpreted as instances of generalization decrement (Kaye et al. 1988; Kaye et al. 1988).

4. Simulations of the model confirm that exposure to the context alone before exposure to the CS results in relatively weak associations being formed between context and CS, while exposure to the context after exposure to the CS weakens the context-CS associations previously formed. But in the former case, the prevention of context-CS associations will allow the process of unitization to proceed further and therefore exert a more profound and long-lasting effect on the associability of the CS with other events. The prediction derivable from this analysis is that the retardation of conditioning produced when latent inhibition is preceded by pre-exposure to the context will take a somewhat unusual form. Conditioning will *initially* proceed rather more rapidly than in a standard latent inhibition group, but will appear to asymptote at a lower level. Precisely such an effect is observable in Hall and Channell's data (Hall and Channell 1985*a*, Figure 2, p. 388), and has been replicated in an unpublished experiment by McLaren.

The reduction in latent inhibition caused by exposure to the context alone after exposure to the CS may be partly outweighed by other factors: this effect will not necessarily be *very* marked when comparison is made with a control group which waits the same length of time between the end of latent inhibition and the beginning of conditioning. Latent inhibition does often show some loss just with the passage of time (Hall and Minor 1984), and it is natural to simulate this by allowing for some forgetting of associations. Such forgetting will also tend to weaken the connections from CS to context, which make an additional contribution to latent inhibition; but exposure to the contextual stimuli alone, even in the absence of the CS, may help to maintain these connections. When the CS elements are retrieved by the context, they will be in a state of activation precisely in the presence of contextual stimuli, and there is no reason why their association with the context should be forgotten. In consequence, when the CS is again presented, it will lower the associability of the contextual stimuli to a greater extent than in any control group. The associability of the entire set of stimuli present at the moment of reinforcement will be lower than it would otherwise have been, and latent inhibition may still be strong.

5. There are, however, two problems here. First, there is the question of whether the habituation of orienting responses to a stimulus can be taken as an index of the decline in its associability which produces latent inhibition (as is assumed by Kaye and Pearce 1984, 1987; see above). Hall and Channell's (1985*b*) data, which appear to show a dissociation between the habituation of orienting responses, which transfers across a change of context, and latent inhibition, which does not, creates problems for this identification. We believe that the resolution of this question must await further data.

The second set of problematic data are those of Kaye *et al.* (1987), which seem to create difficulties for our analysis. In these experiments, the transfer of conditioning from one context to another was measured by the extent to which prior pairing of a CS with shock interfered with new conditioning when the CS was paired with water. This associative interference effect also transferred perfectly across contexts. Now, there is no difficulty in explaining how interference arising from an incompatible, shock-elicited response should have transferred across contexts. But our account appears to predict, as do those of Wagner (1981) and Pearce and Hall (1980), that the CS should have lost associability during the course of conditioning trials with shock, and this source of interference, in effect a latent inhibition effect, should have been disrupted by a change of context. The data of the experiments by Kaye *et al*. provide no evidence of any such latent inhibition, let alone its disruption by a change of context: animals for whom the CS had been previously paired with shock showed a substantial suppression of approach and licking in the first session when the CS was paired with water, but thereafter conditioned rapidly, significantly more rapidly than a latent inhibition group.

The solution is to note that our account follows that of Pearce and Hall (1980) in assuming that the decline in the associability of the CS when it was paired with shock was, in part, a consequence of these CS–shock associations, and will therefore be disrupted at the outset of new conditioning trials when the shock is replaced by water. Latent inhibition is normally context-specific because it depends, in part, on the development of context–CS associations. But to the extent that the latent inhibition produced by pairing a CS with a reinforcer depends on these CS–reinforcer associations, it will be less dependent on context–CS associations and less affected by any change of context. If, in addition, the reinforcer is then changed for a quite different one, of opposite affective sign, latent inhibition will be sufficiently disrupted that one may see no effect of the change of context at all. One virtue of this account is that it explains an otherwise puzzling discrepancy between the results of Kaye *et al*. and those of other experiments where pairing a CS with a weak shock has been shown to retard subsequent conditioning when the same CS is now paired with a stronger shock (Hall and Pearce 1979). Hall and Pearce interpret their results as a latent inhibition effect, and, unlike the interference observed in the study by Kaye *et al*., it is indeed evident as a retardation of the *rate* of new conditioning with the stronger shock. Moreover, again unlike the effect observed in the experiment by Kaye *et al*., it is disrupted by a change of context (Swartzentruber and Bouton 1986; a result which we have confirmed). The puzzle vanishes, however, once one sees that the similarity between the previous weak shock and the new strong shock in Hall and Pearce's experiments will prevent the disruption of latent inhibition observed in experiments by Kaye *et al*. when water is substituted for shock. In the former case, therefore, the associability of the CS will stay low at the start of new conditioning. Thus exactly the same treatment, pairing a CS with a weak shock, will produce latent inhibition when the CS is subsequently paired with strong shock, but little or no *latent inhibition* when the CS is paired with an appetitive reinforcer such as water, even though it will retard conditioning for other reasons.

## References

Baker, A. G. and Mackintosh, N. J. (1977). Excitatory and inhibitory conditioning following uncorrelated presentations of CS and UCS. *Animal Learning and Behavior*, **5**, 315–19.

Baker, A. G. and Mercier, P. (1982). Extinction of the context and latent inhibition. *Learning and Motivation*, **13**, 391–416.

Balaz, M. A., Capra, S., Hartl, P., and Miller, R. R. (1981). Contextual potentiation of acquired behavior after devaluing direct context–US associations. *Learning and Motivation*, **12**, 383–97.

Bateson, P. P. G. and Chantrey, D. F. (1972). Retardation of discrimination learning in monkeys and chicks previously exposed to both stimuli. *Nature*, **237**, 173–4.

Best, M., Gemberling, G. A., and Johnson, P. E. (1979). Disrupting the conditioned stimulus preexposure effect in flavor-aversion learning: effects of interoceptive distractor manipulations. *Journal of Experimental Psychology: Animal Behavior Processes*, **5**, 321–34.

Blough, D. S. (1975). Steady state data and a quantitative model of operant generalization and discrimination. *Journal of Experimental Psychology: Animal Behavior Processes*, **1**, 3–21.

Bouton, M. E. and Bolles, R. C. (1979). Contextual control of the extinction of conditioned fear. *Learning and Motivation*, **10**, 445–66.

Chamizo, V. D. and Mackintosh, N. J. (1989). Latent learning and latent inhibition in maze discriminations. *Quarterly Journal of Experimental Psychology*, **41B**, 21–31.

Channell, S. and Hall, G. (1981). Facilitation and retardation of discrimination learning after exposure to the stimuli. *Journal of Experimental Psychology: Animal Behavior Processes*, **7**, 437–46.

Chantrey, D. F. (1974). Stimulus preexposure and discrimination learning by domestic chicks: effects of varying interstimulus time. *Journal of Comparative and Physiological Psychology*, **87**, 517–25.

Churchill, M., Remington, B., and Siddle, D. A. T. (1987). The effects of context change on long-term habituation of the orienting response in humans. *Quarterly Journal of Experimental Psychology*, **39B**, 315–38.

Dickinson, A. and Shanks, D. (1985). Animal conditioning and human causality judgment. In *Perspectives on learning and memory* (eds. L-G. Nilsson and T. Archer), pp. 167–96. Erlbaum, Hillsdale, NJ.

Durlach, P. J. (1988). Chapter to appear in *Contemporary learning theories* (eds. S. B. Klein and R. R. Mowrer). Erlbaum, Hillsdale, NJ.

Estes, W. K. (1950). Towards a statistical theory of learning. *Psychological Review*, **57**, 94–107.

Forgus, R. H. (1958a). The effects of different kinds of form pre-exposure on form discrimination learning. *Journal of Comparative and Physiological Psychology*, **51**, 75–8.

Forgus, R. H. (1958b). The interaction between form pre-exposure and test requirements in determining form discrimination. *Journal of Comparative and Physiological Psychology*, **51**, 588–91.

Gibson, E. J. and Walk, R. D. (1956). The effect of prolonged exposure to visually presented patterns on learning to discriminate them. *Journal of Comparative and Physiological Psychology*, **49**, 239–42.

Gibson, J. J. and Gibson, E. J. (1955). Perceptual learning: differentiation or enrichment? *Psychological Review*, **62**, 32–41.

Gluck, M. A. and Bower, G. H. (1986). Conditioning and categorization: some common effects of informational variables in animal and human learning, *Proceedings of Cognitive Science Society Conference*.

Green, K. F. and Parker, L. A. (1975). Gustatory memory: incubation and interference. *Behavioral Biology*, **13**, 359–67.

Hall, G. (1980). Exposure learning in animals. *Psychological Bulletin*, **88**, 535–50.

Hall, G. and Channell, S. (1985a). Latent inhibition and conditioning after preexposure to the training context. *Learning and Motivation*, **16**, 381–7.

Hall, G. and Channell, S. (1985b). Differential effects of contextual change on latent inhibition and on the habituation of an orienting response. *Journal of Experimental Psychology: Animal Behavior Processes*, **11**, 470–81.

Hall, G. and Honey, R. (1988). Chapter to appear in *Contemporary learning theories* (eds. S. G. Klein and R. R. Mowrer). Erlbaum, Hillsdale, NJ.

Hall, G. and Minor, H. (1984). A search for context-stimulus associations in latent inhibition. *Quarterly Journal of Experimental Psychology*, **36B**, 145–69.

Hall, G. and Pearce, J. M. (1979). Latent inhibition of a CS during CS–US pairings. *Journal of Experimental Psychology: Animal Behavior Processes*, **5**, 31–42.

Hawkins, R. D. and Kandel, E. R. (1984). Is there a cell-biological alphabet for simple forms of learning? *Psychological Review*, **91**, 375–91.

Hebb, D. O. (1949). *Organization of behavior*. Wiley, NY.

Kamin, L. J. (1968). 'Attention-like' processes in classical conditioning. In *Miami symposium on the prediction of behavior: aversive stimulation* (ed. M. R. Jones), pp. 9–33. University of Miami Press.

Kaye, H., Gambini, B., and Mackintosh, N. J. (1988). A dissociation between one-trial overshadowing and the effect of a distractor on habituation. *Quarterly Journal of Experimental Psychology*, **40B**, 31–47.

Kaye, H. and Pearce, J. M. (1984). The strength of the orienting response during Pavlovian conditioning. *Journal of Experimental Psychology: Animal Behavior Processes*, **10**, 90–109.

Kaye, H. and Pearce, J. M. (1987). Hippocampal lesions attenuate latent inhibition and the decline of the orienting response in rats. *Quarterly Journal of Experimental Psychology*, **39B**, 107–25.

Kaye, H., Preston, G. C., Szabo, L., Druiff, H., and Mackintosh, N. J. (1987). Context specificity of conditioning and latent inhibition: evidence for a dissociation of latent inhibition and associative interference. *Quarterly Journal of Experimental Psychology*, **39B**, 127–45.

Kaye, H., Swietalski, N., and Mackintosh, N. J. (1988). Distractor effects on latent inhibition are a consequence of generalization decrement. *Quarterly Journal of Experimental Psychology*, **40B**, 151–61.

Konorski, J. (1967). *Integrative activity of the brain*. University of Chicago Press.

Lovibond, P. F., Preston, G. C., and Mackintosh, N. J. (1984). Context specificity of conditioning, extinction and latent inhibition. *Journal of Experimental Psychology: Animal Behavior Processes*, **10**, 360–75.

Lubow, R. E. (1973). Latent inhibition. *Psychological Bulletin*, **79**, 398–407.

Lubow, R. E., Rifkin, B., and Alek, M. (1976). The context effect: the relationship between stimulus preexposure and environmental preexposure determines subsequent learning. *Journal of Experimental Psychology: Animal Behavior Processes*, **2**, 38–47.

McClelland, J. L. and Rumelhart, D. E. (1985). Distributed memory and the representation of general and specific information. *Journal of Experimental Psychology: General*, **114**, 159–88.

Mackintosh, N. J. (1975). A theory of attention: variations in the associability of stimuli with reinforcement. *Psychological Review*, **82**, 276–98.

Mackintosh, N. J. (1983). *Conditioning and associative learning*. Oxford University Press.

Mackintosh, N. J. (1987). Neurobiology, psychology and habituation, *Behavioural Research and Therapy*, **25**, 81–97.

Neimark, E. D. and Estes, W. K. (1967). *Stimulus sampling theory*. Holden-Day, San Fr.

Oswalt, R. M. (1972). Relationship between level of visual pattern difficulty during rearing and subsequent discrimination in rats. *Journal of Comparative and Physiological Psychology*, **81**, 122–5.

Pearce, J. M. (1987). A model for stimulus generalisation in Pavlovian conditioning. *Psychological Review*, **94**, 61–73.

Pearce, J. M. and Hall, G. (1980). A model for Pavlovian learning: variations in the effectiveness of conditioned but not of unconditioned stimuli. *Psychological Review*, **87**, 532–52.

Rescorla, R. A. (1971). Summation and retardation tests of latent inhibition. *Journal of Comparative and Physiological Psychology*, **75**, 77–81.

Rescorla, R. A. and Wagner, A. R. (1972). A theory of Pavlovian conditioning: variations in the effectiveness of reinforcement and nonreinforcement. In *Classical conditioning II: current research and theory* (eds. A. H. Black and W. F. Proskay), pp. 64–99. Appleton-Century-Crofts, NY.

Rozin, P. (1976). The evolution of intelligence and access to the cognitive unconscious. In *Progress in psychobiology and physiological psychology*, pp. 245–80. Academic Press, New York.

Rumelhart, D. E., Hinton, G. E., and McClelland, J. L. (1986). A general framework for parallel distributed processing. In *Parallel distributed processing*, Volume 1 (eds. J. L. McClelland and D. E. Rumelhart), pp. 45–76, MIT Press, Cambridge, Mass.

Rumelhart, D. E. and Zipser, D. (1986). Feature discovery by competitive learning. In *Parallel distributed processing*, Volume 2 (eds. J. L. McClelland and D. E. Rumelhart), pp. 151–93. MIT Press, Cambridge, Mass.

Scavio, M. J. Jr (1974). Classical–classical transfer: effects of prior aversive conditioning upon appetitive conditioning in rabbits. *Journal of Comparative and Physiological Psychology*, **86**, 107–15.

Sokolov, Y. N. (1963). *Perception and the conditioned reflex*. Pergamon Press, Oxford.

Sutton, R. S. and Barto, A. G. (1981). Toward a modern theory of adaptive networks: expectation and prediction. *Psychological Review*, **88**, 135–70.

Swartzentruber, D. and Bouton, M. E. (1986). Contextual control of negative transfer produced by prior CS–US pairings. *Learning and Motivation*, **17**, 366–85.

Testa, T. J. and Ternes, J. W. (1977). Specificity of conditioning mechanisms in the modification of food preferences. In *Learning mechanisms in food selection*, (eds. L. M. Barker, M. R. Best, and M. Domjan) pp. 229–53. Baylor University Press, Waco, TX.

Wagner, A. R. (1978). Expectancies and the priming of STM. In *Cognitive processes in animal behavior*, (eds. S. H. Hulse, H. Fowler, and W. K. Honig), pp. 177–209. Erlbaum, Hillsdale, NJ.

Wagner, A. R. (1979). Habituation and memory. In *Mechanisms of learning and motivation* (eds. A. Dickinson and R. A. Boakes), pp. 53–82. Erlbaum, Hillsdale, NJ.

Wagner, A. R. (1981). SOP: A model of automatic memory processing in animal behavior. In *Information processing in animals: memory mechanisms* (eds. N. E. Spear and R. R. Miller), pp. 5–47. Erlbaum, Hillsdale, NJ.

Wagner, A. R. and Rescorla, R. A. (1972). Inhibition in Pavlovian conditioning: application of a theory. In *Inhibition and learning* (eds. R. A. Boakes and M. S. Halliday), pp. 301–36. Academic Press, London.

# 7

## Connections and disconnections: acquired dyslexia in a computational model of reading processes

KARALYN PATTERSON, MARK S. SEIDENBERG, and JAMES L. McCLELLAND

### Introduction

In this chapter we describe a new, parallel distributed processing (PDP) model of visual word recognition and pronunciation, the acquisition of these skills, and their breakdown following brain injury. The model consists of a working, computational simulation of the process of learning to recognize and pronounce written words. In developing this model we were motivated by two general concerns. The first is that, since word recognition is a key component of reading, a comprehensive account of word recognition is critical to an understanding of this important human cognitive skill. A basic characteristic of reading comprehension is that it occurs 'on-line', i.e. essentially as the stimulus is perceived. This characteristic derives in part from the fact that words are recognized rapidly and usually effortlessly; a large amount of research has addressed the types of knowledge and processes that support this capacity, the kinds of information that become available as part of the recognition process, and how this information contributes to other aspects of reading. Furthermore, word recognition presents important developmental issues; learning to read words is among the first tasks confronting the beginning reader, and problems in reading acquisition are typically associated with deficits in this skill. Finally, reading impairments that are a consequence of brain injury are often associated with deficits in word recognition; studies of these acquired forms of dyslexia have provided important evidence concerning the reading process and its neurological realization. As reading researchers, one of our primary goals was to develop a computational model that incorporates much of what is known about these aspects of word recognition.

The other primary motivation for this work was the observation that word recognition provides a domain in which to explore the properties of the connectionist or parallel distributed processing (PDP) approach to understanding human cognition. This approach represents the modern realization of Hebb's (1949) idea that complex human behaviours emerge from the operation of aggregations of simple neuronal processing units. The approach has generated broad interest among cognitive- and neuro-scientists, and has been applied to a wide range of problems in perception, learning, and cognition (e.g. McClelland and Rumelhart 1986; Rumelhart and McClelland 1986a). The first generation of connectionist models illustrated the basic principles and the potential of this approach, but were limited in scope. As a relatively mature area of research, word recognition presented a domain in which to develop a second-generation model capable of simulating a broad range of behavioural phenomena in detail. Such a comprehensive model would provide a basis for assessing the value of the connectionist approach in the development of explanatory theories.

The plan of the paper is as follows. We first provide an overview of the model, describing its basic structure and operation. We then summarize the model's account of the task of naming words aloud. This material is developed in greater detail elsewhere (Seidenberg 1988a; Seidenberg and McClelland 1988a,b), so our treatment of these issues will necessarily be limited. The main focus of this paper concerns our initial explorations of the model's potential to account for certain reading disorders that are observed following brain injury. Although it is by no means a complete theory of word recognition and pronunciation, the model provides a plausible account of some basic phenomena concerning normal performance; we sought to determine whether aspects of pathological performance could be captured in terms of damage to this system. This work represents one of the first attempts to describe and explain pathological performance following brain injury by 'lesioning' a working computational model of normal performance. Although these studies are as yet preliminary in nature, we think that this effort illustrates the utility and potential of the approach.

**Overview of the model**

We conceive of a lexical processing module with the general form illustrated in Fig. 7.1. The long-term goal is an integrated theory that accounts for various aspects of lexical processing involving orthographic, phonological, and semantic information. Such a theory would specify how these types of information are represented in memory, and how they are used in tasks such as deriving the meaning of a word from its written form, deriving the spelling of a word from its meaning or its pronunciation, and deriving a pronunciation from spelling. The implemented model, represented by that part of Fig. 7.1 in heavy outline, is concerned with how readers recognize letter strings and pronounce them aloud. The model consists of a network of interconnected

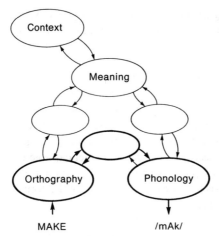

**Fig. 7.1**  General framework for processing of words in reading: the implemented model is in bold outline.

processing units. There are 400 units used to code orthographic information, 200 hidden units, and 460 units used to code phonological information. There are connections from all orthographic units to all hidden units, and from all hidden units to all phonological units. In addition, there is a set of connections from the hidden units back to the orthographic units. The connections between units carry weights that govern the spread of activation through the system. As will become clear below, these weights encode what the model knows about written English, specifically orthographic redundancy (i.e. the frequency and distribution of letter patterns in the lexicon) and the correspondences between orthography and phonology.

**Orthographic and phonological representations**

The orthographic and phonological codes for words (and non-words) are represented as patterns of activation distributed over a number of primitive representational units. Each processing unit has an activation value ranging from 0 to 1. The representations of different entities are encoded as different patterns of activity over these units. The details of these representational schemes are described elsewhere (Seidenberg and McClelland 1988a,b); here we summarize some of their main features.

The phonological representation we employed was the one developed by Rumelhart and McClelland (1986b). The phonemes in a letter string are encoded as a set of triples, each specifying a phoneme and its flankers. The word MAKE, for example, consists of three such triples or 'Wickelphones' (in honor of Wickelgren 1969). The correspondence between Wickelphones and units is one-to-many. Each Wickelphone is encoded as a pattern of activation over a set of units representing phonetic features. Each unit represents a triple of phonetic features, one feature of the first of the three phonemes in each Wickelphone, one feature of the second of the three, and one of the third. For example, there is a unit that represents [vowel, fricative, stop]. This unit should be activated for any word containing a Wickelphone in which this sequence occurs, such as the words POST and SOFT. Word boundaries are also represented in the featural representation, so that there is a unit, for example, that represents [vowel, liquid, word-boundary]; this unit would come on in words like CAR and CALL. In Rumelhart and McClelland's (1986b) scheme, there are 460 units and each Wickelphone activates 16 of them (see their paper for discussion).

The representation used at the graphemic level has similarities with that used at the phonological level, but it consists of 400 units set up according to a slightly different scheme. For each unit, there is a table containing a list of 10 possible first letters, 10 possible middle letters, and 10 possible end letters. These tables are generated randomly, except for the constraint that the symbol for beginning/end of word does not occur in the middle position. When the unit is on, it indicates that the string being represented contains one of the 1000 possible triples that could be made by selecting one member from the first list of 10, one from the second, and one from the third. Each letter triple activates about 20 units. Though each unit is highly ambiguous, over the full set of 400 such randomly constructed units, the probability that any two sequences of three letters would activate all and only the same units in common is effectively zero.

In sum, both the phonological and the orthographic representations can be described as coarse-coded, distributed representations of the sort discussed by Hinton, McClelland, and Rumelhart (1986). The representations allow any letter and phoneme sequences to be represented, subject to certain saturation and ambiguity limits that can arise when the strings get too long. Thus, there is a minimum of built-in knowledge of orthographic or phonological structure. The use of a local context-sensitive coding scheme promotes the exploitation of local contextual similarity as a basis for generalization in the model; that is, what the model learns to do for a grapheme in one local context (e.g. the M in MAKE) will tend to transfer to the same grapheme in similar local contexts (e.g. M in MADE and MATE and, to a lesser extent, M in contexts such as MILE and SMALL). Note that we do not claim that these encoding schemes are fully sufficient for representing all of the letter or phoneme sequences that form words (see Pinker and Prince 1988). However, we are presently applying the model only to monosyllables, for which the representation is adequate (see Seidenberg and McClelland, 1988b, for discussion).

**Processing in the model**

The model takes a letter string as input and yields two types of output: (1) a pattern of activation across the phonological units; and (2) a recreation of the input pattern across the orthographic units. The former can be thought of as the model's computation of a phonological code for the input, and will be discussed in some detail because of its relevance to the word naming task. The latter can be considered a representation of the orthographic input in a short-term sensory store and is critical to our account of lexical decision (Seidenberg and McClelland 1988*a,b*). Each word-processing trial begins with the presentation of a letter string, which the simulation program then encodes into a pattern of activation over the orthographic units, according to the representational assumptions described above. Next, activations of the hidden units are computed on the basis of the pattern of activation at the orthographic level. For each hidden unit, a quantity termed the net input is computed: this is the activation of each input unit times the weight on the connection from that input unit to the hidden unit, plus a bias term unique to the unit. The bias term may be thought of as an extra weight or connection to the unit from a special unit that always has activation of 1.0. The activation of the hidden unit is then determined from the net input using a non-linear function called the logistic function. The activation function must be non-linear for reasons described in Rumelhart, Hinton, and McClelland (1986). It must be monotonically increasing and have a smooth first derivative for reasons having to do with the learning rule. The logistic function satisfies these constraints.

Once activations over the hidden units have been computed, these are used to compute activations for the phonological units and new activations for the orthographic units based on feedback from the hidden units. These activations are computed following exactly the same procedures already described: first the net input to each unit is calculated, based on the activations of all of the hidden units; then the activation of each of these units is computed, based on the net inputs.

**Learning**

When the model is first initialized, the connection strengths and biases in the network are assigned random initial values between $-0.5$ and $+0.5$. This means that each hidden unit computes an entirely arbitrary function of the input it receives from the orthographic units, and sends a random pattern of excitatory and inhibitory signals to the phonological units and back to the orthographic units. This also means that the network has no initial knowledge of spelling patterns or of correspondences between spelling and sound. Thus, the model is effectively *tabula rasa*; the abilities to re-create the orthographic input and generate its phonological code arise as a result of learning from exposure to letter strings and the corresponding strings of phonemes.

Learning occurs in the model in the following way. An orthographic string is presented and processing takes place as described above, producing first a pattern of activation over the hidden units, then a feedback pattern on the orthographic units and a feedforward pattern on the phonological units. At this point these two output patterns produced by the model are compared to the correct, target patterns that the model should have produced. The target for the orthographic feedback pattern is simply the orthographic input pattern; the target for the phonological output is the pattern representing the correct pronunciation of the presented letter string. A real-world counterpart of this second procedure would be a child seeing a letter string and hearing a teacher or other person say its correct pronunciation.

For each graphemic and phonemic unit, the difference between the correct or target activation of the unit and its actual activation is computed. The learning procedure adjusts the strengths of all of the connections in the network in proportion to the extent to which this change will reduce a measure of the total error, $E$. This algorithm is the 'back-propagation' learning procedure of Rumelhart, Hinton, and Williams (1986). Readers are referred to Rumelhart *et al.* for an explanation of how the weights are modified. The most important feature is that the rule changes the strength of each weight in proportion to the size of the effect that changing it will have on the error measure. Large changes are made to weights that have a large effect on $E$, and small changes are made to weights that have a small effect on $E$.

**The training corpus**

The model was trained on all of the monosyllabic words consisting of three or more letters in the Kucera and Francis (1967) word count, minus proper nouns, foreign words, abbreviations, and words that are formed by the addition of a final -s or -ed inflection. This is not a complete list of the uninflected monosyllabic words in English; for example, the word FONT is one of many that do not appear in Kucera and Francis. Nevertheless, the corpus provides a reasonable approximation of the set of monosyllables in the vocabulary of an average American reader. To this list we added a number of words that had been used in some of the experiments that we planned to simulate. The resulting corpus contained 2897 words.

The training regime was divided into a series of 250 epochs. In each epoch, each word had a probability of being presented that was a logarithmic function of its Kucera and Francis frequency. The most frequent word (THE) had a probability of about 0.93; words occurring once per million had probabilities of about 0.05. Thus, the expected value of the number of presentations of a word over 250 epochs ranged from about 230 to about 12. Since the sampling process is in fact random, about 5 per cent of the lowest-frequency items will have occurred less than six times during training.

This sampling method is not intended to mimic the experience of children learning to read in American culture. In the model, all words are available for sampling throughout training, with frequency represented by the probability of selection on a given learning trial. In actual experience, however, frequency derives in part from age at acquisition; words that are higher-frequency for adults tend to be learned earlier by children. Moreover, our treatment of frequency only approximates the differences in familiarity that are relevant to skilled readers, for two reasons. First, there are known inaccuracies in standard frequency norms (Gernsbacher 1984), especially in the lower-frequency range. Second, our encoding of frequency greatly underweights the advantage of higher-frequency words relative to words of lower frequency. In the Kucera and Francis (1967) count, for example, frequencies range from about 70 000 to 1; with the logarithmic compression used in our model, the ratio of highest-frequency word to lowest- is only about 16 to 1.

**Characterizing the model's performance**

The model produces patterns of activation across the orthographic and phonological units as its output. For word naming, we assume that the pattern over the phonological units serves as the input to a system that constructs an articulatory-motor program, which in turn is executed by the motor system, resulting in an overt pronunciation response. In reality, we believe that these processes operate in a cascaded fashion: the response is triggered when the articulatory-motor program has evolved to the point where it is sufficiently differentiated from other possible motor programs. Thus, activation would begin to build up first at the orthographic units, propagating continuously from there to the hidden and phonological units and from there to the motor system.

The simulation model simplifies this procedure. Activations of the phonological units are computed in a single step, and the construction and execution of articulatory-motor programs are unimplemented. Activations computed in this manner can be shown to correspond to the asymptotic activations that would be achieved in a cascaded process (Cohen, Dunbar, and McClelland 1988). We use the phonological error score—the sum of the squared differences between the target activation value for each phonological unit and the actual activation computed by the network—to relate the model's performance to experimental data on latency and accuracy of word-naming responses. The error score is a measure of how closely the pattern computed by the net matches the correct pronunciation (or any other specified pronunciation). In general, after training the error score is lower for the correct pronunciation than for any other.

Even though the correct phonological code may be the best match to the pattern of activation over the phonological units, there is still considerable variation in error scores, and we assume that lower error scores are correlated with faster and more accurate responses under time pressure. The rationale for the accuracy assumption is simply that a low error score signifies a pattern produced by the network that is relatively clear and free from noise, providing a better signal on which the articulatory-motor programming and execution processes can operate. The rationale for the speed assumption is that in a cascaded system, patterns that are relatively clear (low in error) at asymptote reach a criterion level of clarity relatively quickly. Simulations demonstrating this point are presented in Cohen, Dunbar, and McClelland (1988).

The error score should not be viewed as a literal measure of the accuracy of an overt response made by the network. The error scores can never actually reach zero, since the logistic function used in setting the activations of units prevents activations from ever reaching their maximum or minimum values. With continued practice, error scores simply get smaller and smaller, as activations of units approximate more and more closely to the target values of 1 and 0. This improvement continues well beyond the point where the correct answer is the best match to the pattern produced by the network.

We also calculate an orthographic error score, analogous to the phonological error score, which provides a measure of the familiarity and redundancy of a letter string. This measure plays an important role in our account of lexical decision performance, but will not be considered further here (see Seidenberg and McClelland 1988a,b).

In sum, when presented with letter strings, the model produces orthographic and phonological codes which provide the basis for performing tasks such as lexical decision and naming. We characterize the model's performance in terms of error scores calculated for different types of stimuli after different amounts of training, and relate these to human performance on these tasks. Because the model contains such a large pool of words, we can perform very close simulations of many empirical phenomena reported in the literature, often using the identical stimuli as in a particular experiment.

### Summary of the model's performance

Seidenberg and McClelland (1988a,b) describe a broad range of behavioural phenomena simulated by the model. Here we briefly summarize results from simulations of the task of naming words and non-words aloud. We focus on naming because the acquired forms of dyslexia discussed below are typically associated with impairments on this task. The problem of learning to read single words aloud in English is largely determined by properties of the writing system. The alphabetic writing system for English is a code for representing spoken language; units in the writing system—letters and letter patterns—largely correspond to speech units such as phonemes. However, the correspondence between the written and spoken codes is notoriously complex; many correspondences are inconsistent (e.g. -AVE is usually pronounced as in GAVE, SAVE, and CAVE, but there is also HAVE) or wholly arbitrary (e.g. -OLO- in COLONEL, -PS in CORPS). These inconsistencies derive from several sources: there is a competing demand that the orthography preserve morphological information; there are diachronic changes in pronunciation; there is lexical borrowing and historical accident. In fact, the English orthography partially encodes several types of information (orthographic, phonological, syllabic, morphological) simultaneously. Thus, English provides an example of what can be termed a quasiregular system: a body of knowledge that is systematic but admits many exceptions (Seidenberg 1988a). In such systems the relationships among entities are statistical rather than categorical.

During the training phase, the model is exposed to a significant fragment of written English. The effect of the learning rule is that the model picks up on facts about orthographic–phonological correspondences and encodes them in terms of the weights on connections between units. Eventually, the weights achieve values that permit the model to produce the correct output for almost any word in the training set, despite the quasiregular character of the writing system. By 'correct' we mean that the error score for the correct pronunciation is typically very much smaller in magnitude than the error score for an incorrect pronunciation. As already mentioned, even when the best fit is the correct phonological code, the size of the error score varies; i.e. the model performs better on some stimuli than on others. How well it performs on a given stimulus depends on factors such as the frequency of the word and its similarity to other words in the corpus. We evaluate the model by comparing its performance on different types of words to that of human subjects.

Consider two classes of words that have been studied in a large number of behavioural experiments. Regular words such as MUST, LIKE, and CANE contain spelling patterns that recur in a large number of words, always with the same pronunciation. MUST, for example, contains the ending -UST; all monosyllabic words that end in this pattern rhyme (JUST, DUST, etc.). The words sharing the critical spelling pattern are termed the neighbours of the input string (Glushko 1979). Neighbours have been primarily defined in terms of word-endings, also termed rimes (Treiman and Chafetz 1987) or bodies

(Patterson and Morton 1985), although other aspects of word structure also matter (Taraban and McClelland 1987; Kay 1987). Exception words such as HAVE, SAID, and LOSE contain a common spelling pattern which in this particular word is pronounced irregularly. That is, since -AVE is usually pronounced as in GAVE and SAVE, the word HAVE is characterized by an exceptional spelling-to-sound correspondence. In terms of orthographic structure, regular and exception words are similar: both contain spelling patterns that recur in many words. Whereas regular words are thought to obey the pronunciation 'rules' of English, exception words do not. Given that these two word classes are similar in orthographic structure, and that they can be equated for other factors such as length and frequency, then differences between them in terms of processing difficulty must be attributed to the one dimension along which they differ, regularity of spelling–sound correspondences.

Studies examining the processing of such words have yielded the following results. First of all, there are frequency effects: higher-frequency words are named more quickly than lower-frequency words. In addition, regularity effects–faster naming latencies for regular words compared to exceptions—are substantial with lower-frequency items, but may be small or non-existent for higher-frequency words (Andrews 1982; Seidenberg et al. 1984; Seidenberg 1985b; Waters and Seidenberg 1985; Taraban and McClelland 1987). In short, there is a frequency by regularity interaction. In Taraban and McClelland's study, the difference between lower-frequency regular and exception words was a statistically significant 32 ms, while the difference for higher-frequency words was a non-significant 13 ms.

To examine the model's performance on these types of words, we used the identical stimulus set studied by Taraban and McClelland (1987, Experiment 1). Figure 7.2 presents the model's performance on this set of high- and low-frequency regular and exception words after different amounts of training. Each data point represents the mean phonological error score for the 24 items of each type used in the Taraban and McClelland experiment. Training reduces the error scores for all words following a negatively accelerated trajectory. Throughout training, there is a frequency effect: the model performs better on the words to which it is exposed more often. Note that although the test stimuli are dichotomized into high- and low-frequency groups, frequency is actually a continuous variable and it has continuous effects in the model. Early in training, there are large regularity effects for both high- and low-frequency items; in both frequency classes, regular words produce smaller error scores than exception words. Additional training reduces the regularity effect for higher-frequency words, to the point where it is eliminated by 250 epochs. However, the regularity effect for lower-frequency words remains. Figure 7.3 demonstrates the similarity of results from Taraban and McClelland's adult subjects and from the model.

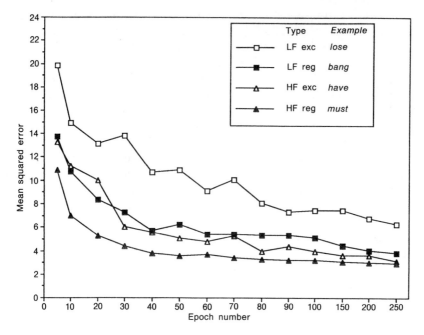

**Fig. 7.2** The model's mean phonological error scores at various stages in training for the words used by Taraban and McClelland (1987).

The frequency-by-regularity interactions obtained in two additional studies, with different sets of stimulus words (Seidenberg 1985*b*, Experiment 2; Seidenberg *et al.* 1984*a*, Experiment 3), have been recreated with equal success by the model's performance (see Seidenberg and McClelland 1988*b*). Indeed, following simulations of 14 conditions from eight experiments comparing regular and exception words, Seidenberg and McClelland obtained a correlation of 0.915 between the experimental data (difference in naming latency between regular and exception words) and the model's performance (difference in phonological error score between regular and exception words).

The model is revealing about the behavioural phenomena in two respects. First, it is clear that in the model the frequency by regularity interaction results because the output for both types of higher-frequency words approaches asymptote before the output for the lower-frequency words. Hence the difference between the higher-frequency regular and exception words is eliminated, while the difference between the two types of lower-frequency words remains. This result suggests that the interaction observed in the behavioural data is attributable to a kind of 'floor' effect due to the acquisition of a high level of skill in de-coding common words. In the model, the differences between the two types of lower-frequency words would also

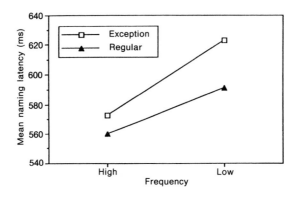

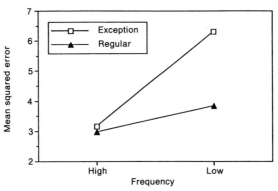

**Fig. 7.3**  Results of the Taraban and McClelland (1987) study (top panel) and the model's performance at 250 epochs (lower panel)

diminish if training were continued for more epochs. This aspect of the model provides an explanation for Seidenberg's (1985) finding that there are individual differences among skilled readers in terms of regularity effects. The fastest subjects in his study showed no regularity effect, even for words that are 'lower' in frequency according to standard norms. The model suggests that the fastest readers may have encountered lower-frequency words more often than the slower subjects, with the result that these words effectively become 'high-frequency' items.

Second, the model provides a theoretical link between effects of frequency and regularity. Both effects are due to the fact that connections that are required for correct performance have been adjusted more frequently in the required direction for frequent or regular items than for infrequent or irregular items. This holds for frequent words simply because they are presented more often. It holds for regular words because they make use of the same connections as other, neighbouring, regular words. Hence, regularity effects are frequency effects: both derive from the effects of repeated adjustment of connection weights in the same direction.

Not only in its simulation of frequency and regularity effects but, more generally, the model's performance is determined by the connection weights which reflect the aggregate effects of many individual learning trials with the items in the training set. In effect, learning results in the recreation within the network of significant aspects of the structure of written English. Because the entire set of weights is used in computing the phonological codes for all words, and because all of the weights are updated on every learning trial, there is a sense in which the output for a given word is a function of training on all words in the set. Differences between words derive from facts about the writing system distilled during the learning phase. The main influence on the phonological output is the number of times the model was exposed to the word itself; after a sufficient amount of training, this is the only factor relevant to performance on 'high-frequency' words. Performance on less-frequent words, however, is also affected by exposure to other words. Words that resemble one another in spelling–sound correspondences have mutually beneficial effects on the weights; words that are similar in spelling but dissimilar in pronunciation have mutually inhibitory effects on the weights. Performance is then determined by the cumulative effects of training on the weights.

To see this more clearly, consider the following experiment. We test the model's performance on the low-frequency regular word TINT; with the weights from 250 epochs, it produces an error score of 8.92. We train the model on another word, adjusting the weights according to the learning algorithm, and then re-test TINT. By varying the properties of the training word, we can determine which aspects of the model's experience exert the greatest influence on the weights relative to the target. In effect, we can simulate the phonological priming effects studied by Meyer, Schvaneveldt, and Ruddy (1974), Hillinger (1980), Tanenhaus, Flanigan, and Seidenberg (1980), and others. For example, Meyer et al. observed that lexical decision latencies to a target word such as ROUGH were facilitated when preceded by the rhyming prime TOUGH but inhibited when preceded by the similarly spelled non-rhyme COUGH. For the purposes of the simulation, we examined the cumulative effects of a sequence of ten prime (learn)—target (test) trials. The primes were a rhyming orthographic neighbour (MINT), a non-rhyming orthographic neighbour (the exception word, PINT), a word with the same consonants but a different vowel (TENT), and an unrelated control (RASP). The data are presented in Fig. 7.4.

The results indicate, first, that overlap in the ends of words (word-bodies or rimes) has greater impact than overlap in word-beginnings. Thus, priming TINT with MINT has greater impact than priming TINT with TENT (it also has greater impact than priming with a word such as TINS or TILT). The model supports the common assumption that the terminal segments of words

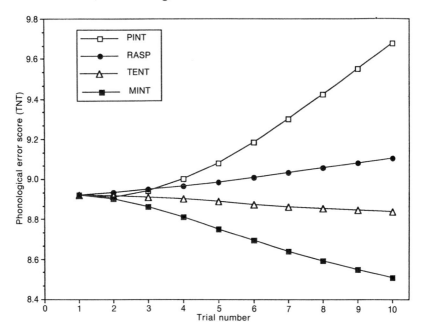

**Fig. 7.4** Effects on the phonological error score for TINT of training with MINT, PINT, TENT or RASP.

are especially critical to naming (Glushko 1979; Meyer, Schvaneveldt, and Ruddy 1974; Seidenberg *et al.* 1984a; Patterson and Morton 1985; Brown 1987; Treiman and Chafetz 1987). This fact derives from properties of the learning algorithm and the training corpus. Word-bodies turn out to be salient because there is more redundancy at the ends than at the beginnings. The learning algorithm picks up on these regularities, which have a large impact on the weights. Importantly, these same characteristics of the model also dictate that the effective relationships between words are not limited to word-bodies. These units happen to be especially salient, but they are not the only aspects of word structure relevant to processing. Thus, in the priming experiment, both TENT and RASP have small effects on the weights relevant to TINT, as do many other words. Experimental data by Kay (1987) confirm the relevance to naming of neighbourhoods defined over word-initial segments.

The other important point is that the model encodes facts about the consistency of spelling–sound correspondences. Thus, priming TINT with MINT has a large positive effect on the weights, but priming with PINT has complementary negative effects. It is clear, then, why the model performs better on regular words than on exceptions. The model's training on MINT and HINT and LINT and PRINT, matching in both spelling pattern and pronunciation, pushes the values of the weights in the same direction. The exception word PINT suffers because the weights come to reflect the fact that words ending in -INT typically rhyme with MINT. Having been exposed to PINT and its pronunciation, the model produces the correct phonological code for PINT; however, this code yields a larger error score than for a comparable regular word, owing to the impact of training on the gang of words like MINT.

The impact of the model's experiences during training can be evaluated not only by presenting words from the training vocabulary but by presenting novel words. Non-words have played an important role in experimental considerations of how people convert print to sound, because such stimulus items can be constructed along any dimensions that the experimenter fancies. In a widely cited study, Glushko (1979) demonstrated that readers are quicker to pronounce non-words (like TIFE) derived from a word-body whose neighbourhood has a regular, consistent pronunciation (LIFE, KNIFE, WIFE, etc.) than to pronounce nonwords (like TIVE) with an inconsistent neighbourhood (FIVE v. GIVE). As Seidenberg and McClelland (1988b) have shown, the significant 22 ms difference obtained in Glushko's Experiment 2 is mirrored by a significant difference of over two points in the model's phonological error scores for these two types of non-word.

The foregoing description of the model's performance in word naming has focused primarily on regularity effects. This is partly due to the prominence of this issue in the literature on reading over the past decade or so, and partly because regularity effects are particularly germane to certain types of reading disorders, to which we now turn. Before doing so, however, we wish to emphasize that evaluations of the model's naming performance are by no means restricted to the contrast between regular and exception words. Seidenberg and McClelland (1988a,b) and Seidenberg (1988a) present successful simulations of experiments on many other characteristics of words, and the reader is referred to these papers for a picture of the full scope of the model.

## Acquired dyslexia

We turn now to questions concerning the impairments of word naming characteristic of certain forms of acquired dyslexia. We have suggested that the model provides a good characterization of a broad range of phenomena related to the naming performance of skilled readers, and that it provides an integrated explanation for these phenomena in terms of the consequences of learning. As a learning model, it also speaks to the issue of how these skills are acquired. Furthermore, the model provides an interesting perspective on the kinds of impairments characteristic of developmental and acquired dyslexias. Developmental dyslexia, which could be seen as a failure to acquire the knowledge that underlies word recognition and naming, is discussed in Seidenberg and McClelland (1988). Acquired dyslexia, arising from damage to a fully developed normal system, is discussed here.

Acquired dyslexia refers to impairments in reading processes observed following brain injury in people who were previously normal readers. Several different types of acquired dyslexia have been identified, each characterized by impairments to selected aspects of processing (for recent reviews, see Coltheart 1985; Ellis and Young 1988). Many of these impairments relate to the process of naming words aloud; in fact, word-naming performance has provided the primary basis for distinguishing among different varieties of acquired dyslexia. These impairments presumably reflect damage to part(s) of the neural machinery responsible for word recognition and pronunciation. Since our model provides a computational account of some of this machinery, it should be possible to simulate word-naming impairments by selectively damaging the model. In this section we report some preliminary experiments of this sort.

Acquired forms of dyslexia have primarily been discussed in the context of a class of 'dual-route' models. As the name implies, these accounts emphasize the idea that two different procedures or mechanisms are required in order to account for naming performance. The mechanisms are distinguished in terms of the types of knowledge representations involved and the types of letter strings to which these are suited. One mechanism involves rules encoding the reader's knowledge of the correspondences between spelling and pronunciation characteristic of written English. These mapping rules can be used to construct a correct pronunciation of any letter string that obeys them—specifically, regular words such as MUST and regular non-words such as NUST; the rule-based procedure will generate incorrect pronunciations for words that violate the rules (e.g. exceptions such as HAVE). This mechanism has been termed a 'non-lexical' or 'subword-level' process because the rules involve generalizations concerning spelling–sound correspondences rather than knowledge of whole specific words. The other mechanism involves stored representations of the pronunciations of known words. The idea here is that the reader identifies a familiar word (directly on the basis of its spelling, and possibly further by consulting its meaning) and then accesses a stored representation of its pronunciation. This mechanism could apply to all known words, but would fail in the case of novel strings such as non-words, which lack representations in memory. This mechanism has been termed a 'lexical' or 'word-level' process because the relevant knowledge representations concern the pronunciations of individual words. Further descriptions of dual-routine accounts of word naming can be found in Patterson, Marshall, and Coltheart (1985).[1]

The major theoretical alternative to the dual-routine model, analogy theory, carved things up slightly differently. Analogy theories proposed by Glushko (1979), Marcel (1980), Humphreys and Evett (1985) and others contain a single type of knowledge representation relevant to pronunciation: they eliminated the separate rule-based knowledge about correspondences between graphemes and phonemes, leaving only the lexical representations, which were thought to be employed in naming both words and non-words. As Patterson and Coltheart (1987) noted, however, these models implicitly preserved the distinction between two phonological procedures in naming: while a word could be named by accessing a stored phonological represen-tation, the pronunciation of a non-word still had to be created by segmenting known words and cobbling together the phonology of the individual segments comprising the non-word.

In summary, most theorizing about how readers (of English) translate orthography to phonology has assumed that different naming mechanisms are required for the correct pronunciation of exception words on the one hand and non-words on the other. One of the main contributions of the Seidenberg and McClelland (1988a,b) model is that it accomplishes this translation process with a single mechanism employing weighted connections between units. All items—regular and irregular, word and non-word—are pronounced using the knowledge encoded in the same sets of connections. This model also differs from dual-routine accounts in that there are no rules specifying the regular spelling–sound correspondences of the language, and there is no lexicon in which the pronunciations of words are listed. The model also differs from proposals by Glushko (1979) and Brown (1987) in that there are no lexical nodes representing individual words and no influences from orthographic neighbours at the time of processing a word. Where the model agrees with these accounts is in regard to the notion that regularity effects result from a conspiracy among known words. In the present model, this conspiracy is realized in the setting of connection strengths. Words with similar spellings and pronunciations produce overlapping, mutually beneficial changes in the connection weights.

Some of the evidence thought to support the distinction between two naming processes came from studies of normal readers pronouncing various types of letter strings. However, this general class of theories perhaps took even greater comfort from the neuropsychological literature. In particular, the patterns of reading performance in two 'varieties' of acquired dyslexia, phonological and surface dyslexia, have been considered to provide crucial evidence. Phonological dyslexic patients (Beauvois and Derouesné 1979; Shallice and Warrington 1980; Patterson 1982) show a dissociation between word and non-word naming; in some cases (e.g. Funnell 1983), the dis-sociation can be dramatic, with around 90 per cent success on words of any class or length but total failure to read aloud even the simplest non-words. Surface dyslexic patients (Marshall and Newcombe 1973; Shallice and Warrington 1980; Coltheart *et al.* 1983) show a dissociation between regular and exception word naming. Though performance on exception words has not, in any case thus far recorded, been at zero, once again the dissociation can be substantial: for example, about 90 per cent success on low-frequency regular words compared with 40 per cent on low-frequency exception words (Bub, Cancelliere, and Kertesz 1985) or, distinguishing amongst 'levels' of regularity, around 80 per cent correct on regular words v. 35 per cent on very irregular words (Shallice, Warrington, and McCarthy 1983).

If phonological dyslexia could be considered to reflect almost total disruption of the routine for subword-level translation, and surface dyslexia could be considered to indicate severe disruption of the routine for word-level translation, it is easy to see why these neuropsychological dissociations have been emphasized, nay treasured, by dual-routine theories. Accordingly, they represent a challenge to any theory proposing a single process by which all letter strings, whether regular words, exception words or non-words, are converted from orthography to phonology. Failure to account for these patterns would weaken this proposal, while a demonstration that such dissociations could arise within a truly single-routine theory like the model outlined here would constitute a powerful argument against the need for postulating multiple routines.

We shall have nothing to say about phonological dyslexia because we have only just begun to consider how the model might account for it. The pattern of reading performance observed in surface dyslexia, on the other hand, seems ideally suited to one kind of evaluation of the model. Some of the earliest studied cases of surface dyslexia (e.g. Marshall and Newcombe 1973) appeared to use their impaired oral reading skill to make sense of the printed word, yielding slow responses, multiple responses, and generally poor performance. More interestingly, three recent studies of patients with impaired comprehension (for both speech and reading) reveal (1) a high degree of accuracy in naming regular words and non-words; and (2) word-naming latencies at least within the range of age-matched controls. The description of 'reading without semantics' has been offered for the first of these cases (Shallice, Warrington, and McCarthy 1983) and is equally appropriate for the other two cases (Bub, Cancelliere, and Kertesz 1985; McCarthy and Warrington 1986). Reading without semantics is of course precisely what the Seidenberg and McClelland model does. Therefore it seems highly relevant to an evaluation of the model to ask the following question: after the model has been trained to the high level of successful 'oral reading' performance described earlier, if it is now damaged in various ways, will we observe the characteristics of surface dyslexic reading?

The remainder of this chapter is largely devoted to exploring this question. Before we begin, it may be helpful to have a slightly more expanded description of reading performance by surface dyslexic patients. As emphasized for neuropsychological impairments in general (Caramazza 1986), and for this pattern of impaired reading in particular (Patterson, Marshall, and Coltheart 1985), no two patients are identical and so a syndrome label should be taken as a loose descriptive device rather than a precise classification. In fact, the naming performance of patients described as surface dyslexics varies greatly. With these caveats in mind, we began by assuming that the following features, observed in what are perhaps the most 'pure' and certainly the best-studied surface dyslexic patients, provided a starting point for our explorations of damage to the model:

1. Most central, and already mentioned, is the patients' significantly greater success in naming of words (like PINE) that have regular, typical spelling-to-sound correspondences than of words (like PINT) with exceptional or atypical spelling-to-sound correspondences.

2. Accuracy in naming non-words can be relatively intact, or at least within the (widely varying: Masterson 1985) range of non-word reading skill shown by normal subjects.

3. At least some surface dyslexic patients' accuracy in word naming mimics a characteristic, discussed earlier, of normal subjects' latencies in word naming: an interaction between frequency and regularity. In the best demonstration of this interaction (by Bub, Cancelliere, and Kertesz 1985), the patient showed an advantage on regular over exception words of 15 per cent for high-frequency words but 50 per cent for low-frequency words.

4. The most common type of reading error is the regularization of an exception word, e.g. PINT—/pint/ rhyming with HINT, COME—/kOm/ rhyming with DOME, etc. (Note: pronunciations will be rendered here not in the international phonetic alphabet but, rather, in terms of the phonemic encoding scheme used in the model, taken from Rumelhart and McClelland (1986*b*), and reproduced here as Table 7.1.) All patients thus far reported do make errors of some other types, such as occasional errors on regular words (e.g. HORSE—/hWs/, BASE—/pAs/) and non-regularization errors on exception words (e.g. FLOOD—/flOd/, LOSE—/lUs/) (all examples from Shallice, Warrington, and McCarthy 1983). The majority of errors, however, are strict regularizations.

5. Finally, as already mentioned, the patients' reading speed can be roughly normal.

In the following sections, we report experiments in which we observed the effects of different types of damage to the simulation model on performance with different types of words and non-words. We shall only be considering the oral reading performance (not lexical decision) of surface dyslexic patients; accordingly, when we talk about output from the model, this will always refer to error scores calculated over the phonological output units. The primary goal of the experiments was exploratory: how would the model perform when different components were damaged? A second goal was to determine whether damage to the model would produce the types of errors characteristic of

**Table 7.1**   *The phonemic categorization system used in the model, plus a pronunciation key*

| | | Place | | | | | |
|---|---|---|---|---|---|---|---|
| | | Front | | Middle | | Back | |
| | | V/L | U/S | V/L | U/S | V/L | U/S |
| Interrupted | Stop | b | p | d | t | g | k |
| | Nasal | m | — | n | — | N | — |
| Continuous | | | | | | | |
| consonant | Fric. | v/D | f/T | z | s | Z/j | S/C |
| | Liq/SV | w/l | — | r | — | y | h |
| Vowel | High | E | i | O | ^ | U | u |
| | Low | A | e | I | a/α | W | */o |

*Key:* N = ng in *sing*; D = th in *the*; T = th in *with*; Z = z in *azure*; S = sh in *ship*; C = ch in *chip*; E = ee in *beet*; i = i in *bit*; O = oa in *boat*; ^ = u in *but* or schwa; U = oo in *boot*; u = oo in *book*; A = ai in *bait*; e = e in *bet*; I = i_e in *bite*; a = a in *bat*; α = a in *father*; W = ow in *cow*; * = aw in *saw*; o = o in *hot*.

Reproduced from Rumelhart and McClelland (1986*b* Table 5, p. 235).

surface dyslexic patients. Ultimately, we would like to achieve simulations of specific cases of surface dyslexia, capturing both their qualitative and quantitative aspects, but we have not done so as yet. In the final section of the paper we discuss some of the issues that need to be addressed if additional research is to achieve this ultimate goal.

One final introductory comment: the model was developed on the basis of, and has been extensively evaluated relative to, data from normal readers. By comparison, these explorations of the neuropsychological implications of the model are at an embryonic stage. At many points in what follows, we shall have to say (or, rather, to save the reader from boredom, we shall hope that it is generally understood) that much more work on this approach is needed before a comprehensive story can be told. Our justification for offering this somewhat premature account is that, as we have already suggested, neuropsychological dissociations could be considered a major challenge to this kind of model which eschews separate routines, rule-based systems and other notions that have played a central role in cognitive neuropsychology. Even if premature, then, it seems useful to indicate some of the ways in which the model might respond to this challenge.

### Overview of methods

The general procedure involved in these explorations was as follows. All lesion studies were done using the weights created after 250 epochs of training, when the model had reached the nearly asymptotic level of performance illustrated earlier. All experiments were concerned with effects of damage ('lesions') to the system; in a later section we discuss other types of pathology that might be simulated. Lesions were made at the three different locations within the model where changes take place as a result of learning: weights on the connections from orthographic input units to hidden units ('early' weights); the hidden units themselves; and weights on the connections from hidden units to phonological output units ('late' weights). Damage was inflicted by zeroing a proportion of the connections or units at the lesion site. In the first, parametric, study to be reported, the proportions of damaged connections or units tested were 0.1, 0.2, 0.4 and 0.6. Damage was introduced probabilistically; with a damage value of 0.4, for example, the output from a random 40 per cent of the specified connections or units was zeroed. For any given lesion experiment, then, we shall be looking at performance for a particular combination of location and level of damage.

Although all representations and processes within the model are distributed (such that the model never, for example, assigns a single hidden unit to a particular word), it is by no means the case that all units are activated. In fact, in the processing of any given word, the majority of hidden units are not activated by the input; on average, about 24 of the 200 hidden units will be activated for any word. The result of this, when combined with probabilistic damage, is high variability from one lesion test to the next. In order to produce a larger pool of data yielding a more stable and less idiosyncratic picture of the model's behaviour when damaged, all lesion experiments for any stimulus set at any particular location and level of damage consisted of ten tests.

The data from a lesion experiment will consist of two measures. The first is the phonological error scores (means and standard deviations) for different pronunciations of the stimulus words being tested. Typically only two pronunciations of each word were tested; for the exception word PINT, for example, the pronunciations of primary interest were the correct one /pInt/ and the regularization /pint/. These mean phonological error scores will represent averages both over words within the set being tested ($N$ to be specified for each experiment) and over tests ($N = 10$). The second measure concerns the relative error scores for the two pronunciations of a given word on a given test. If the model is performing correctly, then it should of course 'prefer' the pronunciation /pInt/ to the pronunciation /pint/. If, when damaged, it yields a lower score for the alternative pronunciation, we call this a reversal. We counted as reversals any cases where the alternative score was at least one full point lower than the score for the correct pronunciation. This measure will be given as reversal rate, meaning the percentage of occasions in a particular lesion experiment where an alternative pronunciation was preferred.

Arguments have been offered elsewhere (earlier in this chapter and in Seidenberg and McClelland 1988) for the adequacy of the phonological error score as a measure of naming performance by normal readers; and the impressive similarity between functions derived from the model and those from real subjects (as illustrated above) supports this rationale. There are, however, two aspects of this error score which make it less than ideal for lesion studies. The first is a substantive issue: the error score combines accuracy and latency in a single measure. While this may offer a reasonable characterization of normal readers, operating at relatively full efficiency with a minimum of errors and a maximum of speed, it is not necessarily so satisfactory for pathological data. If, for example, one patient reads slowly and makes many errors while another reads quickly with (approximately) the same error rate, then no single speed–accuracy trade-off function will characterize both. In the model, a high error score could represent a fast, wrong reading, a slow, correct reading, or a slow, wrong reading; when trying to relate the model's performance to patients, it would be informative if we could discriminate among those alternative interpretations. With the present measure, we cannot.

The other problem is a purely practical, procedural one: the error score represents the degree to which the pattern of activation over the phonological output units differs from the ideal pattern for the specified phonological code. In general, for simulations of normal data (but note that it may not always be safe to assume that the model in its normal, undamaged state 'knows' the correct pronunciation for all words; in fact, it does not), it will be adequate to specify only the correct pronunciation. But as soon as we wish to simulate error-prone patients, then in order to discover what sorts of pronunciation errors the model may make when it has been lesioned, we are required to specify every pronunciation of interest in order to identify the pronunciation yielding the lowest error score. This nuisance is admittedly of concern to the authors rather than to the readers of this chapter. We mention it here only to explain why, for many of the lesion studies to be reported below, we test two pronunciations of each word rather than many.

### Experiment 1: the effect of different locations and levels of damage

To provide a basic introduction to the way in which the model's performance degrades under conditions of damage, we begin with a parametric exploration of the three locations and four levels of damage mentioned above. The stimulus items for this experiment, all four-letter words from the model's vocabulary, were the 16 regular words and 16 exception words listed in Table 7.2. The two sets were approximately balanced for both Kucera and Francis frequency and orthographic error scores; thus we can be reasonably

**Table 7.2**   *The 16 regular and 16 exception words used in Experiment 1, with their correct and alternative pronunciations, mean frequencies\* and mean orthographic and phonological error scores from performance of the undamaged model after 250 epochs of training*

| Regular | COR | OTH | Exception | COR | REG |
|---|---|---|---|---|---|
| COVE | /kOv/ | /kUv/ | MOVE | /mUv/ | /mOv/ |
| TINT | /tint/ | /tInt/ | PINT | /pInt/ | /pint/ |
| BEAD | /bEd/ | /bed/ | DEAD | /ded/ | /dEd/ |
| FOUL | /fWl/ | /fOl/ | SOUL | /SOl/ | /sWl/ |
| HOWL | /hWl/ | /hOl/ | BOWL | /bOl/ | /bWl/ |
| LEAF | /lEf/ | /lef/ | DEAF | /def/ | /dEf/ |
| HOOP | /hUp/ | /hup/ | HOOD | /hud/ | /hUd/ |
| LAKE | /lAk/ | /lak/ | LOSE | /lUz/ | /lOz/ |
| FILE | /fIl/ | /fil/ | FOOT | /fut/ | /fUt/ |
| PASS | /pas/ | /pos/ | POST | /pOst/ | /p∗st/ |
| DAMP | /damp/ | /domp/ | COUP | /kU/ | /kWp/ |
| PINE | /pIn/ | /pin/ | POUR | /pOr/ | /pWr/ |
| BEND | /bend/ | /bEnd/ | PEAR | /pAr/ | /pEr/ |
| SKIN | /skin/ | /skIn/ | TOMB | /tUm/ | /tom/ |
| MEET | /mEt/ | /mAt/ | MONK | /m∧nk/ | /monk/ |
| DEAL | /dEl/ | /del/ | AUNT | /ant/ | /∗nt/ |

40.1 X̄ frequency                                  45.6
5.8 X̄ orthographic error score             6.1
4.1 X̄ phonological error score             4.8

*From Kucera and Francis 1967.

confident that any differences in behaviour between the two sets should be genuinely attributable to regularity of spelling-to-sound correspondences. Also shown in Table 7.2 are the two pronunciations tested for each word. For the exception words, the alternative (to the correct, or COR) pronunciation was of course the regularization (REG). For regular words, it is not always obvious what the alternative should be, but we attempted to make these other (OTH) pronunciations as plausible as possible, for example choosing a pronunciation of the vowel or vowel combination which occurs in other words.

The mean phonological error scores for the two pronunciations of the words in the two sets are shown in Fig. 7.5 (regular) and Fig. 7.6 (exception). The abscissa in each graph represents level of damage, from none (performance of the model in its normal state) to proportion of damage $= 0.6$. For both regular and exception words, COR phonological error scores rise in a monotonic, indeed essentially linear, fashion with increasing level of damage. The effect of level of damage is much more striking than that of

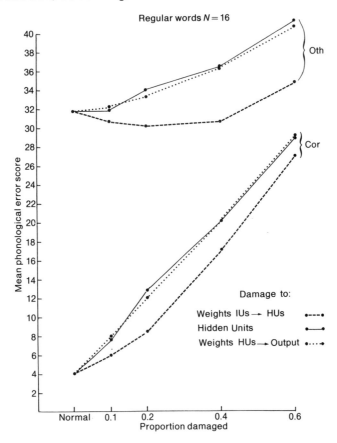

**Fig. 7.5** The model's mean phonological error scores for correct and other pronunciations of regular words under normal conditions and with various locations and levels of damage.

location of damage: in fact, considering only the COR means, location appears to be relatively inconsequential. Damage to early weights consistently yields slightly lower scores than damage to either hidden units or late weights; but means for these latter two locations are virtually indistinguishable.

Three further aspects of the results in Figs 7.5 and 7.6 need to be highlighted:

1. Error scores for REG and OTH pronunciations also rise as a function of damage, but very much less dramatically than those for COR. This is probably not a ceiling effect because it is possible to obtain considerably higher error scores (on other types of words or with additional damage). As a result of this difference in rate of increase, the error scores for the correct

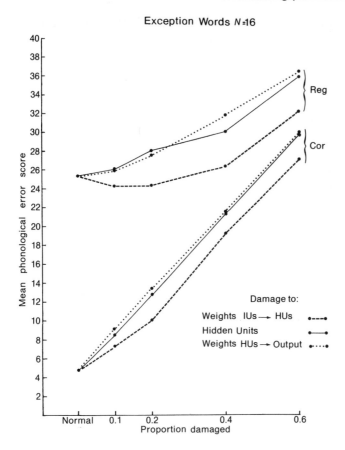

**Fig. 7.6**  The model's mean phonological error scores for correct and regularized pronunciations of exception words under normal conditions and with various locations and levels of damage.

and for the alternative pronunciations begin to converge at higher levels of damage, especially for exception words.

2. With regard to the two classes of words, COR scores for the regular words are consistently, though only marginally, lower than COR scores for the exception words; OTH scores for the regular words, on the other hand, are quite a bit higher than REG scores for the exception words. (This can be seen more easily in Table 7.3 where mean values are listed.) The net result is that there is a smaller difference between COR and REG scores for exception words than between COR and OTH scores for regular words.

3. Where location of damage has a notable effect is not on the means but on the standard deviations of the COR scores. Of particular interest, because

the corresponding means are so similar, is the fact that damage to hidden units is associated with high variability in COR scores, while damage to connections between hidden units and output units produces very much lower standard deviations. These standard deviations are shown beside their corresponding means in Table 7.3.

**Table 7.3**  *Results from Experiment 1 for regular and exception words with different proportions of damage to hidden units or to connections from hidden units to output units: means and standard deviations of phonological error scores for the two different pronunciations, and reversal rates—the proportion of occasions on which the REG or OTH pronunciation yielded a lower error score than the COR pronunciation*

|  | Proportion damaged | | | |
|  | 0.1 | 0.2 | 0.4 | 0.6 |
| --- | --- | --- | --- | --- |
| *Damage to hidden units* | | | | |
| Regular words | | | | |
| mean (s.d.) error COR | 7.6  (3.8) | 12.8  (5.9) | 20.2  (7.9) | 28.9  (8.6) |
| mean (s.d.) error OTH | 31.9 (11.1) | 34.0 (10.7) | 36.4 (11.3) | 41.2 (10.8) |
| reversal rate | 0 | 0 | 2.5% | 7.5% |
| Exception words | | | | |
| mean (s.d.) error COR | 8.4  (4.0) | 12.7  (5.3) | 21.3  (7.6) | 29.7  (8.1) |
| mean (s.d.) error REG | 26.0  (8.8) | 28.0  (8.7) | 30.0  (9.1) | 35.8 (10.2) |
| reversal rate | 1.3% | 2.5% | 16.3% | 23.8% |
| *Damage to connections from hidden units to output units* | | | | |
| Regular words | | | | |
| mean (s.d.) error COR | 7.9  (2.5) | 12.0  (3.1) | 20.2  (3.8) | 29.0  (3.8) |
| mean (s.d.) error OTH | 32.2 (10.7) | 33.4  (9.8) | 36.3  (8.3) | 40.6  (6.7) |
| reversal rate | 0 | 0 | 0 | 0 |
| Exception words | | | | |
| mean (s.d.) error COR | 9.2  (2.4) | 13.4  (2.7) | 21.5  (3.2) | 29.9  (3.6) |
| mean (s.d.) error REG | 26.0  (7.9) | 27.5  (7.4) | 31.8  (7.2) | 36.4  (6.7) |
| reversal rate | 0 | 0 | 1.3% | 8.3% |

The importance of these three points is revealed when we turn to the other measure of interest. Table 7.3 shows reversal rates under conditions of damage to hidden units and to late weights, the two locations which yielded virtually identical mean error scores. The first point (convergence between scores for correct and for alternative pronunciations with increasing level of damage) means that while small amounts of damage yield few if any occasions on which the alternative pronunciation produces a lower score, higher levels of damage produce a number of preferences for the alternative pronunciation. The second point (less distance between COR and REG error scores for exception words than between COR and OTH error scores for regular words) means that any combination of location and level of damage which produces reversals at all produces higher reversal rates for exception than for regular words. The third point (higher variability around the mean for damage to hidden units than for late weights) has the outcome of substantial reversal rates when hidden units are disrupted, but low reversal rates with zeroing of late weights. When the effects of these three points are considered together, the complete picture is a notable number of reversals only for exception words and only given higher levels of damage to hidden units.

The interpretations of both the difference between regular and exception words and the effect of increasing level of damage are reasonably obvious. Even when 60 per cent of the normally encoded information at some level is unavailable, the model generally prefers the correct pronunciation of regular words because the correspondences embodied in regular words are in essence overlearned in the model. Exception words are more vulnerable to damage, but they are sufficiently well learned via distributed representations that their COR pronunciations are typically preferred so long as damage level is low. When about half of the hidden units are inactivated, however, pronunciations reflecting overlearned REG correspondences begin to be more attractive for some exception words on some tests.

The interpretation of the location effect is less obvious. Recall that it is not the case that lesioning late weights results in better performance (i.e. lower mean error scores) than lesioning hidden units: it simply results in more consistent, less variable performance. It is clear why this should have the effect that it has on reversal rates: given that the COR means are always lower than the REG means, it is only when the COR scores vary considerably around the mean that some of them will turn out to be higher than the corresponding REG scores. But why is such variability associated only with damage to hidden units and not with damage to late weights? We suggest that while all representations are distributed, some representations are more distributed than others. There are only 200 hidden units, and on average only about 24 of these are activated for any given word. With 60 per cent probabilistic damage, one infliction of damage could by chance knock out a number of the relevant 24 units, while the next lesion might happen to hit none of the crucial units: thus, high variability from one test to the next. By contrast, the number of connections from hidden units to output units germane to any given word is much larger. Each of the 20-odd hidden units relevant to a word is connected to all 460 phonological units; if the model were performing without error, 16 of these phonological units would be activated for each phoneme in the correct pronunciation. Zeroing the weights on 60 per cent of these connections will indeed have a deleterious effect on performance; but because the 'knowledge' at this level is distributed over such a large number of connections, any random 60 per cent loss will produce deleterious effects similar to any other.

There are marked differences in reversal rates for individual exception words within the set, but we defer discussion of this until Experiment 4, where we consider the variables that make words prone or resistant to regularization.

In summary of Experiment 1, increasing levels of damage at all three locations produces steady increments in the phonological error scores associated with correct pronunciations of known regular and exception words. Higher levels of damage at the location of the hidden units yield a significant number of tests on which the model 'prefers' the regularized pronunciation of an exception word to the correct pronunciation, just as surface dyslexic patients often do in oral reading. Accordingly, most of the remaining lesion experiments will concentrate on this location and level of damage.

**Experiment 2: lesions and novelty**

In earlier sections of this chapter we discussed how the model in its normal state performs both on words in its vocabulary and on novel stimuli (non-words). Experiment 1 demonstrated how the model in various damaged states performs on regular and exception strings, but only ones from its premorbid vocabulary. The purpose of Experiment 2 was to examine how the model deals with novelty once it has been damaged. As explained in the introduction to lesioning the model, at least some surface dyslexic patients (e.g., Bub, Cancelliere, and Kertesz 1985; McCarthy and Warrington 1986) show normal accuracy in non-word reading, though other reported cases of surface dyslexia are either at the bottom end of the range of normal performance (e.g. Kay and Lesser 1985) or frankly impaired at non-word naming (e.g. Masterson 1985).

For our initial exploration of novelty, the stimulus items were triplets consisting of an exception word, a regular word, and a non-word, matched for orthographic 'body' or rime: for example, COME, HOME, and NOME. This design enabled us to test the model's performance using the identical two pronunciations of each body within a triplet: the stimulus items ($N=20$ triplets) with their alternative pronunciations are shown in Table 7.4. The regular pronunciation of a body will of course be considered the correct pronunciation for both the regular word and the non-word members of the triplet but the incorrect pronunciation of the exception word; correspondingly, the irregular pronunciation will be correct for the exception word but

**Table 7.4**  *Stimulus items for Experiment 2: triplets of exception words, regular words and non-words matched for body, with the two alternative pronunciations tested for each triplet*

| Exception word | Regular word | Non-word | Pronunciation of body | |
|---|---|---|---|---|
| | | | Regular | Exception |
| PUT | CUT | DUT | /ʌt/ | /ut/ |
| PINT | HINT | RINT | /int/ | /Int/ |
| GROSS | CROSS | BROSS | /*s/ | /Os/ |
| CASTE | HASTE | NASTE | /Ast/ | /ast/ |
| TOUCH | COUCH | BOUCH | /WC/ | /ʌC/ |
| BOWL | HOWL | POWL | /Wl/ | /Ol/ |
| COME | HOME | NOME | /Om/ | /ʌm/ |
| STEAK | BLEAK | SHEAK | /Ek/ | /Ak/ |
| GIVE | FIVE | MIVE | /Iv/ | /iv/ |
| DEAF | LEAF | NEAF | /Ef/ | /ef/ |
| SOUL | FOUL | DOUL | /Wl/ | /Ol/ |
| PEAR | GEAR | MEAR | /Er/ | /Ar/ |
| GLOVE | GROVE | BLOVE | /Ov/ | /ʌv/ |
| BULL | DULL | TULL | /ʌl/ | /ul/ |
| SWEAT | TREAT | SNEAT | /Et/ | /et/ |
| LOSE | NOSE | BOSE | /Oz/ | /Uz/ |
| BLOWN | CROWN | TROWN | /Wn/ | /On/ |
| FLOOD | BROOD | FROOD | /Ud/ | /ʌd/ |
| POST | LOST | FOST | /*st/ | /Ost/ |
| HAVE | GAVE | BAVE | /Av/ | /av/ |

incorrect for both the regular word and non-word. Reversals will then be instances of phonological error scores REG < IRR for exception words and IRR < REG for regular words and non-words. In order to make reversals a meaningful concept for the non-words, it is obviously necessary to ensure that in its normal, undamaged state, the model prefers the REG to the IRR pronunciation of all of the non-words. The original set of triplets ($N = 30$) turned out to contain 10 items where this was not the case. These have been eliminated, yielding 20 triplets.

Table 7.5 shows the mean phonological error scores (and standard deviations) for the two pronunciations of the 20 items in each word set, both for undamaged performance and with damage to hidden units, $p = 0.6$ (where $N$/cell = 10 runs × 20 items). With the model in healthy condition, performance differs as a function of word class in two ways. First, mean phonological error scores for the COR pronunciations (which are, remember, REG for regular words and non-words but IRR for exception words) have the ordering of regular words < exception words ≪ non-words; this of course reflects what

**Table 7.5**   *Results for Experiment 2. Columns correspond to: (1) the mean phonological error scores for the correct pronunciation of the stimulus items; (2) the standard deviations associated with Column 1 means; (3) the mean phonological error scores for the other pronunciation (regular for the exception words, irregular for the regular words and non-words); (4) s.d.'s for Column 3 means; (5) the difference between the means in Columns 3 and 1; (6) the percentage of tests (N = 200) on which a particular item had a lower error score for OTH than for COR*

|  | (1) | (2) | (3) | (4) | (5) | (6) |
|---|---|---|---|---|---|---|
|  | X̄ COR | (s.d.) | X̄ OTH | (s.d.) | OTH–COR | Reversals (%) |
| *Undamaged* |  |  |  |  |  |  |
| regular | 4.4 | (1.8) | 28.9 | (9.8) | 24.5 | — |
| exception | 5.1 | (2.5) | 26.9 | (11.5) | 21.8 | — |
| non-word | 11.4 | (4.2) | 24.6 | (9.5) | 13.2 | — |
| *Damage HU's p=0.6* |  |  |  |  |  |  |
| regular | 27.1 | (8.0) | 36.8 | (9.2) | 9.7 | 9 |
| exception | 28.1 | (7.7) | 33.7 | (9.6) | 5.6 | 24 |
| non-word | 29.2 | (8.1) | 35.2 | (9.4) | 6.0 | 21 |

the model knows about these three types of letter string. Second, mean error scores for the OTH pronunciations have the reverse ordering, non-words < exception words < regular words. Once again, this is to be expected, reflecting as it were the model's confidence in its preferred pronunciation. The net result, also shown in Table 7.5, is that the difference between OTH and COR pronunciations is biggest for regular words and smallest for non-words.

Turning to damaged performance, we see that the ordering of error scores for correct pronunciations of the three word classes is maintained, but only just: the discrepancies among them are now small. In particular, the major advantage (in undamaged performance) for familiar lexical items over unfamiliar strings is all but lost. The difference between OTH and COR means is much reduced in all three conditions; most interestingly, the exception words, which yielded a difference score not very dissimilar to regular words under normal conditions, show a difference score virtually identical to the non-words after lesioning.

Table 7.5 also shows reversal rates (percentage of tests on which OTH < COR) for the three string types. Experiment 1 taught us the importance of variability to reversal rates, and its role can be seen again here, not in the standard deviations *per se* (which are quite constant across word class under damaged conditions) but in terms of the standard deviations relative to the OTH–COR difference score. For regular words, where this difference score is larger than 1 s.d., the reversal rates are low; for exception words and non-words, where the difference score is less than 1 s.d., the reversal rates are substantially higher.

The reversal rates for the regular and exception words merely replicate (albeit with different stimulus items) those reported for Experiment 1 (Table 7.3). The interesting finding from Experiment 2 is the notable number of reversals for non-words. This aspect of the model's performance seems to constitute a good match for some surface dyslexic patients but not others. The patients studied by Bub, Cancelliere, and Kertesz (1985) and McCarthy and Warrington (1986) were both asked to read aloud Glushko's (1979) list of 43 'exception' pseudowords, which are very similar to the non-words used here. These two patients showed normal accuracy of non-word reading (indistinguishable, in fact, from Glushko's university-student subjects), with few irregular pronunciations (e.g BLEAD—/bled/ rather than /blEd/): 4/43 (9 per cent) and 3/43 (7 per cent), respectively. On the other hand, a surface dyslexic patient studied by Kay and Lesser (1985) made some outright errors in his non-word reading, and his acceptable responses included a somewhat larger proportion (19 per cent) of irregular pronunciations. A question for future exploration is whether other features of the model's lesioned performance have a greater resemblance to Kay and Lesser's patient than to the Bub, Cancelliere, and Kertesz and McCarthy and Warrington patients.

The relatively high and approximately equal reversal rates for exception words and non-words are intriguing in their suggestion that damage can destabilize the model's performance on two different types of items in roughly the same way (at least as assessed by this somewhat gross measure, simple preference for an alternative plausible pronunciation). The exception words are familiar orthographic sequences to the model, but embody letter–sound correspondences that are atypical. The non-words offer correspondences which (at least most often, over the range of known words) are typical; but since the non-words are not familiar orthographic sequences, the model is much less confident about an appropriate pronunciation for them. Only for items that are both familiar and regular does the damaged model retain a reliable preference for the 'correct' pronunciation.

## Experiment 3: frequency effects

The most notable feature of surface dyslexic oral reading, the tendency to regularize words with an irregular spelling-to-sound correspondence, is strongly modulated by frequency for at least some reported patients. M.P., the case studied by Bub, Cancelliere, and Kertesz (1985), made few regularization errors or, indeed, errors of any kind in oral reading of high-frequency exception words. As word frequency declined, her error rate increased steadily, and virtually all her errors were regularizations. Such dramatic frequency effects do not, however, characterize all surface dyslexic patients. For H.T.R. (Shallice, Warrington, and McCarthy 1983), regularity seems to have been such a powerful determinant of reading success that with highly irregular words (e.g. SUEDE, UNIQUE or BUSINESS) she mispronounced the majority of words whatever their frequency. On the other hand, for mildly irregular words (more like the 'exception' words that we have been testing here, e.g. DREAD, CROW), H.T.R.'s success showed some sensitivity to frequency. Experiment 3 was an attempt to determine whether the model's tendency to produce regularization errors (reversals) is modulated by word frequency.

This evaluation was made using three sets of exception words; their frequency characteristics are listed in Table 7.6. In the first set, rather than

**Table 7.6**   *Description of the word sets used to assess frequency effects after damage*

| Word set | (*N*) | X̄ Frequency | Frequency range |
|---|---|---|---|
| (1) Very high frequency words | (20) | 1859.8 | 424–5146 |
| (2) Glushko words | | | |
| low | (10) | 14.6 | 2–36 |
| low–medium | (8) | 69.3 | 51–88 |
| medium–high | (8) | 218.1 | 108–424 |
| high–very high | (9) | 1643.9 | 630–3941 |
| (3) Body-matched pairs | | | |
| lower-frequency member | (11) | 167.6 | 5– 938 |
| higher-frequency member | (11) | 1046.8 | 230–3292 |

comparing different levels of frequency, we simply selected the 20 virtually highest-frequency exception words in the model's vocabulary, words like ARE, HAVE, ONE, WERE, SAID, WHAT. The question is whether such exalted frequency values 'protect' words from reversing. The second set consisted of 35 items from Glushko's (1979) list of exception words; these are 4–5 letter words with reasonably common spelling patterns (i.e. no orthographically weird words are included), all of which, of course, are in the model's vocabulary. For purposes of evaluating frequency effects, the 35 items were divided into four frequency bands, as shown in Table 7.6. Finally, we selected 22 items consisting of 11 'body'-matched pairs with one higher- and one lower-frequency member in each pair; examples of these items with their K–F frequencies in parentheses are GOOD (807)–HOOD (7) and FOUR (359)–POUR (9). As can be seen in Table 7.6, there was considerable overlap in frequency between the two sets as a whole; none the less, within each matched pair, there was always a substantial discrepancy in frequency. The highest frequency item is the lower set, WHERE (938), was matched with THERE (2724).

Table 7.7 presents mean error scores (and s.d.'s) for the COR and REG pronunciations for each list, plus reversal rates. It appears that frequency is not the major determinant of susceptibility to reversal in the model. It has

**Table 7.7**    *Mean (s.d.) phonological error scores for COR and REG pronunciations of the various frequency lists with damage to hidden units p=0.6, plus reversal rates*

| Word set | X̄ COR | (s.d.) | X̄ REG | (s.d.) | Reversals (%) |
|---|---|---|---|---|---|
| (1) Very high frequency words | 29.5 | (8.4) | 34.7 | (9.0) | 29 |
| (2) Glushko words | | | | | |
| low | 32.0 | (8.1) | 35.0 | (8.1) | 37 |
| low–medium | 30.2 | (7.4) | 36.3 | (10.7) | 28 |
| medium–high | 29.6 | (8.6) | 34.8 | (9.9) | 31 |
| high–very high | 28.4 | (8.2) | 35.3 | (10.0) | 26 |
| (3) Body-matched pairs lower–frequency member | 29.8 | (8.0) | 30.7 | (8.0) | 46 |
| higher–frequency member | 28.8 | (8.1) | 31.6 | (7.9) | 35 |

some influence: in the set of body-matched words (list 3), the lower-frequency members reversed more often than the higher-frequency members, and within the four frequency bands of the Glushko words (set 2), the low-frequency items showed the highest reversal rate. On the other hand, considering all word sets in Table 7.5, there are several comparisons where lists with large-frequency differences yield essentially identical reversal rates, for example the very high frequency words and the Glushko low–medium words, or the higher-frequency items of set 3 and the Glushko low words. It is clear (1) that being very common does not protect a word from reversing when the model is damaged; and (2) that we shall have to look to some variable(s) other than frequency if we want to discover the basis for susceptibility to reversal. That is precisely what we shall do next, in Experiment 4.

**Experiment 4: preferred pronunciations, phonemic features, and regularizations**

As indicated in the introduction to lesioning the model, the current form of output from the model (phonological error scores) requires any pronunciation of interest for a given letter string to be explicitly tested. Under damaged conditions, the model may, as we have already seen, prefer the regularized pronunciation of an exception word; but this only informs us that the regularization is *a* preferred pronunciation, not that it is *the* preferred pronunciation; another pronunciation could, under the same lesioned conditions, yield a still lower error score. Regularizations as alternative pronunciations derive from some pre-suppositions about the principles underlying translation from orthography to phonology. For a more theoretically neutral exploration of the question of preferred pronunciations, we tested a small set of exception words by varying the vowel segments of each word to include every possible vowel pronunciation within the model's phonemic coding scheme. Vowels seemed a sensible choice since they tend to have more variable letter–sound correspondences than do consonants.

The model's phonemic coding scheme, taken from Rumelhart and McClelland's (1986) past-tense verb learning model and illustrated earlier in Table 7.1, codes vowels in terms of three dimensions: place (front, middle, back), length (long, short), and height (high, low). Thus, for any given word, there are $3 \times 2 \times 2 = 12$ possible vowel pronunciations, which can be illustrated with respect to the test word PINT. The correct pronunciation is of course /pInt/, where the vowel is middle, long and low. There are then four pronunciations which differ from the correct one by a single vowel feature: /pAnt/ and /pWnt/ move the place from middle to front and from middle to back, respectively, without changing length or height; /pant/ changes the length without affecting place or height; and /pOnt/ changes height only. Five pronunciations involve changes in two of the three features: for example, /pent/ involves a change in both place and length, /pˆnt/ in both height and length, and so on; and two vowel pronunciations involve a change in all three dimensions.

The exception words used for this evaluation were the first 10 words from the set of 16 listed in Table 7.2. As in other experiments, we did an initial test with the model in its normal, undamaged condition and then 10 runs with damage to hidden units, $p = 0.6$. Instead of the usual two error scores to be compared, each test in this experiment yields 12 error scores for each word, corresponding to the 12 possible pronunciations of the vowel. For this experiment, then, we must distinguish between reversal rate (proportion of occasions on which the single alternative corresponding to the regularized pronunciation yielded the lowest error score). Of course it is possible for more than one alternative (indeed, in principle, for all 11 alternatives) to produce error scores lower than the correct pronunciation; but for simplicity's sake, and because we are interested in actual preferences, we shall only discuss data concerning the lowest score for each word on each test.

Table 7.8 displays the phonological error scores (means and s.d.'s), under both normal and damaged conditions, for COR pronunciations and for pronunciations differing from COR by ONE, TWO, or THREE vowel features. It is clear that the model is highly sensitive to phonemic distance, as

**Table 7.8**  *Phonological error scores (means and standard deviations) for a set of 10 exception words tested against all possible pronunciations of the vowel segment*

| | Normal | | | | Damaged | | |
| | (N) | X̄ | (s.d.) | (N) | X̄ | (s.d.) | Lowest score (%) |
| --- | --- | --- | --- | --- | --- | --- | --- |
| COR | (10) | 4.3 | (1.3) | (100) | 30.8 | (7.3) | 44 |
| ONE | (40) | 18.5 | (2.5) | (400) | 36.0 | (8.4) | 37 |
| TWO | (50) | 32.6 | (3.3) | (500) | 40.6 | (8.8) | 17 |
| THREE | (20) | 46.4 | (4.0) | (200) | 44.8 | (9.0) | 2 |

Each word has one correct pronunciation, four pronunciations differing from correct by ONE phonemic feature in the model's coding scheme for vowels, five pronunciations differing by TWO features, and two pronunciations differing by all THREE features. The table shows the model's normal performance and also with damage to hidden units, $p = 0.6$. The last column indicates the proportion of damaged tests for which the lowest phonological error score corresponded to the correct pronunciation or to pronunciations differing by ONE, TWO or THREE features.

measured by number of features differing between correct and alternative pronunciations. Especially when undamaged, but also when lesioned, the model's error scores are monotonically related to the number of features altered.

Such differences in error scores, and their associated standard deviations, translate themselves into reversal rates in the way that we have come to expect. As shown in the final colume of Table 7.8, with lesioning, the COR pronunciation yielded the lowest score on only 44/100 tests; thus overall reversal rate was 56 per cent. Of these 56/100 tests resulting in a reversal, the preferred pronunciation was substantially more likely to be a ONE-feature change than a TWO-feature change and was very unlikely indeed to be a pronunciation differing from COR by THREE features.

This result has important consequences for the interpretation of our lesioning results. First of all, it essentially solves a puzzle concerning regularization rates for specific exception words. As mentioned at the end of Experiment 1, the probability that the damaged model will prefer a regularized pronunciation of an exception word varies substantially across different exception words. Because monosyllabic exception words in English by no means constitute an unlimited pool, the same words tend to turn up repeatedly; for example, each of the 14 words in Table 7.9 happens to have

**Table 7.9**  *For a set of 14 exception words: the number of times each has been tested with damage to hidden units, $p = 0.6$; the word's overall regularization rate; and the number of vowel features (in the model's phonemic coding scheme) by which the regularized pronunciation differs from the correct pronunciation.*

| Word | ($N$ tests) | Regularization rate (%) | No. of features differing between COR and REG |
|------|-------------|-------------------------|-----------------------------------------------|
| HOOD | (70) | 57 | ONE |
| BULL | (50) | 56 | ONE |
| COME | (70) | 54 | ONE |
| GLOVE | (50) | 52 | ONE |
| SOME | (50) | 50 | ONE |
| GOOD | (50) | 46 | ONE |
| FOOT | (50) | 40 | ONE |
| DEAF | (60) | 23 | TWO |
| SOUL | (60) | 18 | TWO |
| HEAD | (60) | 17 | TWO |
| FLOOD | (40) | 15 | TWO |
| POST | (60) | 7 | THREE |
| PINT | (60) | 5 | THREE |
| BOTH | (40) | 0 | THREE |

been examined under conditions of damage to hidden units, $p = 0.6$, in no less than four and, for some words, in as many as seven different tests. For these particular words, then, there are very stable estimates of their tendency to regularization. We spent a considerable amount of time and effort attempting to determine what factor(s) might account for the marked variation in regularization rate listed in Table 7.9. Our third experiment demonstrated that frequency was not the crucial variable, and a number of other explorations (such as orthographic neighbourhood: what proportion of words with that 'body' have a regular or an irregular spelling-to-sound correspondence) similarly failed to explain these dramatic differences in reversal rate. As the final column of Table 7.9 indicates, the determining factor is almost certainly the number of vowel features, in the model's phonemic coding scheme, by which the regularized pronunciation differs from the correct pronunciation.

It might be worth adding the reassuring note that this discovery of the major factor contributing to reversals in no way compromises our crucial finding of higher reversal rates for exception than for regular words. Recall that in

Experiment 2, regular and exception words were matched for body and tested with the same two pronunciations. This means that the distance in phonemic vowel features between the correct and the alternative pronunciation was identical for the regular and exception words in Experiment 2. None the less, damage resulted in a substantial difference between the word classes in reversal rate.

The second important implication of this discovery concerns the model's success in simulating the reading performance of surface dyslexic patients. Regularization of the word PINT is often used in descriptions of such patients, partly because it is in fact a frequent error by real patients and partly because investigators of reading disorders thought that they understood why it should be such a frequent error. In the terminology of Henderson (1982) and Patterson and Morton (1985), PINT is a heretic word: all of the 12 other monosyllabic words ending in -INT are pronounced regularly, as in MINT. If a neurological injury could selectively disrupt some component of the system for retrieving pronunciations of whole familiar words, forcing a patient to rely on some other procedure involving grapheme–phoneme mapping rules or analogies with other known words, it seemed obvious that PINT should then be pronounced /pint/. As it happens, though, the vowel in /pint/ differs from /pInt/ not by ONE or by TWO but by THREE phonemic features. Therefore, although the patient data suggest that this ought to be a common regularization error, the model virtually never prefers /pint/ to /pInt/. Note that this is not to say that the damaged model always prefers the correct pronunciation for PINT. In fact, in Experiment 4 /pInt/ yielded the lowest score on only 5/10 tests. The preferred pronunciation in these reversals was, however, not the regularization /pint/, differing from /pInt/ by THREE features, but rather the pronunciation /pAnt/, differing from /pInt/ by only ONE feature.

The obvious next step was to return to the reading data from surface dyslexic patients to see whether their reading performance might be influenced by this variation of phonemic feature distance which so strongly constrains the model's preferred pronunciations. An error corpus from each of two patients, H.T.R. (Shallice, Warrington, and McCarthy 1983) and K.T. (McCarthy and Warrington 1986) was subjected to the following analysis. In order to make the data set as similar as possible to the results from the model, we included only monosyllabic words in which the patient's error was restricted to the vowel segment of the word. This produced an error set of $N = 61$ for H.T.R. and $N = 88$ for K.T. Each error was coded in terms of the distance (ONE, TWO or THREE features) between the correct pronunciation and the patient's reading response to the word. The reversal errors by the model in Experiment 4 ($N = 56$) were coded in the same way. The results, scored as a percentage of responses corresponding to ONE, TWO or THREE features changed, are shown in Table 7.10.

**Table 7.10** *(1) The proportions of the model's reversals and of the patients' errors (on the vowel segment of monosyllabic words only) that involve a change in ONE, TWO or THREE phonemic vowel features. (2) The percentage of the errors in (1) corresponding to exact regularizations of the exception target word. (3) As in (2), but restricted to words for which the regularization differs from the correct pronunciation by just ONE feature*

|  | Model | H.T.R. | K.T. |
|---|---|---|---|
| (N) | (56) | (61) | (88) |
|  | (%) | (%) | (%) |
| (1)  ONE | 66.1 | 59.0 | 52.2 |
|      TWO | 30.4 | 31.1 | 31.8 |
|      THREE | 3.6 | 9.8 | 15.9 |
| (2)  % regularizations | 19.6 | 78.8 | 81.8 |
| (3)  % regularizations for words where regularized pronunciation is a ONE-feature change | 30.8 | 79.2 | 90.2 |

Much to our surprise, the patients' behaviour in this regard is very well simulated by the model. H.T.R. and, in particular, K.T. are a little more likely than the model to produce responses differing from the correct pronunciation by THREE features (for example, they both read PINT as /pint/!); but the similarities in these values are much more striking than the differences. In fact, this outcome goes beyond mere simulation. It is a prediction from the model to the data, and constitutes an analysis of the patient data that, we claim, no one would have thought of doing without the model's prediction. What this outcome means is that while PINT—/pint/ may be a frequent surface dyslexic reading error, it is not a typical one. Just as in the damaged model, typical reading errors by the patients (at least these two patients) involve a change in just a single phonemic feature.

Although the behaviour of the model and the patients concur closely in this regard, there is in fact one major difference between them. Remember that the 56 observations for the model in this analysis include not just regularizations but all reversals. Likewise, the 61 and 88 errors for H.T.R. and K.T., respectively, are the patient equivalent of reversals: they include not just regularizations but any reading error where the patient's pronunciation was (only) a misreading of the vowel. We can therefore now ask: for the model and for the patients, what proportion of these reversal errors correspond to the single alternative that happens to be the regularized pronunciation of that exception word? As shown in the line of Table 7.10 labelled '% regularizations', this proportion is high for the two patients but low for the model. Although the patients and the model make roughly the same proportions of errors involving ONE- or TWO-feature changes, the patients appear to differentiate among the various options at each level, selectively favouring the pronunciation corresponding to the exact regularization. For the model, on the other hand, all alternatives within each level seem to be more or less equivalent: the regularization has no special status.

Since the word sets used in this comparison between H.T.R., K.T., and the model were not the same, they do not contain the same proportion of words for which the regularized pronunciation is ONE, TWO or THREE features different from the correct pronunciation. Given the dependence of errors on closeness of phonemic features, such unmatched lists will mean unequal 'opportunities' for regularization. As the last line of Table 7.10 demonstrates, however, the picture is only slightly altered if we restrict the comparison to the subset of words within each of these sets where the regularization involves a ONE-feature change. Maximizing the likelihood of regularization in this way increases the model's proportion of reversals that are regularizations from roughly 20 per cent to 30 per cent; but the comparable values for H.T.R. and K.T., respectively, are 80 per cent and 90 per cent.[2]

This difference in tendency to regularization may in fact be a reflection of a more general difference: the model is much more likely that the patients to produce errors which are 'implausible' realizations of the vowel, in the sense that no existing word in English embodies that pronunciation of the vowel grapheme. The patients do make such errors; for example, H.T.R. read SOUL as /sYl/ and BALD as /bOld/, and K.T. read ROOK as /rok/. There are no English words in which OU is pronounced /Y/, A is pronounced /O/ or OO is pronounced /o/. For want of any better description or account, such errors by surface dyslexic patients have typically been described as 'visual' or 'orthographic' (see, for example, Coltheart et al. 1983), and indeed these three examples from the two patients demonstrate why: /sYl/, /bOld/ and /rok/ actually correspond to the phonology of the real words SOIL, BOLD, and ROCK, each of which is orthographically similar to the target word engendering the error response. But, of course, one cannot be sure that these responses represent visual confusions by the patient: they could arise in the process of translation from orthography to phonology just as we assume the patients' regularization errors do.

The point germane to this discussion is that such errors with implausible grapheme–phoneme vowel correspondences are relatively rare in the patients' error corpora: in the subsets of errors being considered here, only $4/61 = 6.6$ per cent of H.T.R.'s errors and $3/88 = 3.4$ per cent of K.T.'s errors were of this type. By contrast, looking at the reversal errors by the model in Experiment 4, $34/56 = 60.7$ per cent of these have implausible correspondences. (Note: this is 34 tokens, i.e. actual instances of reversal, but only 20 types, i.e. different pronunciations.) For example, as already mentioned, the model's most common reversal error for PINT (preferred on 4/10 tests) was /pAnt/; in no real English word is the single vowel I pronounced /A/. Since regularizations never represent implausible correspondences (on the contrary, they represent the most typical correspondence, which is why they are called regular), we suggest that the apparent difference between the model and the patients in regularization rate may be wholly or partly attributable to a difference in the likelihood that the vowel correspondence will be a legitimate one.

This characteristic of the model's lesioned performance clearly does not provide a good match for the behaviour of real patients. The next step in our investigations, but going beyond the scope of this chapter, will be to explore the basis of this difference between model and patient performance. Below we consider some directions that this investigation could take.

### Summary of the lesioning experiments

Like other connectionist models of cognitive processing where the effects of damage have been investigated (e.g. Sejnowski and Rosenberg 1986; Hinton and Shallice, personal communication), the model described here performs in a reasonable manner when lesioned. Phonological error scores, the model's way of indicating its response to a stimulus item, increase monotonically with amount of damage. These augmented scores could be taken to reflect an increase in the proportion of incorrect naming responses, or an increase in the latency of responses, or both. Future work on the model will attempt to differentiate between these two aspects of any oral reading response. The precise location of damage (connections from input units to hidden units; hidden units *per se*; connections from hidden units to output units) has relatively little effect on the size of the error scores; but these locations have differential effects on the variability of error scores, and accordingly on the main measure of interest here: the likelihood that the model will 'prefer' a pronunciation other than the correct one for a given word. Damage to hidden units yields the maximum discrepancy in error rate between regular and exception words.

As Morton and Patterson (1980) insisted for another variety of acquired reading disorder, we must emphasize that there is no precise, fixed characterization of reading performance which qualifies as surface dyslexia. Certain striking features of a patient's overall pattern of reading skill prompt us to use the label 'surface dyslexia'; but each patient is unique. Attempts to simulate the abstract entity called surface dyslexia must be tempered by reminders that real patients are not abstractions. As already noted, some surface dyslexic patients show marked frequency modulation of their success in reading irregular words, while others do not; some patients have an essentially normal ability to read nonsense words, while others do not. Such specific features are only meaningful in relation to the particular patient's precise processing profile. The same approach must be taken in evaluating the model's performance. It does not greatly matter (though it is of course interesting to know) whether the model shows significant frequency effects in exception word performance after lesioning. What matters is an account of why and under what circumstances one expects to find frequency effects, and whether the presence or absence of an effect fits with other things that we know about the model's or the patient's performance.

With this caveat in mind, plus a reminder of our initial warning about the early stage of these explorations of damage to the model, we suggest that this approach to the study of reading disorders—'lesioning' a working computational model—shows considerable promise. Moreover, several aspects of the initial damage experiments leave us optimistic that the particular model we have been using, or something very much like it, has considerable potential to provide a detailed account of acquired reading disorders. The first result from these experiments is the demonstration that the model can in fact produce the types of errors characteristic of surface dyslexic readers. This is important because the model lacks the non-lexical spelling–sound rules previously thought to be responsible for these errors. The second finding is that both patient and model errors are related to the distance between the correct pronunciation and the error in terms of number of phonemic features. We consider this finding to be important because it shows that the attempt to simulate impaired performance can deepen our understanding of the phenomena. In this case, the relevance of phonemic features to patient errors was not recognized until we attempted to simulate their performance.

A third result of the simulations is that they may offer a different interpretation for the 'visual' errors sometimes noted in surface dyslexic patients. The model produced errors such as PINT→/pAnt/, which do occur (though not commonly) in the error corpora of the surface dyslexic patients H.T.R. and K.T. discussed above, and which occur more frequently in other reported cases. It was thought that such an error '. . . could not arise simply through phonological reading' (Coltheart et al. 1983, p. 480) because the single vowel letter I is never pronounced /A/ in an English word. Moreover, if the naming response is treated as the real word PAINT, then its orthographic overlap with the stimulus word PINT is considerable. Therefore, such errors have been called 'visual' or 'orthographic' or, even more literally in the case of PINT→/pAnt/, a letter addition error (Coltheart et al. 1983). Our comment on this topic is merely speculative, especially as the model produces these errors with greater frequency than is observed in most patients; but the fact that the model yielded such errors with a completely intact orthographic encoding system suggests that 'visual' errors need not be 'visual' in origin.

We can summarize the relationship between the model's damaged performance and that of patients in the literature as follows. The performance of the patients who have been categorized as surface dyslexic varies in systematic ways. As a broad generalization, following the description in Shallice and McCarthy (1985), the patients can be divided into two types. Type I patients, including H.T.R. (Shallice, Warrington, and McCarthy 1983), M.P. (Bub *et al.* 1985) and K.T. (McCarthy and Warrington 1986) exhibit the following characteristics:

1. Accuracy of regular word naming is at or near normal levels.
2. Naming latencies are within normal limits.
3. Accuracy in non-word naming is normal.
4. Most errors are regularizations of exception words.
5. Language comprehension and semantic knowledge are severely impaired.

Type II patients, a more heterogeneous lot than Type I, include J.C. and S.T. (Marshall and Newcombe 1973), P.T. (Kay and Lesser 1985) and E.S.T. (Kay and Patterson 1985). These cases exhibit the following characteristics:

1. Naming is poorer for exception than for regular words, but performance on regular words is also impaired.
2. Naming latencies are abnormally slow, and the patient may make a series of attempts to name a single word.
3. Non-word naming is impaired (where tested).
4. Regularization errors do not necessarily account for the majority of errors.
5. There is no marked impairment of semantic knowledge.

Shallice and McCarthy (1985) argue for a qualitative distinction between these two patterns, and they term the first pattern 'semantic dyslexia', reserving the label 'surface dyslexia' for Type II.

Although we began these explorations with the goal of simulating Type I cases, because both they and the model read without semantics, our damage experiments in fact yielded a profile more reminiscent of Type II patients. Our account of these patients cannot be considered complete, because it is likely that they do use partial semantic information derived from the orthographic input to assist the generation of a pronunciation. A more comprehensive account would explain this compensatory strategy and the extent to which it contributes to Type II performance.

The damaged performance of the model clearly does not provide a good fit to the Type I patients. However, it would be inappropriate to conclude that these patients' performance is inconsistent with the model or cannot be simulated by it. Although the types of damage that we have explored do not produce error scores in the normal range for regular words and non-words alongside impaired performance on exception words, this is not to say that such a pattern is an impossible one for the model. First, there are questions about the implementation of the model that need to be explored. Second, the model suggests several other potentially interesting bases for impaired performance that have not been investigated as yet. It is worth considering briefly these directions for future research.

As Seidenberg and McClelland (1988*a,b*) note, several properties of the model seem to be theoretically important. These include the notion that orthographic and phonological representations are distributed, the intermediate level of hidden units, the way the learning rule determines the connection weights, and the idea that naming involves a direct mapping from orthography to phonology. Seidenberg and McClelland also discuss several details of the implemented model that are less theoretically relevant, such as the specifics of the orthographic and phonological encoding schemes, or the particular stimulus set used in training. They argue that the model's ability to capture detailed aspects of normal performance is unlikely to be contingent on these aspects of the implementation. However, we cannot as yet determine exactly how these specifics relate to the effects that we have (and have not!) obtained in regard to surface dyslexia.

For example, there are known limitations to the phonological encoding scheme used in this model and in Rumelhart and McClelland (1986) (see Pinker and Prince 1988; Lachter and Bever 1988). Similarly, it is not clear whether the model's treatment of lexical frequency is adequate; words were sampled during the training phase on the basis of a logarithmic transformation of their Kucera and Francis frequencies. Frequencies in the Kucera and Francis analysis range from about 67 000 to 1; in our scheme the range is only about 16 to 1. The results to this point suggest that these and other aspects of the implementation have little impact on the model's ability to simulate normal performance; however, these limitations may be more important when we turn to making detailed predictions about the exact errors produced by patients. To take one example, the compression of word frequencies may be related to the absence of marked frequency effects in the model's impaired performance. Before any firm conclusions can be drawn, it will be necessary to evaluate versions of the model using different phonological encoding schemes, indices of frequency, amounts of training, etc.

A more severe limitation of the model is that we have not yet implemented procedures for converting the output that it computes into real pronunciations. But this is a limitation on what has been done, not on what can be done. Lacouture (1988), for example, has developed a naming model that computes phonological codes much like the present model. It also exhibits the main types of phenomena concerning, for example, frequency and regularity effects. In Lacouture's model, however, the computed phonological code acts as the input to an autoassociative mechanism, which serves to complete the partially specified phonological code. This pattern completion process could be seen as similar to the process of assembling an articulatory motor program.

The observations from these initial explorations with lesioning suggest to us that it will be important to examine other ways in which the model's performance can degrade. In particular, we need to consider the possibility that the impaired performance characteristic of Type I patients, such as H.T.R. and M.P., does not derive from damage to knowledge representations at all. The computations performed by the model could be impaired in a variety of ways that do not involve damage to representations. For example, the model computes output by passing activation through the network. We have damaged the system by eliminating connections or units. Imagine, instead, that the model is fully intact, but the net activations of units are incorrectly computed. One characteristic of the implemented model, for example, is that the activation coming into a unit (which is a weighted sum of the activations along the lines coming into it) is passed through a logistic function to yield a net activation between 0 and 1. We could then ask what would happen to performance if activations of hidden units were pathologically limited to a level such as 0.8, preventing output units from being fully activated. What kind of articulatory code would be assembled on the basis of this damped output?

We suggest that this line of inquiry is worth pursuing because there is already some evidence that the kinds of errors characteristic of surface dyslexia can be produced by a system that is wholly undamaged. Consider the following experiment, which we have recently completed. Normal university-student subjects are asked to name words such as the ones presented to the model or to a patient like H.T.R. However, we impose a response deadline, such that subjects must initiate pronunciation earlier than normal. Under these conditions, subjects produce naming latencies that are roughly normal but they make substantially more errors. Moreover, these errors include the following (taken from the actual corpus of responses):

*regularizations*:  PINT→/pint/; PLAID→/plAd/; STEALTH→/stElth/;
 DONE→/dOn/
*'visual' errors*:  TROUGH→tough; BREAD→beard; WALL→well
*other errors*:  BUSH→/bish/; BURY→/bErE/; DROUGHT→/drOt/;
 BATH→/bEth/

We assume that these errors arise simply because the deadline forces subjects to begin assembling a pronunciation before the computation of the phonological code is completed. In our implemented model, the activations of output units are computed on a single sweep; in a more realistic model, the activations would build up over time (cf. McClelland 1979; Cohen, Dunbar, and McClelland 1988; Seidenberg and McClelland 1988*b*). The effect of the deadline would be realized by initiating the assembly process before the phonological nodes had reached asymptotic levels of activation. A similar outcome would obtain if nodes were pathologically prevented from reaching these levels.

We are not suggesting that performance under deadline conditions fully mimics the performance of any surface dyslexic. For one thing, the maximum error rate obtained for a normal subject in the deadline condition was 20 per cent, much lower than would be seen in a patient. This might be expected because imposing a deadline that encourages early assembly is not equivalent to a pathological condition that prevents units from reaching asymptotic levels of activation. However, the experiment does show that the types of errors that have been observed in neuropsychological case studies can be produced by subjects whose knowledge representations are intact; the relevance of this observation for accounts of surface dyslexia is a matter worth considering further.

Along the same lines, it is also worth considering whether Type I patients might begin to assemble pronunciations prematurely because their access to semantic information is grossly impaired. The naming task requires that the subject produce the correct pronunciation of a word. The demands of the task change somewhat when the stimuli include non-words, which lack a certifiably 'correct' pronunciation. There may be some trials on which normal subjects check the phonological code computed on the basis of orthography (as in our model) against a phonological code computed on the basis of the orthography→meaning→phonology 'route' implied by Fig. 7.1. Since the meaning-based routine is not available to Type I surface dyslexics (i.e. semantic dyslexics), it would never be checked. The absence of any feedback from other parts of the lexical system might result in relatively rapid use of the pathway from orthography to phonology; the subject has 'nothing to lose' by initiating pronunciation, so to speak.

Finally, one other possibility should be mentioned. Perhaps the simulation results are telling us that something very like the model we have proposed is relevant to normal performance but not to all cases of surface dyslexia. Perhaps the knowledge representations of patients such as H.T.R. and M.P. are damaged to the point where they no longer support pronunciation at all. The patients are none the less asked to pronounce words and non-words. Under these conditions they may utilize other types of knowledge relevant to pronunciation. It is possible that readers have formed some explicit generalizations about the correlations between spelling and pronunciation, perhaps stored in the form of 'rules'. These generalizations could arise in several ways. For example, they could be the detritus of the learning process; children are often taught to read by introducing explicit pronunciation rules. The 'rules' could also reflect generalizations about the properties of a complex computational mechanism like the one in our model. We ourselves often resort to such generalizations in summarizing the behaviour of the model. These generalizations are not accurate in detail and they do not reflect the actual underlying computational mechanisms. It is quite possible that our self-knowledge of complex perceptual and cognitive processes consists of generalizations of this type. When the normal naming mechanism is impaired, then it is possible that patients rely upon this knowledge which, though of limited applicability, is sufficient to yield correct pronunciations of common spelling patterns.

If this conjecture is correct, we are back to a modified 'dual-route' model as the account of naming *disorders*. There is a normal naming mechanism, like the one in the implemented model; there is a second type of knowledge, definitely 'non-lexical', which supports the naming behaviour of at least some surface dyslexics. It remains to be seen how this account, offered here as speculation, will fare in the light of future evidence. Note, however, that while this account involves two naming mechanisms, it differs from the 'dual-route' model in critical respects. The main assumption of the dual-route model is that separate mechanisms are necessary in order to pronounce exception words on the one hand and non-words on the other (Coltheart 1987). Hence, both routines play a role in normal performance. Our model, in which a single mechanism supports the pronunciation of all types of letter strings, challenges this 'central dogma' of dual-route theories (Seidenberg 1988*b*). This second type of knowledge merely comes into play when the normal system is non-functional. Thus, even this version of the model cannot be taken as an implementation of the dual-route account.

**Conclusions**

As indicated in the introduction to lesioning the model, the possibility of an account of acquired dyslexia within the model of oral reading that we have discussed is of some considerable theoretical significance. Surface dyslexia, especially in conjunction with its contrasting pattern of impaired reading, phonological dyslexia, has suggested to many that there must be at least two separable routines for the translation of orthography to phonology. Dual-routine theories have already been challenged by the demonstration that the undamaged model can learn to read regular words, exception words and non-words with a single procedure. Such theories will be in further contention if patterns of acquired dyslexia are reproducible by means of damage to the model. Note that the preceding sentence and the first sentence of this paragraph use the modest words 'if' and 'possibility': we are not claiming that the model can now offer such an account, only that it looks promising and well worth further exploration.

By way of summary, the model in its current state does a good job of accounting for what we might term the first-order phenomena in naming, the performance of normal subjects in reading different types of words, and non-words. The model provides the only quantitative account of normal performance; moreover the fit between simulation and behavioural data is quite close. The model also accounts for the second-order phenomena, such as the types of errors observed in cases of surface dyslexia. The unresolved questions concern third-order predictions, regarding the exact proportions of errors of different types, and the different patterns of performance associated with surface dyslexia. It is not surprising that it is at this level that questions arise concerning limitations of the implemented model. Although substantive questions remain to be addressed, we think that these initial efforts have opened an interesting line of inquiry that is likely to contribute to a deeper understanding of reading and its disorders.

## Acknowledgement

We are grateful to Rosaleen McCarthy for providing us with a corpus of reading errors for the patient K.T., studied by McCarthy and Warrington (1986).

## Notes

1. Most recent versions of dual-routine models actually posit three pronunciation processes, the 'non-lexical' or 'subword-level' procedure mentioned above, and two 'lexical' procedures that involve accessing stored representations of word pronunciations. These representations, it is argued, can be accessed in two ways: either directly (by a procedure that transcodes from orthography to lexical phonology) or indirectly (from orthography to semantic representations and then to lexical phonology). The hypothesis of a direct lexical but non-semantic procedure has been based partly on patterns of acquired reading disorders (see for example Schwartz, Saffran, and Marin 1980; Funnell 1983) but also on results from normal subjects concerning the interrelationships between naming of words and naming of pictures (see Durso and Johnson 1979, for relevant data and Warren and Morton 1983, for discussion). The main point germane to the present discussion is that in all these accounts, at least two procedures are considered necessary to accomplish successful naming of regular words, exception words, and non-words. The model described here does not reject the notion that written words might be pronounced with reference to their meanings; as Fig. 7.1 suggests, a word could be named by a two-stage process in which meaning is computed from the orthographic input, and the pronunciation from meaning. In contrast to dual- (or triple-) routine models, however, this 'lexical' pathway is not necessary for the pronunciation of any type of letter string. In sum, the model squeezes three routines into two, with the added caveat that the primary procedure for translating from orthography to phonology is sufficient for all types of letter strings.

2. Since this chapter was written, the model has been augmented with a new procedure for assessing its output. The procedure compares the model's output not just to the correct (specified) pronounciation but also to all other pronounciations that can be created by replacing a single phoneme in that word with some other phoneme; it then reports the best match. Since this search only covers a subset of the possible

phonological patterns, we cannot guarantee that the best match among this set of comparisons is the best possible match; but the procedure does provide more comprehensive information regarding the model's 'preferred pronunciations'. Using this procedure, Seidenberg and McClelland (1988b) demonstrated that the trained and undamaged model makes errors (i.e. cases where the best fit to the computed pattern is a pronunciation other than the correct one) on only 2.7 percent of the 2897 words in its training vocabulary. The new procedure is of particular value in assessing output from the lesioned model; for example, one can readily determine whether the incorrect best match for an exception word is an exact regularization. Recent simulations using the new procedure suggest that the high levels of damage (60 percent of hidden units) used in most of our initial experiments may not in fact provide the best approximation to surface dyslexia. Although the overall error rate is certainly higher when more hidden units are silenced, the proportion of errors corresponding to exact regularizations actually decreases. In a test using the exception words from Taraban and McClelland's (1987) experiment with 20 percent of hidden units zeroed, nearly half (47 percent) of the model's errors were exact regularizations. Although this is still a somewhat lower regularization rate than that shown by the surface dyslexic patients in Table 7.10, it is a step in the right direction; future explorations may provide still closer approximations.

## References

Andrews, S. (1982). Phonological recoding: is the regularity effect consistent? *Memory & Cognition*, **10**, 565–75.

Beauvois, M. F. and Derouesné, J. (1979). Phonological alexia: three dissociations. *Journal of Neurology, Neurosurgery and Psychiatry*, **42**, 1115–24.

Brown, G. D. A. (1987). Resolving inconsistency: a computational model of word naming. *Journal of Memory and Language*, **26**, 1–23.

Caramazza, A. (1986). On drawing inferences about the structure of normal cognitive systems from the analysis of patterns of impaired performance: the case of single-patient studies. *Brain and Cognition*, **5**, 41–66.

Bub, D., Cancelliere, A., and Kertesz, A. (1985). Whole-word and analytic translation of spelling to sound in a non-semantic reader. In *Surface dyslexia: neuropsychological and cognitive studies of phonological reading* (eds. K. E. Patterson, J. C. Marshall, and M. Coltheart). Erlbaum, London.

Cohen, J., Dunbar, K., and McClelland, J. L. (1988). On the control of automatic processes: a parallel distributed processing model of the Stroop effect. AIP technical report 40, Department of Psychology, Carnegie-Mellon University, Pittsburgh, PA.

Coltheart, M. (1985). Cognitive neuropsychology and the study of reading. In *Attention and performance XI* (eds. M. I. Posner and O. S. M. Marin). Erlbaum, Hillsdale, NJ.

Coltheart, M. (1987). Functional architecture of the language-processing system. In *The cognitive neuropsychology of language* (eds. M. Coltheart, G. Sartori, and R. Job). Erlbaum, London.

Coltheart, M., Masterson, J., Byng, S., Prior, M., and Riddoch, J. (1983). Surface dyslexia. *Quarterly Journal of Experimental Psychology*, **35A**, 469–95.

Durso, F. T. and Johnson, M. K. (1979). Facilitation in naming and categorizing repeated pictures and words. *Journal of Experimental Psychology: Human Learning and Memory*, **5**, 449–59.

Ellis, A. W. and Young, A. W. (1988). *Human cognitive neuropsychology*. Erlbaum, London.

Funnell, E. (1983). Phonological processes in reading: new evidence from acquired dyslexia. *British Journal of Psychology*, **74**, 159–80.

Gernsbacher, M. A. (1984). Resolving 20 years of inconsistent interactions between lexical familiarity and orthography, concreteness and polysemy. *Journal of Experimental Psychology: General*, **113**, 256–81.

Glushko, R. J. (1979). The organization and activation of orthographic knowledge in reading aloud. *Journal of Experimental Psychology: Human Perception and Performance*, **5**, 674–91.

Hebb, D. O. (1949). *Organization of behavior*. Wiley, New York.

Henderson, L. (1982). *Orthography and word recognition in reading*. Academic Press, London.

Hillinger, M. L. (1980). Priming effects with phonemically similar words: the encoding-bias hypothesis reconsidered. *Memory & Cognition*, **8**, 115–23.

Hinton, G. E., McClelland, J. L., and Rumelhart, D. E. (1986). Distributed representations. In *Parallel distributed processing*, Volume 1 (eds. D. E. Rumelhart and J. L. McClelland). MIT Press, Cambridge, Mass.

Humphreys, G. W. and Evett, L. J. (1985). Are there independent lexical and nonlexical routes in word processing? An evaluation of the dual-route theory of reading. *The Behavioral and Brain Sciences*, **8**, 689–740.

Kay, J. (1987). Phonological codes in reading: assignment of sub-word phonology. In *Language perception and production* (eds. A. Allport, D. MacKay, W. Prinz, and E. Scheerer). Academic Press, London.

Kay, J. and Lesser, R. (1985). The nature of phonological processing in oral reading: evidence from surface dyslexia. *Quarterly Journal of Experimental Psychology*, **37A**, 39–81.

Kay, J. and Patterson, K. (1985). Routes to meaning in surface dyslexia. In *Surface dyslexia: neuropsychological and cognitive studies of phonological reading* (eds. K. E. Patterson, J. C. Marshall, and M. Coltheart). Erlbaum, London.

Kucera, H. and Francis, W. N. (1967). *Computational analysis of present-day American English*. Brown University Press, Providence, Rhode Island.

Lachter, J. and Bever, T. G. (1988). The relation between linguistic structure and associative theories of language learning. *Cognition*, **28**, 195–247.

Lacouture, Y. (1988). A connectionist model of the lexicon. Unpublished PhD thesis, McGill University.

McCarthy, R. and Warrington, E. K. (1986). Phonological reading: phenomena and paradoxes. *Cortex*, **22**, 359–80.

McClelland, J. L. and Rumelhart, D. E. (1986). *Parallel distributed processing*, Volume 2. MIT Press, Cambridge, Mass.

Marcel, T. (1980). Surface dyslexia and beginning reading: a revised hypothesis of the pronunciation of print and its impairments. In *Deep dyslexia* (eds. M. Coltheart, K. Patterson, and J. C. Marshall). Routledge and Kegan Paul, London.

Marshall, J. C. and Newcombe, F. (1973). Patterns of paralexia: a psycholinguistic approach. *Journal of Psycholinguistic Research*, **2**, 175–99.

Masterson, J. (1985). On how we read non-words: data from different populations. In *Surface dyslexia: neuropsychological and cognitive studies of phonological reading* (eds. K. E. Patterson, J. C. Marshall, and M. Coltheart). Erlbaum, London.

Meyer, D. E., Schvaneveldt, R. W., and Ruddy, M. G. (1974). Functions of graphemic and phonemic codes in visual word recognition. *Memory & Cognition*, **2**, 309–21.

Morton, J. and Patterson, K. (1980). A new attempt at an interpretation, or, an attempt at a new interpretation. In *Deep dyslexia* (eds. M. Coltheart, K. Patterson, and J. C. Marshall). Routledge and Kegan Paul, London.

Patterson, K. E. (1982). The relation between reading and phonological coding: further neuropsychological observations. In *Normality and pathology in cognitive functions* (ed. A. W. Ellis). Academic Press, London.

Patterson, K. and Coltheart, V. (1987). Phonological processes in reading: a tutorial review. In *Attention and performance XII: the psychology of reading* (ed. M. Coltheart). Erlbaum, London.

Patterson, K., Marshall, J. C., and Coltheart, M. (1985). *Surface dyslexia: neuropsychological and cognitive studies of phonological reading.* Erlbaum, London.

Patterson, K. and Morton, J. (1985). From orthography to phonology: an attempt at an old interpretation. In *Surface dyslexia: neuropsychological and cognitive studies of phonological reading* (eds. K. Patterson, J. C. Marshall, and M. Coltheart). Erlbaum, London.

Pinker, S. and Prince, A. (1988). On language and connectionism: analysis of a parallel distributed processing model of language acquisition. *Cognition*, **28**, 73–194.

Rumelhart, D. E., Hinton, G. E., and McClelland, J. L. (1986). A general framework for parallel distributed processing. In *Parallel distributed processing*, volume 1 (eds. D. E. Rumelhart and J. L. McClelland). MIT Press, Cambridge, Mass.

Rumelhart, D. E., Hinton, G. E., and Williams, R. J. (1986). Learning internal representations by error propagation. In *Parallel distributed processing*, volume 1 (eds. D. E. Rumelhart and J. L. McClelland). MIT Press, Cambridge, Mass.

Rumelhart, D. E. and McClelland, J. L. (1986a). *Parallel distributed processing*, Volume 1. MIT Press, Cambridge, Mass.

Rumelhart, D. E. and McClelland, J. L. (1986b) On learning the past tenses of English verbs. In *Parallel distributed processing*, Volume 2 (eds. D. E. Rumelhart and J. L. McClelland). MIT Press, Cambridge, Mass.

Schwartz, M. F., Saffran, E. M., and Marin, O. S. M. (1980). Fractionating the reading process in dementia: evidence for word-specific print-to-sound associations. In *Deep dyslexia* (eds. M. Coltheart, K. Patterson, and J. C. Marshall). Routledge and Kegan Paul, London.

Seidenberg, M. S. (1985). The time-course of phonological code activation in two writing systems. *Cognition*, **19**, 1–30.

Seidenberg, M. S. (1988a). Visual word recognition and pronunciation: A computational model and its implications. In *Lexical representation and process* (ed. W. D. Marslen-Wilson). MIT Press, Cambridge, Mass., in press.

Seidenberg, M. S. (1988b). Cognitive neuropsychology and language: the state of the art. *Cognitive Neuropsychology*, **5**, 403–26.

Seidenberg, M. S. and McClelland, J. L. (1988a). A distributed, developmental model of visual word recognition and pronunciation: acquisition, skilled performance, and dyslexia. In *From reading to neurons: toward theory and methods for research on developmental dyslexia.* MIT Press/Bradford Books, Cambridge, Mass.

Seidenberg, M. S. and McClelland, J. L. (1988b). A distributed, developmental model of visual word recognition and naming. *Psychological Review*, in press.

Seidenberg, M. S., Waters, G. S., Barnes, M. A., and Tanenhaus, M. K. (1984). When does irregular spelling or pronunciation influence word recognition? *Journal of Verbal Learning and Verbal Behavior*, **23**, 383–404.

Sejnowski, T. J. and Rosenberg, C. R. (1986). *NETtalk: a parallel network that learns to read aloud.* Baltimore: Johns Hopkins University EE and CS Technical Report JHU/EECS-86/01.

Shallice, T. and McCarthy, R. (1985). Phonological reading: from patterns of impairment to possible procedures. In *Surface dyslexia: neuropsychological and cognitive studies of phonological reading* (eds. K. Patterson, J. C. Marshall, and M. Coltheart). Erlbaum, London.

Shallice, T. and Warrington, E. K. (1980). Single and multiple component central dyslexic syndromes. In *Deep dyslexia* (eds. M. Coltheart, K. Patterson, and J. C. Marshall). Routledge and Kegan Paul, London.

Shallice, T., Warrington, E. K., and McCarthy, R. (1983). Reading without semantics. *Quarterly Journal of Experimental Psychology*, **35A**, 111–38.

Tanenhaus, M. K., Flanigan, H., and Seidenberg, M. S. (1980). Orthographic and phonological code activation in auditory and visual word recognition. *Memory & Cognition*, **8**, 513–20.

Taraban, R. and McClelland, J. L. (1987). Conspiracy effects in word recognition. *Journal of Memory and Language*, **26**, 608–31.

Treiman, R. and Chafetz, J. (1987). Are there onset- and rime-like units in printed words? In *Attention and performance XII: the psychology of reading* (ed. M. Coltheart). Erlbaum, London.

Warren, C. and Morton, J. (1982). The effects of priming on picture recognition. *British Journal of Psychology*, **73**, 117–29.

Waters, G. S. and Seidenberg, M. S. (1985). Spelling-sound effects in reading: time course and decision criteria. *Memory & Cognition*, **13**, 557–72.

Wickelgren, W. A. (1969). Context-sensitive coding, associative memory, and serial order in (speech) behaviour. *Psychological Review*, **76**, 1–15.

# 8

## Rules and connections in human language
### STEVEN PINKER and ALAN PRINCE

### Introduction

Everyone hopes that the discoveries of neuroscience will help explain human intelligence, but no one expects such an explanation to be done in a single step. Neuroscience and cognitive science, it is hoped, will converge on an intermediate level of 'cognitive architecture', which will specify the elementary information processes arising as a consequence of the properties of neural tissue and serving as the building blocks of the cognitive algorithms that execute intelligent behaviour. This middle level has proven to be elusive. Neuroscientists study firing rates, excitation, inhibition, and plasticity; cognitive scientists study rules, representations, and symbol systems. Although it's relatively easy to imagine ways to run cognitive symbol systems on digital computers, how they could be implemented in neural hardware has remained obscure. Conversely, it is easy to get neural networks to execute simple forms of associative learning, but learning a language or engaging in logical reasoning is quite another thing. Any theory of this middle level faces a formidable set of criteria: it must satisfy the constraints of neurophysiology and neuroanatomy, yet supply the right kind of computational power to serve as the basis for cognition.

Recently there has been considerable enthusiasm for a theory that claims to do just that. *Connectionist* or *parallel distributed processing* (*PDP*) models try to model cognitive systems using networks of large numbers of densely interconnected units. The units transmit signals to one another along weighted connections; they 'compute' their output signals by weighting each of their input signals by the strength of the connection it comes in on, summing the weighted inputs, and feeding the result into a non-linear output function, usually a threshold. Learning consists of adjusting the strengths of connections and the threshold values, usually in a direction that reduces the discrepancy between an actual output and a 'desired' output provided by a set of 'teaching' inputs (Feldman and Ballard 1982; Hinton, McClelland, and Rumelhart 1986). These are not meant to be genuine neural models. Though some of their properties are reminiscent of the nervous system, others, such as the teaching and learning mechanisms, have no neural analogue, and much of what we know of the topology of neural connectivity plays no role (Crick and Asanuma 1986). However, their proponents refer to them as 'brain-style' or 'brain-metaphor' models, and they have attracted enormous interest among psychologists and neuroscientists alike. Much of this interest comes from demonstrations that show how the models can exhibit rule-like behaviour without containing rules. The implication is that PDP networks eventually might be consistent with both neurophysiology and with a revised, but adequate theory of cognition, providing the long-sought bridge.

## A connectionist model of language acquisition

The most dramatic and frequently cited demonstration of the rule-like behaviour of PDP systems comes from a model of the acquisition of the past tense in English (Rumelhart and McClelland 1986). It addresses a phenomenon that has served as textbook example of the role of rules in cognitive behaviour (Berko 1958). Young children use regular (*walked*) and irregular (*broke*) verbs early on, but then begin to generalize the regular -*ed* ending, saying *breaked* and considerably later, *broked* as well. By kindergarten they can convert a nonsense word *jick* provided by an experimenter into *jicked*, and easily differentiate the three different phonological variants of the regular suffix: -*t* for words ending in an unvoiced consonant (*walked*), -*d* for words ending in a voiced phoneme (*jogged*), or -*ed* for words ending in a *t* or *d* (*patted*). According to the traditional explanation of the developmental sequence, children first memorize past forms directly from their parents' speech, then coin a rule that generates them productively.

Remarkably, Rumelhart and McClelland's network model exhibits the same general type of behaviour (and also several other developmental phenomena), but has no rules at all. It has no representations of words, regular versus irregular cases, roots, stems, or suffixes. Rather, it is a simple two-layer network, with a set of inputs units that are turned on in patterns corresponding to the verb stem, a set of output units that are turned on in patterns corresponding to the verb's past-tense form, and connections between every input unit and every output unit. All that happens in learning is that the network compares its own version of the past-tense form with the correct version provided by a 'teacher', and adjusts the strengths of the connections and the thresholds so as to reduce the difference (see the appendix to this chapter, where the design and operation of the Rumelhart–McClelland model are explained in detail). Rumelhart and McClelland suggest, and many are quick to agree, that this shows the viability of associationist theories of language acquisition, despite their virtual abandonment by linguists 25 years ago (Chomsky 1959). A system can show rule-like behaviour without actually containing rules; perhaps the more sophisticated PDP version of associationism can serve as the basis of a revised theory of the psychology of language at the same time as its underlying mechanisms are tuned to be more faithful to neurophysiology.

Of course, the fact that a computer model behaves intelligently without rules does not show that humans lack rules, any more than a wind-up mouse shows that real mice lack motor programs. In a recent paper (Pinker and Prince 1988), we have argued that the Rumelhart–McClelland model is incorrect on empirical grounds. Our arguments complement those of Fodor and Pylyshyn (1988) and Lachter and Bever (1988), who come to similar conclusions about other PDP models of language and cognition (see Pinker and Mehler 1988). The evidence comes from a number of sources: the nature of children's language, as observed both in experiments and naturalistic studies; regularities in the kinds of words and sentences people judge to be natural-sounding or ill-formed in their colloquial speech; and the results of the simulation runs of the models themselves. If true, the implications are important, for they bear on the claims that associative networks can explain human rule-governed intelligence. We review here the most prominent evidence, which falls into three groups: the design of the model, its asymptotic performance (which ought to approximate adults' command of everyday English), and its child-like intermediate behaviour. (We suggest that readers unfamiliar with the model examine the appendix, where it is briefly described.)

### Evidence for the linguistic constructs left out of the Rumelhart–McClelland model

The Rumelhart–McClelland model owes its radical look to the fact that it has nothing corresponding to the formal linguistic notions 'segment', 'string', 'stem', 'affix', 'word', 'root', 'regular rule', or 'irregular exception'. However, in standard psycholinguistic theories these entities are not mere notational conveniences, but constructs designed to explain facts about the organization of language. By omitting the constructs without adequate substitutes, the R–M model is inconsistent with these facts.

1. *Strings and segments.* According to standard theories, a word's phonologi-cal representation contains a *string* of segments (phonemes), each segment decomposed into features that correspond to aspects of the articulation or sound of the segment (e.g. voiced/unvoiced, nasal/oral, front/back). Rumel-hart and McClelland, in contrast, use a completely 'distributed' representation (see Hinton *et al.* 1986), in which a word is a (simultaneous) pattern of activation over a single vector of units. This leads to an immediate problem for them: representing linear order. If each unit simply represented a phoneme or feature, the model would not be able to distinguish words in which the same

sounds appear in different orders, for example *apt*, *pat*, and *tap*. Thus R and M are led to use context-sensitive units, each of which encodes the presence of a substring of *three* adjacent phonological features in a word. For example, 'unvoiced–unvoiced–voiced' and 'fricative–stop–low_vowel' are two of the context-sensitive features activated for the word *stay*. The input and output vectors each consist of 460 of these units; by activating subsets of them, it is possible to define unique patterns for the common English verbs.

There is good evidence that people don't use context-sensitive units of this kind, however. First, trisegmental units cannot uniquely encode all linguistic strings: though such units may work for English, the won't work generally. For example, the Australian language Oykangand contains distinct words *algal* and *algalgal*. These decompose into the very same set of context-sensitive features, and hence the model is incapable of distinguishing them. Second, the features make the wrong predictions about psychological similarity. Pairs of strings that differ in terms of the order of two phonemes, such as *slit* and *silt*, are judged to sound similar, and indeed confusions among them are the probable cause of certain changes in the history of English such *brid* to *bird* or *thrid* to *third*. However, if the *atomic* units of description correspond to (what we usually thing of as) triples, then ⟨abc⟩ and ⟨acb⟩, as atoms, are entirely distinct (one mustn't be misled by the fact that we, the theorists, use three-letter mnemonic abbreviations for them). Without introducing arbitary tricks into the model, it is impossible to account for perceived similarities between words defined by them (Pinker and Prince 1988; Lachter and Bever 1988). Third, the model makes the wrong prediction about the kinds of rules that should be easy to learn, hence prevalent in languages, and those rules that should be absent from languages. It is as easy for the model to learn bizarre, cross-linguistically non-existent rules for forming the past tense (such as reversing the order of the phonemes of the stem, which involves the simple association of each input unit ⟨abc⟩ with the output unit ⟨cba⟩; or changing every phoneme to the next one in English alphabetical order; or adding a *g* to the end of a word if it begins with *st* but a *p* if it begins in *sk*) as it is to learn common rules (e.g. do nothing to the stem; add a *d* to the stem).

The basic problem is that in their simple associationist architecture, the same units must represent both the decomposition of a string into phonetic components and the order in which the components are concatenated. These are conflicting demands and ultimately the units can satisfy neither successfully. The Rumelhart–McClelland representational system is a case study in the difficulty of meeting the known constraints on cognitive structure. The actual units of phonological structure—from phonetic features, to segments, to syllables and stress-groups—are reasonably well understood. Abandoning them in favour of a unit—the feature triplet—that demonstrably has no role in linguistic processes is sure to lead to major empirical problems.

2. *Morphology and phonology*. The R–M model computes a one-step mapping from the phonological features of the stem to the phonological features of the past-tense form. This allows it to dispense with many of the rules and abstract representations one finds in familiar theories of language. But there is overwhelming evidence that the mapping is actually computed in several layers. Consider the pattern of differences in the suffixes in *walked, jogged*, and *patted*, which are contingent on the last phoneme of the stem. These differences are not unique to the past-tense form: they also occur in the passive participle (*he was kicked, he was slugged, he was patted*) and in adjectives (*sabre-toothed, long-nosed, one-handed*). They also occur with different suffixes altogether, such as the plural (*hawks, dogs, hoses*) or the possessive (*Pat's, Fred's, George's*). They even occur in simple words lacking inflection: there are words like *ax* and *act*, with two unvoiced consonants in a row, and words like *adze*, and two voiced consonants in a row, but no words pronounced like *acd* or *agt*, with an unvoiced consonant followed by a voiced consonant or vice-versa. The obvious explanation is that the *t–d–ed* pattern has nothing to do with the past tense at all; it belongs to a different system—phonology—that adjusts words and strings so as to conform to the sound pattern of English, regardless of how the words or strings were formed. (Basically, the phonological rules here force consonant clusters at the ends of words to be either consistently voiced or consistently unvoiced, and they insert a vowel between adjacent consonants if they are too similar.) The regular past-tense pattern, belonging to the 'morphological' system, is simply that /d/ gets added to the end of a verb; the threefold variation is handled by a different phonological component. By collapsing the distinction into a single component, the model cannot account for the fact that the pattern of threefold variation follows from general constraints on the language as a whole.

3. *Stem and affix*. Linguistic processes tend to 'copy' stems with only minor modifications—*walk/walked* is a pervasive pattern; *go/went* is extremely rare. In some languages, the stem is copied twice, a phenomenon called 'reduplication': the past of *go* would be *gogo*. Similarly, the identity of an affix tends to be preserved across its variants: the endings for *jog* and *pat* are *-d* and *-ed*, respectively, not *-d* and *-ob* or *-iz* and *-gu*. A subtle but important property of network models is that there is no such thing as pure copying, just modifiable connections between one set of units and another set. Only the consistency of the pairings among units can affect the operation of the model, not what the units stand for (the labels next to the units are visible to the theorist, but not to the model). Hence the prevalence of copying operations in linguistic mappings is inexplicable; the network model could just as easily learn rules that change all a's to e's, all b's to c's, and so on.

4. *Lexical items*. In standard psychological theories, a word has an 'entry' in a

'mental lexicon' that is distinct from its actual sound. This is necessary because of homophones such as *ring* and *wring* or *lie* (prevaricate) and *lie* (recline). Crucially, homophones can have different past-tense forms, for example, *rang* and *wrung*, or *lied* and *lay*. The R and M model, because it simply maps from phonological units to phonological units, is incapable of handling such words.

A natural reaction to this phenomenon might be to suppose that the past-tense form is associated with meaning as well as with sound; perhaps the different semantic feature representations of the meanings of *ring* and *wring* can be directly associated with their different past-tense forms. Somewhat surprisingly, it turns out that meaning is almost completely irrelevant to the past-tense form; such forms are sensitive to distinctions at a level of representation at which verb roots are distinct but meaningless symbols. For example, verbs like *come, go, do, have, set, get, put, stand,* . . . , each have dozens of meanings, especially in combination with 'particles' like *in, out, up,* and *off,* but they have the same irregular past-tense forms in each of these semantic incarnations. This even occurs when these stems appear in combination with meaningless prefixes—*stood/understood, get/forget, come/ overcame* (though the prefixes are meaningless, they must be real prefixes, appearing in other words: *overcome* or *become,* which contain intuitively recognizable prefixes, are transformed to *overcame* and *became,* but *succumb,* which sounds similar but lacks a genuine prefix, is not transformed into *succame*). Conversely, synonyms need not have the same kind of past-tense forms: compare *hit/hit* versus *strike/struck* versus *slap/slapped,* which have similar meanings, but different kinds of past tenses. Thus, the similarity space relevant to the irregular past tenses has no semantic dimensions in it; all that matters is gross distinctness ('*wring* is not the same word as *ring*'), not actual meaning.

Even the distinction between a 'verb' and a 'verb root' is psychologically significant. Somewhat to the puzzlement of non-scientific prescriptive grammarians, people find it natural to say *broadcasted,* not *broadcast, joy-rided,* not *joy-rode, grandstanded,* not *grandstood, high sticked* (in ice hockey), not *high-stuck.* The reason is that 'irregularity' is a property attached to verb roots, not verbs. For each of these verbs, speakers have a sense, usually unconscious, that they were derived from nouns (*a joy-ride, a high stick,* etc.). Since it makes no sense for a noun to be marked in a person's mental dictionary as having an irregular 'past-tense form', any verb that is felt to be derived from nouns or adjectives automatically becomes regular, hence *joy-rided.*

What all these examples suggest is that the mental processes underlying language are sensitive to a system of representation—traditionally called 'morphology'—at which there are lawful regularities among entities that are neither sounds nor meanings, specifically, lexical items, stems, affixes, roots, and parts-of-speech.

5. *Regular versus irregular pasts.* A revolutionary aspect of the Rumelhart–McClelland model is that the regular and irregular past-tense alternations are collapsed into a single network. This is an example of one of the frequently claimed advantages of connectionist systems in general: that rule-governed cases, partially rule-governed cases, and isolated exceptions are all treated uniformly (McClelland and Rumelhart 1985). But of course this is only an advantage if people show no clear-cut distinction between rule-governed and exceptional behaviour. In the case of the past-tense system, however, qualitative differences can be documented. Consider these four:

(a) Irregular verbs cluster into 'family resemblance groups' that are phonologically similar: *blow/blew—grow/grew—throw/threw; take/took —shake/shook; sting/stung—fling/flung—stick/stuck.* Regular verbs have nothing in common phonologically; any string can be a regular verb.

(b) Irregular pasts can be fuzzy in their naturalness or acceptability, depending on how similar they are to the central tendency of a cluster: *wept, knelt, rent,* and *shod* sound stilted to many speakers, especially speakers of American English. In the extreme case, irregular past-tense forms can sound totally bizarre: *Last night I forwent the pleasure of grading papers,* or *I don't know how she bore it* have a very strange sound to most ears. In contrast, regular verbs, unless they are similar to an irregular cluster, have no gradient of acceptability based on their phonology: even phonologically unusual stems such as *genuflect* yield past-tense forms that sound as natural in the past tense as they are in the present tense; *she eked out a living* is no worse-sounding than *she ekes out a living; they prescinded* no worse than *they prescind* (even if one has no idea what *prescind* means).

(c) There are no sufficient conditions for a verb to be in any irregular class: though *blow* becomes *blew* in the past, *flow* becomes *flowed;* though *ring* becomes *rang, string* becomes *strung* and *bring* becomes *brought.* In contrast, a sufficient condition for a verb to be regular is that it not be irregular; if it is regular, its past-tense form is 100 per cent predictable.

(d) Most of the irregular alternations can only apply to verbs with a certain structure: the pattern in 'send/sent', namely to change a *d* to a *t*, requires that there be a *d* in the stem to begin with. The regular rule, which adds a *-d* to the stem, regardless of what the stem is, can cover all possible cases by its very nature.

These differences, though subtle, all point to the same conclusion. There is a psychologically significant difference between regular and irregular verbs: the former seem to be governed by an all-or-none process—a rule—that applies across the board except where specifically preempted by the presence of an irregular past-tense form; the latter consist of several memorized lists of similar-sounding words forming fuzzy family resemblance classes.

## The model's degree of success

Despite the optimistic claims of success for the model, its actual performance is limited in significant ways. After 80 000 training trials (about 200 presentations, each of 420 pairs of verb stems and their correct past-tense forms), the model is given 72 new verbs in a test of its ability to generalize. It made errors on 33 per cent of these verbs. In some cases, it emitted no response at all; in others, it offered a single incorrect form; in still others, it offered both a correct and an incorrect form, unable to decide between them (these cases must count as errors: a crucial aspect of the psychology of language is that irregular forms preempt regular ones in people's speech—not only do people say *went* and *came*, but they avoid saying *goed* and *comed*).

The model's errors can be traced to several factors. First, it associates past-tense features with specific stem features; it has no concept of an abstract entity 'stem' independent of the features it is composed of. Hence if there are gaps in the phonological space defined by the stems that the model was trained on, it could fail to generalize to newly presented items occupying those gaps and emit no response at all, even to common words such as *jump* or *warm*. Second, the model soaks up any degree of regularity in the training set, leading it to overestimate the generality of some of the vowel changes found among English irregular verbs, and resulting in spurious overregularizations such as *shipped* as the past of *shape* or *brawned* as the past of *brown*. Third, the model has no way of keeping track of separate competing responses, such as *type* and *typed*; hundreds of mutually incompatible features associated with a stem are all activated at once in the output feature vector, with no record of which ones cohere as target responses. Though Rumelhart and McClelland constructed a temporary, separate response-competition module to extract a cohesive response, the module could not do so effectively, producing blended hybrids such as *typeded* for *type*, *membled* for *mail*, and *squakt* for *squat*.

## Children's language

The most dramatic aspect of the past-tense model is its apparent ability to duplicate the stages that children pass through: first using *ate*, then both *ate* and *eated* (and occasionally *ated*), finally *ate* exclusively. This is especially surprising because nothing changes in the model itself; it just responds passively to the teacher's input.

For this reason, it turns out that the model's changes are caused by changes in its input. Rumelhart and McClelland note that high-frequency verbs tend to be irregular and vice versa. Children, they reasoned, are likely to learn a few high-frequency verbs first, then a large number of verbs, of which an increasing proportion would probably be regular. Hence in simulating children with their model, they defined two stages. In the first stage they fed in 10 high-frequency verbs (two regular and eight irregular), paired with their correct past-tense forms, 10 times each. In the second stage they fed in 420 high-frequency and medium-frequency verb pairs, 190 times each, of which 336 (80 per cent) were regular. Frequencies were determined by published statistics of a large corpus of written English. The model responded accordingly: in the first stage, the regular pattern was only exemplified by two verbs, only one more than each of the eight irregular patterns, and the model in effect recorded 10 separate patterns of associations between stem and past. Thus it performed perfectly on the irregular verbs. In the second stage, there was a huge amount of evidence for the regular pattern, which swamped the associations specific to the irregular verbs, resulting in 'overgeneralization errors' such as *breaked*. Finally, as the 420-word corpus was presented over and over, the model was able to strengthen connections between features unique to irregular stems and features unique to its past forms, and to inhibit connections to the features of the regular ending, so as to approach correct performance.

The prediction, then, is that children's overgeneralization should also be triggered by changes in the ratio of irregular to regular forms in their vocabularies. The prediction is completely false. Figure 8.1 shows data from four children at six different stages of development; overgeneralization typically occurs in the stage marked 'III'. The proportion of regular verbs in the children's vocabularies remains essentially unchanged throughout this period, and there is never a point at which regular verbs predominate (Pinker and Prince 1988). The same is true of token frequencies, and of frequencies in parental speech (Slobin 1971). The cause of the onset of overgeneralization is not a change in vocabulary statistics, but some endogenous change in the child's language mechanisms. This is also shown by the fact that across a sample of children, use of the regular pattern correlates with general measures of grammatical sophistication, though not with chronological age. The use of irregular past forms, in contrast, correlates with chronological age (Kuczaj 1977). This is exactly what one would expect if, contrary to the predictions of the model, rote (for the irregulars) and rule (for the regulars) were distinct mechanisms, the former depending on sheer quantity of exposure to the language, the latter on mastery of the grammatical system in general.

A second interesting way in which the model appears to mimic children is in the late appearance of doubly marked errors such as *ated*. The model becomes prone to such errors because of response blending: when the responses for *ate* and *eated* each attain a sufficient level of strength at the same time, the model has no way of keeping track of which segments belong to which target and

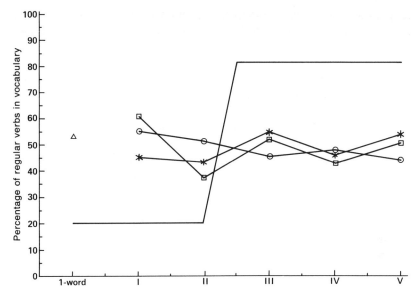

**Fig. 8.1**    Percentage of regular verbs in the vocabulary of the four children over six stages of development, and in the Rumelhart–McClelland model. The model predicts that 'overgeneralization errors', i.e. giving an irregular verb a regular past-tense form, such as *bring/bringed*, would result from a high incidence of regular verbs in the vocabulary, which strengthens the connections for this regular pattern. While the model showed overgeneralization errors after the introduction of a high percentage of regular verbs, there is no evidence that children use a high percentage of regular verbs at any stage that can be correlated with their overgeneralization errors.

blends them. The alternative hypothesis is that children misconstrue *ate* as itself being a stem and mistakenly attach the regular ending to it—basically, they think there are two distinct English verbs, *eat* and *ate* (Kuczaj 1978, 1981). The data favour this hypothesis. Unambiguous blends of irregular vowel changes and the regular ending (e.g. *sepped* for *sip*) are extremely rare in children's speech (Pinker and Prince 1988). However, errors involving a past form misconstrued as a stem are common: children often say *ating, he ates*, and *to ate* (Kuczaj 1981). Moreover, when children are simply asked to convert *eat* to a past-tense form in experiments, they virtually never say *ated*, showing that when children say *ated*, it is because of something they do to an input consisting of *ate*, not an input consisting of *eat*. Apparently, children do not derive inflected forms by haphazardly assembling them out of bits and pieces associated with the stem; they largely respect the integrity of words and the systematic modifications that can be applied to them (Slobin 1985). In sum, the mechanisms invoked by the Rumelhart–McClelland model to account for children's behaviour—lack of distinct mechanisms for memorization and rules, sensitivity to input frequency, and response blending—are inconsistent with the data from developmental psycholinguistics.

## Implications for the nature of human cognitive architecture

The Rumelhart–McClelland model is an extremely important contribution to our understanding of human language mechanisms. For the same reason that its impressive performance at first seemed to vindicate associative networks lacking implemented rules, the empirical flaws revealed by closer scrutiny provide valuable lessons about the kinds of mechanisms that language—and probably many other aspects of cognition—requires.

1. *Elements versus their positions.* Lashley's problem of serial order in behaviour applies in full force to language, and it is not solved by invoking feature units that conflate a feature and its immediate context. Such units cannot encode certain words at all, and they cannot explain patterns of psychological similarity defined by a given feature appearing in different serial positions.

2. *Variables.* A variable is a symbol that can stand for a group of individuals regardless of their individual properties; in arithmetic, '$x + 1 > x$' is true regardless of whether $x$ is even, odd, prime, and so on. Languages use variables in many of their operations; the regular past-tense rule in English, which adds -*d* to the variable 'stem', is a perfect example. Associating response features with the concrete features of a class of inputs is not the same thing as linking them to a symbol or variable that represents the class itself, because the associations are sensitive to the properties of the particular sample of inputs in a way that a genuine variable is not.

3. *Individuals.* Two objects may share all their relevant features, yet may be distinct in the world, hence their representations must be kept distinct in the brain. The case of *lie/lay* v. *lie/lied* shows that it must be possible to represent two identical patterns of features as corresponding to distinct entities. It is not enough to have large numbers of units with different perceptual receptive fields; some structures must be dedicated to representing an entity as simply being a distinct entity *per se*.

4. *Binding.* Vision researchers have recently been made aware of one of the inherent problems of representing objects simply as patterns of activation over feature maps: it is impossible to keep the bindings of two simultaneously presented objects distinct, and a pressured perceiver is liable to illusory

conjunctions whereby a red circle + green square is perceived as a green circle + red square (Treisman and Schmidt 1982). A serial attentional mechanism is invoked in such cases to glue features into objects. Similarly, it is not sufficient that words be produced solely by activating patterns of features associated with an input, because when there are competing targets, there is no way of keeping the competing alternatives from blending. Simple connectionist models of language have this problem, but children's inflectional systems, apparently, do not.

5. *Modularity*. Recently there has been considerable debate about the extent to which the mind is composed of relatively autonomous subsystems or 'modules' (Fodor 1983). Very convincing evidence for decomposition into subsystems has come for vision research, which has made it clear that the visual system is not a single black box but is composed of many partially autonomous subsystems (van Essen and Maunsell 1983; Livingstone and Hubel 1988). This conclusion was suggested by the methodology of 'dissection by psychophysics', even before it was corroborated by neuroanatomical and neurophysiological techniques. Though the neuroanatomy of language is not well understood, the equivalent 'psychophysical' investigations strongly support a functional decomposition of language skill into subcomponents, and any model of language abilities will have to reflect this rather than mapping from input to output in a single link. Furthermore, the internal 'links' are organized in specific ways. In the present case, phonology and morphology reveal themselves as distinct subsystems, and that is only the most obvious cut.

6. *Independence from correlational statistics of the input*. Connectionist networks, like all associationist models, learn by recording patterns of correlation among perceptual features. Language acquisition almost certainly does not work that way; in many cases, children ignore pervasive environmental correlations and make endogenously driven generalizations that are in some cases surprising with respect to the correlational statistics of the input but are consistent with subtle grammatical principles (Pinker 1984, in press). This can be seen in the case of the past tense, where the onset of overgeneralization is clearly independent of input statistics, and the extent of generalization in the adult state (e.g. avoiding it if an irregular form exists; but overriding the irregular form if the verb is derived from a noun root) is not a reflection of any simple correlational property of the input. More generally, to the extent that language is composed of separate subsystems, the role of environmentally driven changes must be quite circumscribed: if a subsystem's inputs and outputs are not connected to the environment, but to other internal subsystems, then they are invisible to the environment and there is no direct way for the connectionist's 'teaching inputs' to tune them to the correct state via incremental changes from a tabula rasa.

Overall, there is a more general lesson. Theories attempting to bridge neuroscience and cognition must be consistent with the data of both. The data of human language in particular are extremely rich, and theories of considerable sophistication and explanatory power have been developed in response to them. Though it may be convenient to impose a revisionist associationist theory on the phenomena of language, such a move is not scientifically defensible. Building the bridge will be more difficult, and more interesting, than it might first appear.

## Appendix

### How the Rumelhart–McClelland model works

Rumelhart and McClelland's model, in its trained state, is supposed to take any stem as input and emit the corresponding past-tense form. They assume that the acquisition process establishes a direct mapping from the phonetic representation of the 'stem' or 'root' (in English, this is usually the same as the infinitival or present-tense form) to the phonetic representation of the past-tense form. The model is shown in Fig. 8.2; of its three components, the centre one, the 'pattern associator', is the most theoretically important.

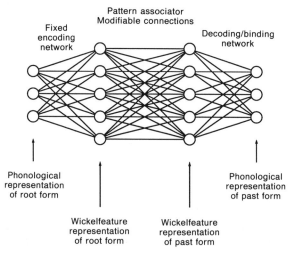

**Fig. 8.2**  The architecture of the Rumelhart–McClelland model.

The model's pattern associator is a simple network with two layers of nodes, one for representing input, the other for output. Nodes in the R–M model may only be 'on' or 'off'; thus the nodes represent binary features, 'off' and 'on' marking the simple absence or presence of a certain property that a word may have. Each stem must be encoded as a unique subset of turned-on input nodes; each possible past-tense form as a unique subset of output nodes turned on.

A problem arises here. A natural assumption would be that words are strings on an alphabet, a concatenation of phonemes. But each item fed to a pattern association network must dissolve into an unordered set of properties (coded as turned-on units). Dedicating each unit to a phoneme would obliterate information about serial order, leading to the confusion of 'pit' and 'tip', 'cat' and 'tack', and so on. To overcome this problem, Rumelhart and McClelland turned to a scheme proposed by Wickelgren (1969), according to which a string is represented as the set of the trigrams (three-character sequences) that it contains. (In order to locate word-edges, it is necessary to assume that word-boundary (#) is a character in the underlying alphabet.) Rumelhart and McClelland call such trigrams *Wickelphones*. Thus a word like 'strip' translates to the following set of Wickelphones : {*ip#, rip, str, tri, #st*}. The word 'strip' is reconstructible from this trigram set. Although certain trigram sets are consistent in principle with more than one string, Rumelhart and McClelland found that all words in their sample were uniquely encoded.

However, Rumelhart and McClelland did not build their model with each node standing for a Wickelphone. There would have been two problems with that scheme. First, the number of possible Wickelphones for their representation of English would have multiplied out to over 43 000 nodes for the input stem, 43 000 nodes for the output past form, and two billion connections between them, too many to handle in their computational model. Second, it was hoped that the model would be able to generalize beyond the word set given to it, and provide past-tense forms for new stems based on their similar representation to the ones trained. Since the phonological regularities (like those involved in past-tense formation) do not treat phonemes as atomic, unanalysable wholes but pertain instead to their constituent phonetic properties like place and manner of articulation, voicing, the height and tenseness of vowels, obstruency (noisiness), and so on, it is necessary that such fine-grained information be present in the network. The Wickelphone is too coarse to support the necessary generalization; for example, any English speaker who had to provide a past-tense form for the hypothetical verb *to Bach* (as in the composer) would pronounce it *bacht*, not *bachd* or *bach-ed*, even though *ch* is not a consonant they have heard used in an English verb. This reaction is based on the similarity of *ch* to *p, k, s*, and so on, all of which share the feature 'unvoiced', and the tacit knowledge that verbs ending in unvoiced consonants have their past-tense suffix pronounced as *t*. Since atomic symbols for phonemes do not provide a mechanical way of exploiting this similarity, a decomposition of phonemes into features is a standard tool of phonology. Rumelhart and McClelland therefore assume a phonetic decomposition of segments into features which are in broad outline like those used by phonologists. Thus, rather than dedicating nodes to Wickelphones, they used what they called 'Wickelfeatures'. A Wickelfeature is a trigram of features, one from each of the three elements of the Wickelphone. For example, the features 'VowelUnvoicedInterrupted' and 'HighStopStop' are two of the Wickelfeatures in the ensemble that would correspond to the Wickelphone 'ipt'. By simplifying the Wickelfeature set in a number of other ways that will not be discussed here, Rumelhart and McClelland pared down the necessary number to 460 (see Rumelhart and McClelland 1986, and Pinker and Prince 1988, for more complete descriptions of the model).

Each node, then, represents a Wickelfeature; Wickelphones themselves play no direct role. A word is represented by a collection of turned-on nodes that correspond to the Wickelfeatures contained in it. This results in a 'distributed' representation: an individual word does not register on its own node, but is analysed as an ensemble of properties, Wickelfeatures. As Fig. 8.1 shows, Rumelhart and McClelland invoke an 'encoder' of an unspecified nature to convert an ordered phonetic string into a set of activated Wickelfeature units.

In the pattern associator, every input node is connected to every output node, giving each input Wickelfeature node the chance to influence every node in the output Wickelfeature set. Suppose that a set of input nodes is turned on, representing an input to the network. Whether a given output node will turn on is determined by weighting each active input link by the strength of that link and comparing that weighted sum to the output node's threshold. The decision is made probabilistically: the nearer the input weighted sum is to the threshold, the more random the decision.

An untrained pattern associator starts out with no pre-set relations between input and output nodes: the link weights are all set to zero. Training involves presenting the network with an input stem and comparing the output pattern actually obtained with the desired pattern for the past-tense form, which is provided to the network by a 'teacher' as a distinct kind of 'teaching' input (not shown in Fig. 8.1). The corresponding psychological assumption is that the child, through some unspecified process, has already figured out which past-tense form is to be associated with which stem form.

The comparison between the actual output pattern computed by the connections between input and output nodes, and the desired pattern provided by the 'teacher', is made on a node-by-node basis. Any output node that is in the wrong state becomes the target of adjustment. If the network ends up leaving a node off that ought to be on according to the teacher, changes are made to render that node more likely to fire in the presence of the particular input at hand. Specifically, the weights on the links connecting active input units to the recalcitrant output unit are increased slightly; this will increase the tendency for the currently active input units—those that represent the input form—to activate the target node. In addition, the target node's own threshold is lowered slightly, so that it will tend to turn on more easily across the board.

If, on the other hand, the network incorrectly turns an output node *on*, the reverse procedure is employed: the weights of the connections from currently active input units are decremented (potentially driving the connection weight to a negative, inhibitory value) and the target node's threshold is raised; a hyperactive output node is thus made more likely to turn off given the same pattern of input node activation. Repeated cycling through input–output pairs, with concomitant adjustments, shapes the behaviour of the pattern associator. This is the 'perceptron convergence procedure' (Rosenblatt 1962) and it is known to produce, in the limit, a set of weights that successfully maps the input activation vectors onto the desired output activation vectors, as long as such a set of weights exists.

In fact, the R–M net, following about 200 training cycles of 420 stem-past pairs (a total of about 80 000 trials), is able to produce correct past forms for the stems when the stems are presented alone, i.e. in the absence of 'teaching' inputs. A single set of connection weights in the network is able to map *look* to *looked, live* to *lived, melt* to *melted, hit* to *hit, make* to *made, sing* to *sang*, even *go* to *went*. The bits of stored information accomplishing these mappings are superimposed in the connection weights and node thresholds; no single parameter corresponds uniquely to a rule or to any single irregular stem-past pair.

The structure of the encoding and decoding networks are not the focus of Rumelhart and McClelland's efforts, but they had to have several special properties for the model to work properly. The input encoder was deliberately designed to activate some incorrect Wickelfeatures in addition to the precise set of Wickelfeatures in the stem: specifically, a randomly selected subset of those Wickelfeatures that encode the features of the central phoneme properly but encode incorrect feature values for one of the two context phonemes. Because of this selective 'blurring', the process that gives rise to it cannot be random noise. Rather, the blurred representation is intended to foster a further kind of generalization of the right sort; blurring the input representations makes the connection weights in the R–M model less likely to be able to exploit the idiosyncrasies of the words in the training set and hence reduces the model's tendency toward conservatism.

The output decoder faces a difficult task. When an input stem is fed into the model, the result is a set of activated output Wickelfeature units characterizing properties of the predicted past-tense form. Nothing in the model ensures that the set of activated output units will fit together to describe a legitimate word or even a unique, consistent, and well-formed string of phonemes. Since the output Wickelfeatures virtually never define such a string exactly, there is no clear sense in which one knows which word the output Wickelfeatures are defining. A special mechanism called the *whole-string binding network* was programmed to provide an estimate of the model's tendencies to output possible words. Basically, this network had one unit standing for every possible string of phonemes less than 20 phonemes long (obviously, the actual set had to be pruned considerably from this astronomically large number of possibilities; this was done with the help of another mechanism that will not be discussed here). Once the set of Wickelfeature units in the past-tense vector is activated, the whole-string units in the binding network 'compete' for them: each whole-string unit has a transient strength value that increases in proportion to the number of activated Wickelfeatures that the word it represents uniquely contains. ('Credit' for activated Wickelfeatures contained in several words is split among the units standing for those words.) Conversely, activated Wickelfeatures that are not contained in a word cause the strength of that word's unit to diminish. Strings whose units exceed a threshold level of strength after this competition process stabilizes are interpreted as the final output of the model.

In sum, the R–M model works as follows. The phonological string is cashed in for a set of Wickelfeatures by an unspecified process that activates all the correct and some of the incorrect Wickelfeature units. The pattern associator excites the Wickelfeature units in the output; during the training phase its parameters (weights and thresholds) are adjusted to reduce the discrepancy between the excited Wickelfeature units and the desired ones provided by the teacher. The activated Wickelfeature units may then be decoded into an output word by a whole-string binding network.

## References

Berko, J. (1958). The child's learning of English morphology. *Word*, **14**, 150–77.

Chomsky, N. (1959). A review of B. F. Skinner's 'Verbal Behavior'. *Language*, **3**, 26–58.

Crick, F. and Asanuma, C. (1986). Certain aspects of the anatomy and physiology of the cerebral cortex. In *Parallel distributed processing: explorations in the microstructure of cognition*. Volume 2: *Psychological and biological models* (eds. J. L. McClelland, D. E. Rumelhart, and the PDP Research Group). MIT Press, Cambridge, Mass.

Feldman, J. A. and Ballard, D. H. (1982). Connectionist models and their properties. *Cognitive Science*, **6**, 205–54.

Fodor, J. (1983). *Modularity of mind*. MIT Press, Cambridge, Mass.

Fodor, J. A. and Pylyshyn, Z. (1988). Connectionism and cognitive architecture: a critical analysis. *Cognition*, **28**, 3–71.

Hinton, G. E., McClelland, J. L., and Rumelhart, D. E. (1986). Distributed representations. In *Parallel distributed processing: explorations in the microstructure of cognition*. Volume 1: *Foundations* (eds. D. E. Rumelhart, J. L. McClelland, and the PDP research group). MIT Press, Cambridge, Mass.

Kuczaj, S. A. (1977). The acquisition of regular and irregular past tense forms. *Journal of Verbal Learning and Verbal Behavior*, **16**, 589–600.

Kuczaj, S. A. (1978). Children's judgments of grammatical and ungrammatical irregular past tense verbs. *Child Development*, **49**, 319–26.

Kuczaj, S. A. (1981). More on children's initial failure to relate specific acquisitions. *Journal of Child Language*, **8**, 485–7.

Lachter, J. and Bever, T. G. (1988). The relation between linguistic structure and associative theories of language learning—a constructive critique of some connectionist learning models. *Cognition*, **28**, 195–247.

Livingstone, M. and Hubel, D. (1988). Segregation of form, color, movement, and depth: anatomy, physiology, and perception. *Science*, **240**, 740–9.

McClelland, J. L. and Rumelhart, D. E. (1985). Distributed memory and the representation of general and specific information. *Journal of Experimental Psychology: General*, **114**, 159–88.

Pinker, S. (1984). *Language learnability and language development*. Harvard University Press, Cambridge, Mass.

Pinker, S. (in press). *Learnability and cognition: the acquisition of argument structure*. MIT Press, Cambridge, Mass.

Pinker, S. and Mehler, J. (eds.) (1988). *Connections and symbols*. MIT Press, Cambridge, Mass.

Pinker, S. and Prince, A. (1988). On language and connectionism: analysis of a parallel distributed processing model of language acquisition. *Cognition*, **28**, 73–193.

Rosenblatt, F. (1962). *Principles of neurodynamics*. Spartan, NY.

Rumelhart, D. E. and McClelland, J. L. (1986). On learning the past tenses of English verbs. In *Parallel distributed processing: explorations in the microstructure of cognition*. Volume 2: *Psychological and biological models* (eds. J. L. McClelland, D. E. Rumelhart, and the PDP research group). MIT Press, Cambridge, Mass.

Slobin, D. I. (1971). On the learning of morphological rules: a reply to Palermo and Eberhart. In *The ontogenesis of grammar: a theoretical symposium* (ed. D. I. Slobin). Academic Press, NY.

Slobin, D. I. (1985). Crosslinguistic evidence for the language-making capacity. In *The crosslinguistic study of language acquisition*. Volume II: *Theoretical issues* (ed. D. I. Slobin). Erlbaum, Hillsdale, NJ.

Treisman, A. and Schmidt, H. (1982). Illusory conjunctions in the perception of objects. *Cognitive Psychology*, **14**, 107–41.

van Essen, D. C. and Maunsell, J. (1983). Hierarchical organization and functional streams in the visual cortex. *Trends in Neurosciences*, **6**, 370–5.

Wickelgren, W. A. (1969). Context-sensitive coding, associative memory, and serial order in (speech) behavior. *Psychological Review*, **76**, 1–15.

# Part III

## Implications for neurobiology

# 9

## Computational neuroscience: modelling the brain.

R. G. M. MORRIS

The organization of this book reflects two different approaches to neural network research. The earlier chapters are primarily concerned with the design of artificial networks for carrying out various psychological tasks. Such networks are often said to be 'neurally-inspired' but not 'neurally-constrained'. They have a brain-like style of processing, in that they consist of large numbers of processing units to which information is presented in a distributed manner, but they are not intended to be simulations of specific parts of the brain. The aim of these PDP models is well captured by the subtitle of Rumelhart and McClelland's (1986) volumes, namely to explore the 'microstructures of cognition'. To those such as Allport (1980), frustrated by years of 'black-box' models in which information is successively subjected to 'processing', 'more-processing', and then 'even-more-processing' but whose inner workings were never explained, PDP models have considerable appeal.

However, many neurobiologists are likely to be sceptical of this strictly psychological approach to neural network modelling. The neuroanatomist who spends hours at the microscope painstakingly working out the detailed connectivity of a particular area of the brain might be a little suspicious of PDP theorists 'inventing' networks to do particular tasks; the neurophysiologist who burns the midnight oil impaling cells with microelectrodes and recording their activity may be surprised by the apparently arbitrary assumptions made concerning the input/output functions of 'simple' processing units made within many PDP models. As noted elsewhere (Crick and Asanuma 1986; Crick 1989), certain of the assumptions made in some PDP models are either unrealistic or downright false—such as 'synaptic' connections which can change from excitatory to inhibitory. One sceptic has gone further, claiming that 'the only thing neural networks have in common with the human brain is the word neural' (Poggio 1988).

It is, therefore, not surprising that a different approach to neural network research is emerging. In this, the networks are explicitly 'brain models' based on real anatomy and constrained, in a bottom-up fashion, by neurophysiological information about their dynamic operation. Such models typically embody concepts from PDP models, such as parallel processing or the use of learning rules such as back-propagation; but they also take advantage of the existence of different cell-types, they may contain elements of serial processing and, in some cases, they exploit such neurobiological concepts as extrinsic neurotransmitter modulation which have no obvious place within extant PDP-models.

To what extent is this approach to neural networks radically different from PDP modelling? Certainly both the aims and constraints differ but, equally, there are aspects of PDP modelling and computational neuroscience which are very similar. One way of summarizing the difference is in terms of Marr's (1982) tripartite scheme of 'computational task', 'algorithm', and 'implementation'. In certain respects, PDP models can be viewed as an effort to discover brain-like algorithms for performing highly specific psychological tasks—such as categorization, past-tense learning, and so on. Real brain models, on the other hand, are also concerned with the implementation of algorithms. PDP modelling will always seem incomplete as a theory of the brain in the absence of implementational details. Computational neuroscience will, however, have difficulty in making sense of how a bit of the brain works unless provided with functional information about what it does.

On this view, argument about the relative merits of PDP modelling and computational neuroscience is sterile, being no more than yet another manifestation of the curious lack of communication which exists between psychology and neurobiology and which has been institutionalized for decades. There are two facets of this failure of communication. First, neurobiologists would be mistaken if they supposed that decisions about the design of a PDP network for performing some psychological function are, in practice, arbitrary. On the contrary, the decision about whether to use a one-layered or a multi-layered network reflects considerable theoretical understanding about the computational capacities of different networks and different learning rules (Rumelhart and McClelland 1986). Moreover, it is no accident that the need to use an error-correcting learning rule and the issue of whether a one- or multilayered network may be required maps quite precisely on to certain classical problems in experimental psychology (see Gluck and Bower 1988; Sutherland and Mackintosh 1971).

The second and opposite facet of this failure of communication is that I share Crick's view that, if our aim is to understand the brain, there is little value in designing and evaluating neural networks whose underlying assumptions about brain organization are known at the outset to be false (cf. Sejnowski *et al.* 1988 who distinguished between 'realistic' and 'simplifying' brain models). This latter criticism is easy to make, but meeting it is more difficult. Faced with the truly massive amount of information we have about the brain, one of the crucial problems facing modellers is to identify features of neural activity which really are involved in information processing and those features having to do with 'mere housekeeping' (e.g. with keeping neurons alive and thus an implementational 'detail' of little processing consequence). This distinction is not always easy to draw. A relevant, and ironic, example is to be found in the history of research on excitatory neurotransmission in the central nervous system. Research in this field has recently culminated in the discovery of one mechanism through which synapses may change in efficacy (see Collingridge and Bliss 1987). Progress in this field was hampered for many years by the widespread belief that the major excitatory neurotransmitter L-glutamate (now implicated in this mechanism) played a strictly metabolic function but had no role in neurotransmission.

The last few years have seen the publication of several neural network models which are explicit brain models. Excellent reviews of these and earlier models are provided by Cowan and Sharp (1988) and by Sejnowski *et al.* (1988). A few examples may help to illustrate the scope of the approach. Pellionisz and Llinas (1979) have proposed that the firing patterns of cerebellar neurons can be understood in terms of tensor network theory. This theory provides a way of understanding how cerebellar Purkinje cells may provide a predictive 'look ahead' of the inputs arriving in cerebellar cortex, and that this serves an important role in the dynamic control of posture and balance. Linsker (1986, 1988) has described how the development of the receptive field properties of cells in the lateral geniculate and primary visual cortex may emerge from an activity-dependent modification of the synaptic weights of topographically projecting pathways. His 'informax' model has certain similarities to ideas about self-organization in the development of retino-tectal projections (Willshaw and von der Malsburg 1976). Bear *et al.* (1987) have described a physiologically plausible implementation of the earlier Bienenstock *et al.* (1982) algorithm for the development of ocular dominance columns in visual cortex. This theory attempts to offer a mechanistic account of the neural events responsible for alterations in ocular dominance during development and in experiments involving reverse suture. Zipser and Andersen (1988) have explored how a three layered network, in which the weights are adjusted by back-propagation during training, may be used to model the control of gaze direction. The network receives information about both the position of an image on the retina and information about eye position relative to the head, and it produces an output which encodes the location of the object in head-centred co-ordinates. This output, held to correspond to the firing patterns of cells in posterior parietal cortex, could serve as an eye-movement command-signal for centring the image of the object on the fovea.

The chapters that follow are all concerned with learning and memory. The topic is clearly central to neural network research because synaptic plasticity is widely believed to be the mechanism through which information is stored in the brain. Two of the chapters (by Rolls, and by Granger and Lynch) outline models which embrace many ideas from PDP models (such as the distributed representation of information). However, they also refer to detailed issues such as the exact patterns of connectivity of feedforward projection fibres from one part of the network to another, and the role of feedback inhibition from basket cells in limiting the firing of the principal cells or in performing competitive learning. Neither model uses back-propagation as the learning rule. Indeed, back-propagation continues to be viewed sceptically by many students of the neurobiology of learning for the simple reason that so many types of learning and memory—particularly recognition memory—occur so rapidly. Even with recent modifications such as 'fast' and 'slow' weights, back-propagation often requires hundreds of iterations before the input produces the desired output.

The other two chapters have a very different scope. My own contribution does not include any formal model. Instead, I contrast two different strategies for investigating the role of synaptic plasticity in learning. The first involves training animals to perform a task and then searching for the morphological, physiological, or biochemical consequences of this training. The second strategy involves identifying a specific type of synaptic plasticity and then investigating whether it plays any role in learning. In the discussion of work following the second of these strategies, I review work on hippocampal long-term potentiation (LTP), a physiological phenomenon first reported in detail by Bliss and Lomo (1973). The chapter summarizes properties of LTP indicating that its underlying mechanisms may be of functional significance and describes behavioural experiments from a number of laboratories which have explored its putative role in learning.

In describing a neural network model of classical conditioning in an invertebrate, Hawkins's chapter begins and ends with expressions of guarded scepticism about PDP models. His model is based on a wealth of detailed anatomical, physiological, and biochemical information about the connectivity and dynamic functioning of identified cells in the abdominal ganglion of *Aplysia*. The model explains certain simple forms of conditioning, such as acquisition, extinction, and discrimination, and it provides an account of certain higher forms also, such as second-order conditioning, blocking, and contingency effects. However, although inspired by psychological theories of these phenomena, Hawkins's model differs from the theories of Rescorla and Wagner (1972) and Mackintosh (1975) in being constrained by *known* properties of neural circuitry. The bold ambition of being biologically realistic is expressed in the form of a series of equations capturing cellular processes such as, for example, how the number of available calcium channels in pre-synaptic terminals (which, in turn, determine transmitter release on to motor neurons and thus motor output) change in response to both sensory activation and the passage of time, how the duration of action-potentials relates to the phosphorylation of potassium channels through a second-messenger triggered by cAMP and so on. These equations are, therefore, mathematical formulations of identified cellular processes. Taken together, they provide a quantitative description of synaptic depression (held to be the basis of both habituation and extinction), pre-synaptic facilitation (responsible for sensitization), and activity-dependent modulation of pre-synaptic facilitation (responsible for classical conditioning). Hawkins refers to these processes as a 'cellular alphabet' out of which higher forms of conditioning emerge.

While this chapter is modest and cautious in style, the reader should not underestimate either the boldness of the claims being made or the truly remarkable discoveries to have emerged from the work of Kandel and his colleagues on *Aplysia* (and upon which Hawkins bases his model). To take an example, Hawkins asserts that his model 'incorporates in very rudimentary forms, the notions of predictability and internal representation' which are so central to modern accounts of conditioning. One of the equations (Equation 8) incorporates features of both the Rescorla–Wagner and the Mackintosh theories of associative conditioning. This equation describes how the amount of cAMP present in a pre-synaptic terminal varies as a function of (1) the accommodation of neural activity in the facilitator neuron (a measure of the predictability of activity in the US pathway) and (2) a variable rate parameter specific to the sensory neuron (whose variation is dependent on reinforcement history). Many psychologists will be surprised by the claim that a phenomenon such as 'predictability', can be reduced to a mathematical equation describing how cAMP varies inside a neuron.

How successful is Hawkins's model? One important virtue is that the mathematical formulation, rigorously expressed in specific equations and implemented on a computer, is an important advance on the qualitative ideas originally put forward by Hawkins and Kandel (1984). A concrete example concerns the problem of contingency effects. It is well established (Rescorla 1968) that if a stimulus A is paired with a US, conditioning is more effective if A predicts all occurrences of the US (Group 1) that if additional presentations of the US occur in the absence of A (Group 2). This contingency effect was not easily explained by Hawkins and Kandel's (1984) earlier qualitative model because it seemed to predict that the additional unpredicted US presentations in Group 2 would, counter-intuitively, lead to added conditioning through the mechanism of presynaptic facilitation. We now know that appropriate contingency effects can be shown in *Aplysia* (Hawkins et al. 1986) and, as described in the chapter, this finding may be partly explained in terms of the faster rate of habituation of the US when it is presented repeatedly. It turns out that the partly habituated US impairs the rate of conditioning on paired A–US trials to a greater extent than can be offset by the contribution due to sensitization on US-alone trials. Experiments to distinguish this account of contingency effects from Rescorla and Wagner's account in terms of conditioning to background cues can now be designed and evaluated in relation to both models.

Another important but more general virtue of Hawkins's model is that it respects the complexity of individual neurons as processing devices. I cannot express the point better than the author himself in his concluding discussion where he compares his model with PDP models:

> . . . network models usually assume that the basic computing unit does something fairly simple, whereas real neurons are much more complex . . . The basic types of cellular plasticity in the model are explained by the probabilistic behaviour of millions of ion channels and enzyme molecules which interact in complex ways to determine the behaviour of the neuron.
>
> (Hawkins, Chapter 10, p. 241).

Thus, in order to understand fully the processing capacities of a neural circuit, we need to understand it at many different levels of analysis—including the cellular level. This perspective is, I suspect, not widely shared by many psychologists who doubt the necessity to be concerned with such 'low-level' implementational details. However, while I share Hawkins's view of the need to refer to the cellular level for a full understanding of mechanism, I am less certain that he has got the mapping between psychological processes and his cellular alphabet quite right. A particular problem, discussed in detail elsewhere (Morris 1989), is that the claim that classical conditioning can be implemented as an alteration in the efficacy of existing neural connections (which is implicit in his model) does not require that all forms of conditioning be explained as a process or algorithm through which existing reflexes are modulated. Hawkins's view that alpha and beta conditioning are not fundamentally different (p. 224) is an inappropriate inference which, I believe, follows from giving undue attention to cellular mechanisms at the expense of properties of conditioning which only *emerge* at the system level.

This point can be expressed in a different way with reference to the functional properties of NMDA receptors (reviewed in detail in Chapter 11). $N$-methyl-D-aspartate receptors are a subtype of excitatory amino acid receptor activated by the excitatory neurotransmitter, L-glutamate. These receptors have the important property of only being active when pre-synaptic activity is coincident with post-synaptic depolarization. It is, therefore, tempting to describe NMDA receptors as 'associative learning receptors' by analogy with the way in which Hawkins sees activity-dependent amplification of presynaptic facilitation as the 'basis' of classical conditioning (his all important Equation 10.8). However, in my view, it would be a mistake to follow this course. What NMDA receptors do is to detect the conjunction of two neural events and to signal this conjunction with a specific ionic messenger (calcium). Their 'function' is fully described by this statement. Whether they play a functional role in experience-dependent alterations of ocular dominance (Bear *et al.* 1987), selective attention (Koch 1987), or certain types of learning (Chapter 11) depends critically upon (1) the circuitry into which they are embedded, and (2) the cellular events triggered by calcium after its entry into the cell. Thus, while the expression of function entails cellular mechanisms, it cannot be described exclusively in cellular terms. For this reason, it seems to me that Hawkins's equations might be better described as a cellular alphabet of plasticity than a cellular alphabet of learning.

Rolls (Chapter 12) outlines a model of the hippocampus in which each of the three stages of the classical trisynaptic circuit performs either of two different network functions. The first stage, the dentate gyrus, is held to perform a recoding function to remove redundancy in the hippocampal input from entorhinal cortex. This is achieved by a competitive learning algorithm implemented via feedback inhibition from basket cells on to the principal cells of the dentate gyrus—the granule cells. The 'sharpened' stimulus is then fedforward to area CA3 via the sparsely connected mossy fibres. Area CA3 is ascribed an autoassociative function by virtue of the extensive recurrent collaterals between CA3 neurons which account for over 70 per cent of the synapses on individual cells. The computational effect of this autoassociation is to build 'episodic' memories by combining information projected into CA3 from different cortical association areas. Finally, information corresponding to individual episodic memories is projected into area CA1 via neural activity on the Schaffer collaterals. Area CA1 is held to be a second competitive learning stage to enable a more efficient recoding of event memories than is possible within CA3. This is necessary because the functional architecture of CA3 is, according to Rolls's model, so organized to maximize the possibility of pattern completion and such organization is not, at an implementational level, appropriate for effective recoding. In any event, the final output from CA1 is a signal which, projected back to cortex via neurons in the subiculum and deep layers of entorhinal cortex, serves to guide long-term information storage in cortex.

Although Rolls's model is sketched only in outline, it none the less represents a valuable step towards understanding hippocampal function. First, it takes particular account of the patterns of connectivity between successive stages of the network, emphasizing the sparse connectivity between individual dentate cells and the CA3 neurons on to which they project, and the much higher connectivity (circa 500 times greater) between individual CA3 neurons. The model makes use of these differences in connectivity in ascribing the roles of pattern separation to the dentate gyrus and autoassociation to CA3 respectively. One way in which these features of the model might be developed further could be (a) by looking at a wider range of different input stimuli and methods of stimulus representation, and (b) in relation to the topography of the perforant path input from different parts of the entorhinal cortex and the very precise lamella organization of the subsequent mossy fibre projection to CA3. Second, the model makes a number of predictions concerning the response properties of hippocampal cells and, towards the end of his chapter, Rolls describes experiments on unit-recording during conditional spatial tasks which support his model. A third interesting feature concerns the role of long-term depression of synaptic efficacy. It has long been realized that matrix memory systems in which synapses can only increase in efficacy would rapidly saturate. Rolls considers two different roles for long-term depression of synaptic weights. He suggests that homosynaptic depression (i.e. depression restricted to synapses which have been activated in a specific way) might play a role in normalization of the synaptic weight vector on each dendrite, while heterosynaptic depression (i.e. depression across all inactive synapses on a dendrite) might play a role in tuning the effectiveness of stimulus categorization. I am inclined to a similar but opposite view! That is, heterosynaptic depression will reduce the synaptic weights at inactive terminals at the same time that active terminals potentiate. Only terminals which are persistently inactive will be driven to their minimal value. The net result will, effectively, be akin to normalization. Conversely, input activity which *might* fire an output cell but which fails to do so because of feedback inhibition realizing the process of competitive learning *should* have its effectiveness weakened. This could be achieved by homosynaptic depression of synaptic weights at terminals active during feedback inhibition. It would be valuable to know more about the mathematical work to which Rolls alludes in his discussion of these aspects of his model. Hopefully, these latter features of the model will stimulate more experimental research on the conditions under which synaptic depression takes place.

Granger and Lynch describe a neural network which has the property of being able to take a second-look at a stimulus or—more literally—a 'second-sniff'. The model concerns pyriform or olfactory cortex and is 'bottom-up' in the sense that it is faithful to the sparseness of the connectivity, the predominantly rostral to caudal flow of feedforward excitatory collateral connections and numerous other properties of pyriform neurons. It also embodies experimentally identified principles of synaptic modifiability, such as the capacity to undergo synaptic potentiation up to some ceiling level in response to inputs patterned at the rat's sniffing frequency. The main findings of the simulation are that multiple samples of the input stimulus (i.e. 'sniffing') gives a serial output whose categorical status changes from coarse-grained to fine-grained over successive sniffs. Put simply, the first sniff indicates the general category of an odour (e.g. a 'fruity' smell) while a second or later sniff gives an output unique to the particular input (e.g. 'banana'). How does it do this?

There are a series of critical propositions. One is that the firing of cells in pyriform cortex puts them into a state where they cannot immediately be fired again by a similar input unless that input is part of a high-frequency burst of activity. This selectivity is achieved as follows: First, cell firing causes a long-lasting after-hyperpolarization which renders the cell unable to fire in response to subsequent single-pulse inputs. Second, inhibitory cells become temporarily refractory after being activated by pyriform cell firing or via feedforward neural input coming along the lateral olfactory tract (LOT) from the olfactory bulb. Thus, a burst input on the LOT causes a series of excitatory postsynaptic potentials (EPSPs) against a background of *both* hyperpolarization *and* refractory feedforward inhibition. Only EPSPs within a burst can accumulate sufficiently to bring the cell to a threshold for synaptic potentiation.

Thus, in 'learning mode' synaptic potentiation occurs on certain postsynaptic cells in response to particular odours. Odour A might give rise to one spatial pattern of potentiation across the pyriform, while odour B will cause a different pattern. A consequence of this potentiation is that, in 'performance mode', odours A' or A″ (similar to A but dissimilar to B) will, on the first sniff, cause a nearly identical pattern of pyriform cell firing to that elicited by A. Thus, the output to A, A', or A″ will differ from that to odours B, B', and B″. This 'categorical response' to odours A, A', and A″ is a consequence of the 'pattern completion' which single layer nets perform so well.

But how does the network distinguish between the similar odours on later sniffs? This part of the model is less completely described but is apparently achieved through appeal to the rostral to caudal flow of collateral feedforward excitatory connections. In the rostral pyriform, the first sniff of odours A and A' will most potently activate 'overlapping' cells which have been maximally potentiated during the learning of A, A', and A″. These cells will then become refractory and, during this period, the second and subsequent sniffs will only be able to fire that subset of non-overlapping cells which are activated by A but not by A', by A' but not by A″ etc., and which have not been potentiated during the earlier learning mode. These cells will then feedforward excitation via diffuse unmyelinated fibres to the caudal pyriform to 'guide' the spatial pattern of potentiation on cells there which happen also to receive a direct input along the LOT. The resulting spatial pattern of potentiation across the caudal pyriform in response to odour A will therefore be a conjunction of input corresponding (1) to odour A itself, and (2) to the differences between odour A and whatever other similar odours were presented during training. In this way, the final output from the caudal pyriform will be a much more fine-grained response to the particular odour differentiating it from other similar odours.

Granger and Lynch's model makes a number of predictions. For example, it predicts that cells in the rostral pyriform should be found which, after training, fire once and are then quiescent and that such cells should show a categorical response to all members of a family of similar smelling odours. Second, it predicts that different response properties should be found for cells in the caudal pyriform. Relevant experiments are underway (Lynch, personal communication, 1988). I do, however, have two worries about the model. First, I do not fully understand how cells in the caudal pyriform come to respond in such a different way to those in more rostral areas and I look forward to seeing more details of the relevant simulations in later papers.

Second, the model can only explain categorization on the basis of stimulus quality and not on the basis of semantic category. I see no way in which cells in any part of the pyriform might come to respond differently to odours as a function of whether they are associated with reward or non-reward. It will be interesting to see whether such differences in response properties emerge in the course of the unit-recording studies currently underway.

## Acknowledgements

I am grateful to Jay Buckingham, Ian Reid, and David Willshaw for their comments on earlier drafts of this introduction.

## References

Allport, D. A. (1980). Patterns and actions: cognitive mechanisms are content specific. In *Cognitive psychology: new directions* (ed. G. Claxton), pp. 26–64. Routledge and Kegan Paul, London.

Bear, M. F., Cooper, L. N., and Ebner, F. F. (1987). A physiological basis for a theory of synapse modification. *Science*, **237**, 42–8.

Bienenstock, E. L., Cooper, L. N., and Munro, P. W. (1982). Theory for the development of neuron selectivity: orientation specificity and binocular interaction in visual cortex. *J. Neurosci.*, **2**, 32–48.

Bliss, T. V. P. and Lomo, T. (1973). Long-term potentiation of synaptic transmission in the dentate area of the anaesthetised rabbit following stimulation of the perforant path. *J. Physiol. (Lond.)*, **232**, 331–56.

Collingridge, G. L. and Bliss, T. V. P. (1987). NMDA receptors—their role in long-term potentiation. *Trends in Neurosci.*, **10**, 288–93.

Cowan, J. D. and Sharp, D. (1988). Neural networks. *Los Alamos Technical Bulletin*, UR-87-4098.

Crick, F. H. C. (1989). The current excitement about neural networks. *Nature*, **337**, 129–32.

Crick, F. H. C. and Asanuma, C. (1986). Certain aspects of the anatomy and physiology of the cerebral cortex. In *Parallel Distributed Processing* (eds. Rumelhart, D. E. and McClelland, J. L.) Vol II, pp. 333–70, Bradford Books, MIT Press, Cambridge.

Gluck, M. and Bower, G. (1988). Evaluating an adaptive network model of human learning. *Journal of Memory and Language*, **27**, 166–95.

Hawkins, R. D. and Kandel, E. R. (1984). Is there a cell-biological alphabet for simple forms of learning? *Psychol. Rev.*, **91**, 375–91.

Hawkins, R. D., Carew, T. J., and Kandel, E. R. (1986). Effects of interstimulus interval on classical conditioning of the siphon withdrawal reflex in *Aplysia*. *J. Neurosci.*, **6**, 1695–701.

Koch, C. (1987). The action of the corticofugal pathway on sensory thalamic nuclei: a hypothesis. *Neuroscience*, **23**, 399–406.

Linsker, R. (1986). From basic network principles to neural architecture. *Proc. Nat, Acd. Sci. USA*, **83**, 7508–12, 8390–4, and 8779–83.

Linsker, R. (1988). Self-organisation in a perceptual network *Computer*, March, 105–17.

Mackintosh, N. J. (1975). A theory of attention: variations in the associability of stimuli with reinforcement. *Psychol. Rev.*, **82**, 276–98.

Marr, D. (1982). *Vision*. W. H. Freeman and Co., San Francisco.

Morris, R. G. M. (1989). Synaptic plasticity, neural architecture and forms of learning. In *Brain organisation and memory: cells, systems and circuits* (eds. J. L. McGaugh, N. M. Weinberger, and G. Lynch). Oxford University Press, New York (in press).

Pellionisz, A. and Llinas, R. (1979). Brain modelling by tensor network theory and computer simulation. The Cerebellum: Distributed processor for predictive coordination. *Neuroscience*, **4**, 323–48.

Poggio, T. quoted in *Time* magazine, 8 August 1988, page 59.

Rescorla, R. A. (1968). Predictability of shock in the presence and absence of CS in fear conditioning. *J. Comp. Physiol. Psych.*, **66**, 1–5.

Rescorla, R. A. and Wagner, A. R. (1972). A theory of Pavlovian conditioning: variations in the effectiveness of reinforcement and nonreinforcement. In *Classical conditioning II: current research and theory* (eds. A. H. Black and W. F. Prokasy). Appleton-Century Crofts, New York.

Rumelhart, D. E. and McClelland, J. L. (1986). *Parallel Distributed Processing*, Vols I and II. Bradford Books, MIT Press, Cambridge.

Sejnowski, T. E., Koch, C., and Churchland, P. (1988). Computational Neuroscience. *Science*, **241**, 1299–306.

Sutherland, N. S. and Mackintosh, N. J. (1971). *Mechanisms of animal discrimination learning*. Academic Press, London.

Willshaw, D. J. and von der Malsburg, C. (1976). How patterned neural connections can be set up by self-organisation. *Proc. Roy. Soc. London. B.*, **194**, 431–45.

Zipser, D. and Andersen, R. A. (1988). A back-propagation programmed network that simulates response properties of a subset of posterior parietal neurons. *Nature*, **331**, 679–84.

# 10

# A biologically realistic neural network model for higher-order features of classical conditioning

## ROBERT D. HAWKINS

Recent advances in computational neuroscience have shown that networks of neuron-like elements with simple learning rules can accomplish impressive cognitive feats (see other chapters in this volume). These networks have similarities to biological nervous systems, but they also have many differences. In this chapter I would like to consider how a real nervous system, that of the marine mollusc *Aplysia californica*, might accomplish some elementary cognitive tasks. Although this nervous system is not capable of speech generation or recognition, it can do more than we might have expected, and it has the advantage that its neural circuitry and physiology are relatively well known.

Research on *Aplysia* and on other invertebrate and simple vertebrate systems over the last two decades has yielded a reasonable understanding of the cellular mechanisms of several simple forms of learning, including habituation, sensitization, classical conditioning, and operant conditioning (for reviews see Carew and Sahley 1986; Byrne 1987; Hawkins, Clark, and Kandel 1987). One result of such research on both *Aplysia* and *Drosophila* is that a mechanism of classical conditioning appears to be an elaboration of a mechanism of a simpler form of learning, sensitization (Duerr and Quinn 1982; Hawkins *et al.* 1983). The results from *Aplysia* are reviewed in Section 1 of this chapter.

The finding that sensitization and classical conditioning appear to be mechanistically related suggested the hypothesis that yet more complex forms of learning might in turn be generated from combinations of an alphabet of the mechanisms of these elementary forms of learning (Hawkins and Kandel 1984). The higher-order features of classical conditioning provide an attractive area in which to investigate this hypothesis, for two reasons. First, these features of conditioning have a cognitive flavour (in the sense that the animal's behaviour is thought to depend on a comparison of current sensory input with an internal representation of the world) and they may therefore provide a bridge between basic conditioning and more advanced forms of learning (Kamin 1969; Rescorla 1978; Wagner 1978; Mackintosh 1983;

Dickinson 1980). Second, some of these features of conditioning have been demonstrated in invertebrates, where a cellular analysis of their mechanisms may be feasible (Sahley, Rudy, and Gelperin 1981; Colwill 1985; Hawkins, Carew, and Kandel 1986; Farley 1987).

In a theoretical paper, Eric Kandel and I suggested how several of the higher-order features of conditioning could be accounted for by combinations of the mechanisms of habituation, sensitization, and classical conditioning in the basic neural circuit for the *Aplysia* gill-withdrawal reflex (Hawkins and Kandel 1984). Since the arguments in that paper were entirely qualitative, however, quantitative modelling seemed desirable. In Sections 2–4 of this chapter, I describe quantitative modelling based on the ideas Kandel and I presented earlier. As in our previous paper, I have restricted myself to cellular processes and circuitry which are known to exist in *Aplysia*, rather than using hypothetical 'neuron-like' elements or algebraic learning rules. Although this decision is somewhat arbitrary, I feel that it is important, since the ultimate goal of neuroscientists is to understand how real neurons and circuits generate complex behaviours. The specific ideas I present are somewhat speculative and may turn out to be wrong, but they illustrate an initial approach to the problem of accounting for cognitive processes in biological terms.

## 1. Behavioural and cellular studies of learning in Aplysia

Studies of learning in *Aplysia* have focused on the defensive withdrawal reflexes of the external organs of the mantle cavity. In *Aplysia* and in other molluscs, the mantle cavity, a respiratory chamber housing the gill, is covered by a protective sheet, the mantle shelf, which terminates in a fleshy spout, the siphon. When the siphon or mantle shelf is stimulated by touch, the siphon, mantle shelf, and gill all contract vigorously and withdraw into the mantle cavity. This reflex is analogous to vertebrate defensive escape and withdrawal responses, which can be modified by experience. Unlike vertebrate withdrawal reflexes, however, the *Aplysia* withdrawal reflex is partly monosynaptic—siphon sensory neurons synapse directly on gill and siphon motor neurons (Fig. 10.1). None the less, this simple reflex can be modified by two forms of non-associative learning, habituation and sensitization, as well as two forms of associative learning classical and operant conditioning. The neural mechanisms of habituation, sensitization, and classical conditioning have been partially analysed at the cellular and molecular levels.

*Habituation*

In habituation, perhaps the simplest form of learning, an animal learns to ignore a weak stimulus that is repeatedly presented when the consequences of

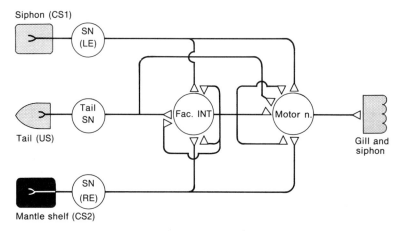

Siphon (CS1)

SN (LE)

Tail SN

Tail (US)

Fac. INT

Motor n.

Gill and siphon

SN (RE)

Mantle shelf (CS2)

**Fig. 10.1**  Partial neuronal circuit for the *Aplysia* gill- and siphon-withdrawal reflex and its modification by tail stimulation. Mechanosensory neurons (SN) from the siphon (LE cluster), mantle (RE cluster) and tail excite gill and siphon motor neurons. The sensory neurons also excite facilitator interneurons which produce pre-synaptic facilitation at all the terminals of the sensory neurons. Approximately 25 siphon sensory neurons, 25 gill and siphon motor neurons, and 5 facilitator interneurons have been identified (Byrne *et al.* 1974; Kupfermann *et al.* 1974; Perlman 1979; Frost *et al.* 1985*b*; Hawkins *et al.* 1981; Mackey *et al.* 1986). Several other interneurons which are not included in this diagram have also been described (Hawkins *et al.* 1981; Byrne 1981; Mackey *et al.* 1987).

the stimulus are neither noxious nor rewarding. Thus, an *Aplysia* will initially respond to a tactile stimulus to the siphon by briskly withdrawing its gill and siphon. But with repeated exposure to the stimulus, the animal will exhibit reflex responses that are reduced to a fraction of their initial value. Habituation can last from minutes to weeks, depending on the number and pattern of stimulations (Carew, Pinsker, and Kandel 1972; Pinsker *et al.* 1970).

At the cellular level, the short-term (minutes–hours) form of habituation involves a depression of transmitter release at the synapses that the siphon sensory neurons make on gill and siphon motor neurons and interneurons (Castellucci and Kandel 1974; Castellucci *et al.* 1970). This depression is thought to involve a decrease in the amoung of $Ca^{++}$ that flows into the terminals of the sensory neurons with each action potential (Klein *et al.* 1980). Since $Ca^{++}$ influx determines how much transmitter is released, a decrease in $Ca^{++}$ influx would result in decreased release (Fig. 10.2(a)). Recent evidence suggests that habituation may also involve depletion of releasable transmitter pools (Bailey and Chen 1985; Gingrich and Byrne 1985).

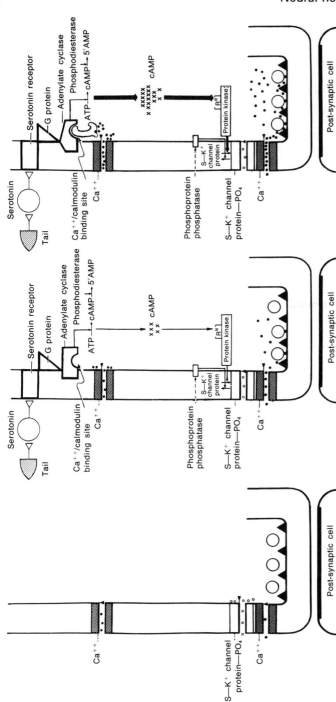

**Fig. 10.2** Cellular mechanisms contributing to habituation, sensitization, and classical conditioning of the *Aplysia* gill- and siphon-withdrawal reflex. (a) Habituation. Repeated stimulation of a siphon sensory neuron, the pre-synaptic cell in the diagram, produces prolonged inactivation of Ca$^{++}$ channels in that neuron (represented by the closed gates), leading to a decrease in Ca$^{++}$ influx during each action potential and decreased transmitter release. (b) Sensitization. Stimulation of the tail produces prolonged inactivation of K$^{+}$ channels in the siphon sensory neuron through a sequence of steps involving cAMP and protein phosphorylation. Closing these K$^{+}$ channels produces broadening of subsequent action potentials, which in turn produces an increase in Ca$^{++}$ influx and increased transmitter release. (c) Classical conditioning. Tail stimulation produces amplified facilitation of transmitter release from the siphon sensory neuron if the tail stimulation is preceded by action potentials in the sensory neuron. This effect may be due to priming of the adenyl cyclase by Ca$^{++}$ that enters the sensory neuron during the action potentials, so that the cyclase produces more cAMP when it is activated by the tail stimulation.

*Sensitization*

Sensitization is a somewhat more complex form of non-associative learning in which an animal learns to strengthen its defensive reflexes and to respond vigorously to a variety of previously weak or neutral stimuli after it has been exposed to a potentially threatening or noxious stimulus. Thus, if a noxious sensitizing stimulus is presented to the neck or tail, the siphon- and gill-withdrawal reflexes will be enhanced, as will inking, walking, and other defensive behaviours (Pinsker *et al.* 1970; Walters, Carew, and Kandel 1981). This enhancement persists from minutes to weeks depending on the number and intensity of the sensitizing stimuli (Pinsker *et al.* 1973; Frost *et al.* 1985*a*).

The short-term (minutes–hours) form of sensitization involves the same cellular locus as habituation, the synapses that the sensory neurons make on their central target cells, and again the learning process involves an alteration in transmitter release—in this case an enhancement in the amount released (Castellucci and Kandel 1976; Castellucci *et al.* 1970). But sensitization uses more complex molecular machinery. This machinery has at least five steps (Figs. 10.1 and 10.2(b)). 1. Stimulating the tail activates a group of facilitator neurons which synapse on or near the terminals of the sensory neurons and act there to enhance transmitter release. This process is called *pre-synaptic facilitation.* 2. The transmitters released by the facilitator neurons, which include serotonin, a small peptide (SCP), and an unknown transmitter, activate an adenylate cyclase which increases the level of free cyclic AMP in the terminals of the sensory neurons. 3. Elevation of free cyclic AMP, in turn, activates a second enzyme, a cAMP-dependent protein kinase. 4. The kinase acts by means of protein phosphorylation to close a particular type of $K^+$ channel and thereby decreases the total number of $K^+$ channels that are open during the action potential. 5. A decrease in $K^+$ current leads to broadening of subsequent action potentials, which allows a greater amount of $Ca^{++}$ to flow into the terminal and thus enhances transmitter release (Kandel and Schwartz 1982; Klein and Kandel 1980; Siegelbaum, Camardo, and Kandel 1982; Castellucci *et al.* 1982; Bernier *et al.* 1982; Hawkins, Castellucci, and Kandel 1981; Kistler *et al.* 1985; Abrams *et al.* 1984; Glanzman, Mackey, and Kandel 1986; Mackey, Hawkins, and Kandel 1986). Recent evidence suggests that sensitization may also involve mobilization of transmitter to release sites, perhaps through $Ca^{2+}$/calmodulin- or $Ca^{2+}$/phospholipid-dependent protein phosphorylation (Gingrich and Byrne 1985; Hochner *et al.* 1986*a,b*; Boyle *et al.* 1984; Sacktor *et al.* 1986). The neural circuit for the gill- and siphon-withdrawal reflex also includes other sites of plasticity that could contribute to sensitization (Jacklet and Rine 1977; Kanz *et al.* 1979; Hawkins, Castellucci and Kandel 1981; Frost and Kandel 1984; Forst, Clark, and Kandel 1985*b*). Finally, in addition to producing sensitization, noxious stimuli can also produce transient *inhibition* of the gill- and siphon-withdrawal reflex (Mackey *et al.* 1987; Marcus *et al.* 1987; Krontiris-Litowitz, Erickson, and Walters 1987). This effect appears to be due in part to activation of FMRFamide neurons which produce pre-synaptic inhibition of the siphon sensory cells by acting through a different second-messenger system, the metabolites of arachidonic acid (Piomelli *et al.* 1987; Mackey *et al.* 1987).

*Classical conditioning*

Classical conditioning resembles sensitization in that the response to a stimulus in one pathway is enhanced by activity in another. In classical conditioning an initially weak or ineffective conditioned stimulus (CS) becomes highly effective in producing a behavioural response after it has been paired temporally with a strong unconditioned stimulus (US). Often a reflex can be modified by both sensitization and classical conditioning. In such cases, the response enhancement produced by classical conditioning (paired presentation of the CS and US) is greater and/or lasts longer than the enhancement produced by sensitization (presentation of the US alone). Moreover, whereas the consequences of sensitization are broad and affect defensive responses to a range of stimuli, the effects of classical conditioning are specific and enhance only responses to stimuli that are paired with the US.

In conditioning of the *Aplysia* withdrawal response, the unconditioned stimulus is a strong shock to the tail that produces a powerful set of defensive responses; the conditioned stimulus is a weak stimulus to the siphon that produces a feeble response. After repeated pairing of the CS and US, the CS becomes more effective and elicits a strong gill- and siphon-withdrawal reflex. Enhancement of this reflex is acquired in less than 15 trials, is retained for days, extinquishes with repeated presentation of the CS alone, and recovers with rest (Carew, Walters, and Kandel 1981). The siphon-withdrawal reflex can also be differentially conditioned using stimuli to the siphon and mantle shelf as the discriminative stimuli. Using this procedure, we have found that a single training trial is sufficient to produce significant learning, and that the learning becomes progressively more robust with more training trials (Carew, Hawkins, and Kandel 1983). We also found significant conditioning when the onset of the CS preceded the onset of the US by 0.5 s, and marginally significant conditioning when the interval between the CS and the US was extended to 1.0 s. In contrast, no significant learning occurred when the CS preceded the US by 2 s or more, when the two stimuli were stimultaneous, or, in backward conditioning, when the US onset preceded the CS by 0.5 s or more (Hawkins, Carew, and Kandel 1986). Thus, conditioning in *Aplysia* resembles conditioning in vertebrates in having a steep interstimulus interval (ISI) function, with optimal learning when the CS precedes the US by approximately 0.5 s (e.g. Gormezano 1972).

What cellular processes give classical conditioning this characteristic stimulus and temporal specificity? Evidence obtained over the past several years indicates that classical conditioning of the withdrawal reflex involves a pairing-specific enhancement of pre-synaptic facilitation. In classical conditioning the sensory neurons of the CS pathway fire action potentials just before the facilitator neurons of the US pathway become active. Using a reduced preparation we have found that if action potentials are generated in a sensory neuron just before the US is delivered, the US produces substantially more facilitation of the synaptic potential from the sensory neuron to a motor neuron than if the US is not paired with activity in the sensory neuron or if the order of the two stimuli is reversed (Hawkins et al. 1983; Clark 1984). Pairing spike activity in a sensory neuron with the US also produces greater broadening of the action potential and greater reduction of the outward current in the sensory neuron than unpaired stimulation, indicating that the enhancement of facilitation occurs pre-synaptically (Hawkins et al. 1983; Hawkins and Abrams 1984). Thus, at least some aspects of the mechanism for classical conditioning occur within the sensory neuron itself. We have called this type of enhancement *activity-dependent amplification of pre-synaptic facilitation*. Similar cellular results have been obtained independently by Walters and Byrne (1983), who have found activity-dependent synaptic facilitation in identified sensory neurons that innervate the tail of *Aplysia*. By contrast, Carew et al. (1984) have found that a different type of synaptic plasticity first postulated by Hebb (1949), which has often been thought to underlie learning, does *not* occur at the sensory neuron–motor neuron synapses in the siphon-withdrawal circuit. Plasticity at other sites in the reflex circuit may, however, also contribute to conditioning (Lukowiak 1986; Colebrook and Lukowiak 1988).

These experiments indicate that a mechanism of classical conditioning of the withdrawal reflex is an elaboration of the mechanism of sensitization of the reflex: pre-synaptic facilitation caused by an increase in action-potential duration and $Ca^{++}$ influx in the sensory neurons. The pairing-specificity characteristic of classical conditioning results because the pre-synaptic facilitation is augmented or amplified by temporally paired spike activity in the sensory neurons. We do not yet know what aspect of the action potential in a sensory neuron interacts with the process of pre-synaptic facilitation to amplify it, nor which step in the biochemical cascade leading to pre-synaptic facilitation is sensitive to the action potential. Preliminary results suggest that the influx of $Ca^{++}$ with each action potential provides the signal for activity, and that it interacts with the cAMP cascade so that serotonin produces more cAMP (Fig. 10.2(c)). Thus, brief application of serotonin to the sensory cells can substitute for tail shock as the US in the cellular experiments, and $Ca^{++}$ must be present in the external medium for paired spike activity to enhance the effect of the serotonin (Abrams 1985; Abrams et al. 1983). Furthermore, serotonin produces a greater increase in cAMP levels in siphon sensory cells if it is preceded by spike activity in the sensory cells than if it is not (Kandel *et al.* 1983; see also Occor, Walters, and Byrne, 1985, for a similar result in *Aplysia* tail sensory neurons). Finally, experiments on a cell-free membrane homogenate preparation have shown that the adenyl cyclase is stimulated by both $Ca^{2+}$ and serotonin, consistent with the idea that the cyclase is a point of convergence of the CS and US inputs (Abrams *et al.* 1985).

## 2. A computational model for higher-order features of classical conditioning

The quantitative model I have developed to simulate various aspects of conditioning incorporates the neural circuit shown in Fig. 10.1 and the cellular processes illustrated in Fig. 10.2. On the cellular level, my model is very similar to the single-cell model of Gingrich and Byrne (1987) for conditioning. Basically, I have attempted to plug a simplified version of Gingrich and Byrne's single-cell model into a small neural circuit, to see whether the resulting circuit properties could account for higher-order features of classical conditioning. Unlike Gingrich and Byrne, I have not tried to fit a particular set of empirical data, since some of the features of conditioning addressed have not yet been tested in *Aplysia*. Rather, my goal is to show that these higher-order features of conditioning could in principle be generated in the manner I suggest.

The cellular processes in my model were made as simple as possible to reduce both free parameters and computation time, and are therefore only approximations of reality. Thus, most of the cellular processes are assumed to be linear, which is probably not accurate. Also, in the version described in this paper, habituation is assumed to be due solely to $Ca^{2+}$ channel inactivation and sensitization to spike broadening, although experimental evidence suggests that transmitter depletion and mobilization are also involved. This choice was not critical, however, since an alternative version based solely on transmitter handling produced similar results for most of the features of conditioning discussed. Free parameters in the model were adjusted by trial and error so that one set of parameters would produce strong conditioning with as many higher-order features as possible. None of the parameter values appeared to be critical within a factor of 2, although this point was not investigated systematically.

Time is modelled as a series of discrete units, which are conceived of as being the same length as the stimulus durations. No attempt has been made to model events (such as the interstimulus interval function) with a greater time resolution. In each time unit *CS1*, *CS2*, the US, or any combination of these stimuli can occur. A stimulus produces one or more action potentials in the corresponding sensory neuron. Stimulus strength is coded by the number of action potentials produced—in most of the simulations shown, *CS1* and *CS2* each have strengths of 1 arbitrary unit and produce one action potential, and the US has a strength of 6 arbitrary units and produces six action potentials. Synaptic depression is assumed to be independent of the number of action potentials produced (this is approximately true since the depression is partially offset by a homosynaptic facilitatory process not modelled here—see Gingrich and Byrne 1985). Thus, if a sensory neuron is activated, the number (*N*) of available calcium channels in that neuron decreases by a fixed percentage:

$$\Delta N = -C1 \times N \tag{10.1}$$

where *C1* is a constant, and this number recovers by another fixed percentage during each time unit:

$$N(t+1) = N(t) + C2(N_{max} - N(t)) \tag{10.2}$$

The duration of each action potential in a sensory neuron is assumed to be proportional to the cAMP level in that neuron plus one:

$$Dur = (1 + C3) \times cAMP \tag{10.3}$$

and calcium influx per action potential is proportional to the action potential duration times the number of available calcium channels:

$$Ca = Dur \times N/N_{max} \tag{10.4}$$

To keep the equations as simple as possible, transmitter release from each sensory neuron is assumed to be linear with calcium influx, and the resultant PSP in both the motor neuron and the facilitator neuron is linear with the total transmitter released by all of the sensory neurons:

$$PSP = C4 \times \sum Ca \tag{10.5}$$

The facilitator neuron fires a number of action potentials equal to the difference between the PSP and a threshold:

$$Spikes = PSP - Thresh \quad \text{if} \quad PSP > Thresh, \text{ 0 otherwise} \tag{10.6}$$

The facilitator neuron threshold is variable, and is set equal to a fraction of the PSP level during the *preceding* time unit:

$$Thresh\ (t) = C5 \times PSP(t-1) \tag{10.7}$$

This has the effect of causing accommodation of facilitator neuron firing during a prolonged input. Spikes in the facilitator release transmitter which causes an increase in cAMP levels in the sensory neurons according to the following equation:

$$\Delta cAMP = C6 \times Spikes \times [1 + (C7 \times Ca(t-1))] \tag{10.8}$$

where $[1+(C7 \times Ca(t-1))]$ represents 'priming' of the adenyl cyclase by calcium influx in the sensory neuron during the *preceding* time unit. cAMP levels then decay by a fixed percentage during each time unit:

$$cAMP(t+1) = C8 \times cAMP(t) \tag{10.9}$$

In the simulations shown in this paper, the initial values are as follows:

$$N = N_{max}$$
$$cAMP = 0$$
$$Thresh = 0$$
$$Ca = 0$$

and the parameter values are as follows:

$$C1 = 0.15$$
$$C2 = 0.005$$
$$C3 = 1.0$$
$$C4 = 7.5$$
$$C5 = 0.9$$
$$C6 = 0.002$$
$$C7 = 15.0$$
$$C8 = 0.9975$$

To minimize computation time, the time unit is 10 s (very similar results were obtained in Fig. 10.3 with a 1 s unit, which is more realistic). With these parameters, the time constant for decay of cAMP levels is approximately 1 h, and the time constant for recovery from calcium channel inactivation is approximately 30 min. The output of the model is the amplitude of the PSP in the motor neuron. I have not specified the function which relates PSP amplitude to behaviour (gill and siphon contraction), but for most purposes this is assumed to be linear.

### 3. Simulations of basic features of conditioning

*Acquisition*

Figure 10.3 shows a simulation of acquisition and extinction of a conditioned response by the model described in Section 2. The results of the simulation are qualitatively similar to results obtained with real *Aplysia* (Carew, Walters, and Kandel 1981), but they have been made quantitatively more dramatic for illustrative purposes. In the hypothetical experiment shown in Fig. 10.3 there is a pre-test, five paired trials with the CS preceding the US by 1 time unit, five extinction trials, and a post-test. The intertrial interval is 5 min. The ordinate shows the amplitude of the PSP produced in the motor neuron each time a

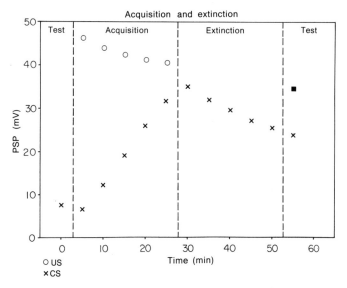

**Fig. 10.3** Simulation of acquisition and extinction. The ordinate shows the amplitude of the PSP produced in the motor neuron each time a stimulus (CS or US) occurs in a hypothetical conditioning experiment with five training trials and five extinction trials. $\bigcirc$ = US, $\times$ = CS, $\blacksquare$ = response to the CS at that time if the five extinction trials are omitted. CS strength = 1 arbitrary unit, US strength = 6 arbitrary units, ITI = 5 min.

stimulus (CS or US) occurs. Conditioning in this simulation is due to activity-dependent amplification of pre-synaptic facilitation of the PSP from the CS sensory neuron to the motor neuron (Equations (10.3), (10.4), (10.5), (10.6), and (10.8)).

Psychologists sometimes distinguish between increasing the amplitude of a pre-existing response to the CS ('alpha conditioning') and learning a new response ('beta conditioning'). In the simulation, conditioning produces an enhancement of a pre-existing PSP in the motor neuron ('alpha conditioning'). However, if there were a threshold PSP amplitude for producing a behavioural response (of, for example, 15 mV), conditioning would lead to the development of a new response to the CS at the behavioural level ('beta conditioning'). These results suggest that there is no fundamental difference between 'alpha' and 'beta' conditioning, but, rather, the apparent difference between the two may depend on how the response is measured.

As in many instances of real conditioning (e.g. Carew, Walters, and Kandel 1981), the acquisition function illustrated in Fig. 10.3 is slightly S-shaped. The initial acceleration (which is more evident with weaker CSs—see Fig.10.14) is due to positive feedback in the calcium priming process: the first conditioning trial produces broadening of the action potential in the sensory neuron and hence an increase in calcium priming of the cAMP cascade on the second conditioning trial (Equations (10.3), (10.4), and (10.8)). This produces greater broadening of the action potential and greater calcium priming on the third trial, etc. The deceleration in acquisition occurs as the response evoked by the CS approaches that evoked by the US. This leads to decreased effectiveness of the US due to accommodation in the facilitator neuron (see the discussion of blocking, below), so that the response to the CS asymptotes at approximately the level of the response to the US.

*Extinction*

Extinction in this model is assumed to have the same cellular mechanism as habituation—synaptic depression due to inactivation of $Ca^{2+}$ channels (Equation (10.1)). Any stimulus (CS or US) thus tends to activate two competing processes in the stimulated sensory neurons: depression, which is intrinsic to those neurons, and facilitation, which is caused by excitation of the facilitator neuron. The net result depends on the balance of these two processes. The parameters in these simulations were chosen so that depression would predominate with repetition of either the CS or the US by itself, leading to gradual extinction or habituation of responding.

Extinction has a number of features in common with habituation, which are simulated by the model. For example, if the CS is not presented for some time following extinction, the animal's response to the CS recovers, indicating that the animal remembers the original training (Carew, Walters, and Kandel 1981). This effect, which is called spontaneous recovery, can be accounted for by recovery from $Ca^{2+}$ channel inactivation (Equation (10.2)). The response to the CS can also be restored by presentation of a strong extraneous stimulus. Pavlov (1927) referred to this phenomenon as 'disinhibition', because he thought that extinction was due to inhibition which the extraneous stimulus removed. In the model described here, however, 'disinhibition' is accounted for by the same cellular process as dishabituation—pre-synaptic facilitation of the sensory neuron.

A conditioned response may lose its strength not only through extinction, but also through the simple passage of time or forgetting. The filled square in Fig. 10.3 shows the small amount of forgetting that would have occurred in this simulation if the five extinction trials had been omitted. Forgetting in the simulation is due to the gradual decline in cAMP levels in the sensory neuron following training (Equation (10.9)).

*Differential conditioning*

The stimulation shown in Fig. 10.3 illustrates the effect of paired training on the response to the CS. However, control procedures are necessary to demonstrate that an increase in responding to the CS is associative in nature.

The model successfully simulates a number of control procedures that have been used in real *Aplysia* (Carew, Walters, and Kandel 1981; Carew, Hawkins, and Kandel 1983; Hawkins, Carew, and Kandel 1986). For example, simulations with the CS and US occurring either by themselves or explicitly unpaired produce little or no increase in responding to the CS (post-test = 62 per cent, 126 per cent, and 84 per cent of pre-test respectively). Moreover, the rank order of effectiveness of various training procedures (Paired > US-alone > No training ≈ Unpaired > CS-alone) is the same in the simulations as in real experiments (Carew, Walters, and Kandel 1981). In the simulations this is because CS-alone training produces habituation, US-alone training produces sensitization, unpaired training produces a combination of the two, and paired training produces an amplification of sensitization.

Figure 10.4 shows a simulation of another type of control procedure, differential conditioning. In this experiment, two CSs which activate different sensory neurons are used (Fig. 10.1). During training, one CS is paired with the US and the other CS is given unpaired with the US. The response to the paired CS shows a large increase, whereas the response to the unpaired CS shows none, demonstrating the associative nature of the learning. In

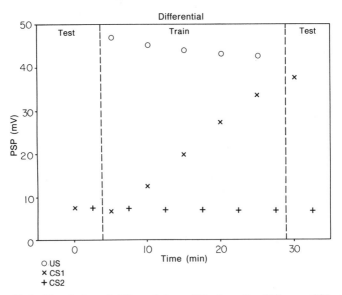

**Fig. 10.4**  Simulation of differential conditioning: ○ = US; × = CS1; + = CS2.

differential conditioning with real *Aplysia*, there is frequently also some increase in responding to the unpaired CS, which can be attributed to the non-associative process of sensitization (e.g. Carew *et al.* 1983). An interesting result of the model is that the relative amounts of conditioning and sensitization depend entirely on the priming factor, $C7$. Thus, differences in the magnitude of that factor could explain why conditioning produces different amounts of sensitization in different animals or different experiments. Another result which is frequently observed in differential conditioning experiments is an initial increase in responding to the unpaired CS, followed by a decrease. This effect is not observed in the simulation shown in Fig. 10.4, in which each CS excites one sensory neuron. However, it can be simulated if the two CSs are assumed to excite overlapping sets of sensory neurons ($CS1 = SN1$, $SN2$ and $CS2 = SN2$, $SN3$—see Fig. 10.5). As previously suggested by Rescorla and

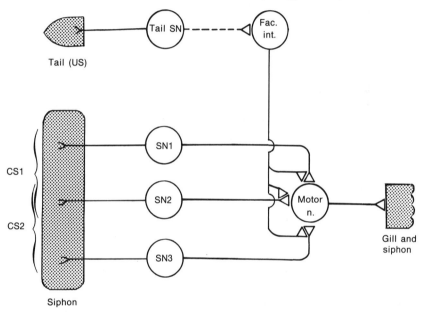

**Fig. 10.5**  Proposed cellular mechanisms of stimulus specificity and generalization. CS1 excites sensory neurons 1 and 2, and CS2 excites neurons 2 and 3. Only those sensory neurons that are active preceding the US undergo the amplfed form of pre-synaptic facilitation. Thus, conditioning of CS1 produces partial, but not complete, generalization to CS2. Some of the synaptic connections shown in Fig. 10.1 have been omitted to simplify the wiring diagram.

Wagner (1972), the shared sensory neuron may be thought of as responding to the stimuli that are always present in the experimental situation (the background stimuli). The use of such compound stimuli in the simulations produces a biphasic learning curve for the unpaired CS, primarily because it produces a similar biphasic curve for the shared sensory neuron ($SN2$), which is in effect 'overshadowed' by $SN1$ (see the discussion of overshadowing below).

*Generalization*

As demonstrated by differential conditioning, animals learn to respond to the conditioned stimulus and not to other irrelevant stimuli. Activity-dependent enhancement of pre-synaptic facilitation readily confers this stimulus specificity: only those sensory neurons that are active preceding the US undergo the amplified form of pre-synaptic facilitation, and thus only the response to the paired conditioned stimulus is selectively enhanced (Fig. 10.4).

Stimulus specificity is not generally complete, however. After conditioning, animals will respond to stimuli other than the conditioned stimulus, and the strength of the response will depend on the degree of similarity between the test stimulus and the conditioned stimulus. The model includes two cellular explanations for stimulus generalization. The first is sensitization: an aversive unconditioned stimulus will produce some enhancement of defensive responses to *all* stimuli, whether they are paired with it or not. This enhancement will simply be greater for the paired stimuli. The second explanation (which is basically similar to those proposed by Bush and Mosteller (1951) and Atkinson and Estes (1963) is that there will be some overlap in the sensory neurons and interneurons excited by different stimuli (Fig. 10.5). Thus, conditioning of one stimulus will produce amplified pre-synaptic facilitation of some (but not all) of the neurons that are excited by a second stimulus, and will therefore produce partial enhancement of the response to the second stimulus. The greater the similarity between the stimuli, the more overlap there will be in the neurons they excite, and consequently the more generalization.

A simulation of generalization based on these ideas is shown in Fig. 10.6. In this simulation, $CS1$ excites sensory neurons 1 and 2 and $CS2$ excites sensory neurons 2 and 3. Conditioning $CS1$ leads to an increase in responding to $CS2$ in part because of sensitization caused by presentation of the US during training, and in part because the two stimuli excite a common sensory neuron that undergoes activity-dependent enhancement of pre-synaptic facilitation during conditioning (Fig. 10.5). Clearly, this mechanism could account for a wider range of generalization if it occurred at sensory interneurons as well as at primary sensory neurons.

## 4. Simulations of higher-order features of conditioning

In addition to the basic features described above, classical conditioning has several higher-order features which are thought to have a cognitive flavour. Some of these were first described by Pavlov and the early students of associative learning; others have been described more recently by Kamin, Rescorla, Wagner, and others who have been interested in the cognitive or

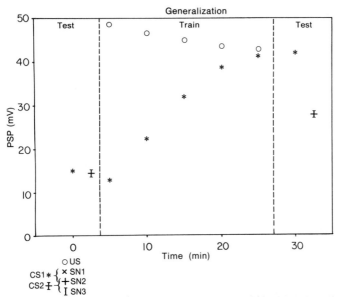

**Fig. 10.6** Simulation of generalization: ○ = US; × = SN1 (sensory neuron 1); + = SN2; I = SN3. CS1 excites SN1 and SN2, and CS2 excites SN2 and SN3.

information-processing aspects of learning. According to this view, in a classical conditioning experiment the animal builds an internal representation of the external world, compares this representation with reality—with the view of the world as validated by current sensory information—and then modifies its behaviour accordingly (Dickinson 1980; Kamin 1969; Mackintosh 1983; Rescorla 1978; Wagner 1978).

In the light of the evidence for a cellular relationship between habituation, sensitization, and classical conditioning, it is interesting to examine the possibility that a cellular alphabet exists for a variety of learning processes. Can combinations of the elementary mechanisms used in habituation, sensitization, and conditioning account for additional higher-order aspects of associative learning without requiring additional cellular mechanisms? Here I shall consider five higher-order features: (1) second-order conditioning; (2) blocking; (3) overshadowing; (4) contingency effects; and (5) pre-exposure effects. The explanations proposed for these phenomena are not meant to be exclusive. Rather, I wish only to indicate how simple cellular processes, such as synaptic depression and facilitation, could be used in different combinatorial ways to contribute to these higher-order features of behaviour.

*Second-order conditioning*

A second-order conditioning experiment has two stages: in Stage I *CS*1 is paired with the US, and then in Stage II a second CS (*CS*2) is paired with *CS*1.

As Pavlov (1927) noted, this procedure can lead to an associative increase in responding to *CS2*. Thus, in effect, as a result of the conditioning in Stage I, *CS1* acquires the ability to act as a US in Stage II. Second-order conditioning is thought to be ubiquitous in everyday life and to bridge the gap between laboratory experiments and complex natural behaviour, which often does not have obvious reinforcers. Second-order conditioning also illustrates the interchangeability of the CS and US, since the same stimulus can serve as either a CS or a US in a conditioning experiment.

Second-order conditioning might be explained by two features of the neural circuit shown in Fig. 10.1. First, in addition to being excited by the US, the facilitator neuron is also excited by the CS sensory neurons. Second, the facilitator neuron produces facilitation not only at the synapses from the sensory neurons to the motor neurons but also at the synapses from the sensory neurons to the facilitator neuron itself. This fact has the interesting consequence that the sensory–facilitator synapses (unlike the sensory–motor synapses) should act like Hebb synapses. According to this idea, firing a sensory neuron just before firing the facilitator produces selective strengthening of the synapses from that sensory neuron to the facilitator. As a result, during Stage I conditioning, *CS1* acquires a greater ability to excite the facilitator, allowing it to act as a US in Stage II.

Figure 10.7 shows a simulation of second-order conditioning based on this

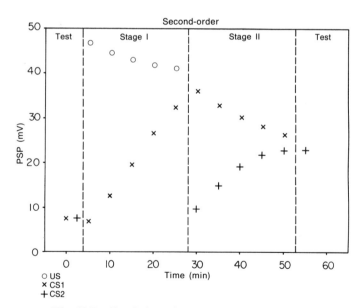

**Fig. 10.7** Simulation of second-order conditioning.

mechanism. During Stage II, the response to $CS2$ increases while $CS1$ undergoes extinction. As controls, $CS2$ does not condition in Stage II if $CS1$ is presented unpaired with the US in Stage I, or if $CS2$ is presented unpaired with $CS1$ in Stage II.

*Blocking*

Like a second-order conditioning experiment, a blocking experiment has two stages. In Stage I, $CS1$ is paired with the US as usual. In Stage II, $CS2$ is added to $CS1$ and the compound stimulus $CS1$, $CS2$ is paired with the US. As Kamin (1969) noted, this procedure generally produces little conditioning of $CS2$, even though good conditioning of $CS2$ occurs if $CS1$ is omitted in Stage II or if $CS1$ was not previously conditioned in Stage I. Thus, simultaneous presentation with a previously conditioned stimulus ($CS1$) 'blocks' conditioning of a naïve stimulus ($CS2$).

The discovery of blocking was very influential in the history of thinking about conditioning, because blocking demonstrates that animals may *not* acquire a conditioned response despite many pairings of the CS and US. This result suggests that conditioning is not simply an automatic outcome of stimulus pairing, but may instead involve cognitive processes. For example, Kamin (1969) proposed that an animal forms expectations about the world, compares current input with those expectations, and learns only when something unpredicted occurs. Because $CS1$ comes to predict the US in the first stage of training, in the second stage the compound $CS1$, $CS2$ is not followed by anything unexpected and, therefore, little conditioning occurs.

Rescorla and Wagner (1972) have formalized this explanation by suggesting that the associative strength of a CS in effect subtracts from the strength of a US with which it is paired (see the Discussion at the end of this chapter). In the neural model, this subtraction function is accomplished by accommodation of firing in the facilitator neuron (Fig. 10.8). Thus, as the synapses from $CS1$ to the facilitator become strengthened during Stage I training, the facilitator fires progressively more during $CS1$ and less during the US, due to accommodation caused by $CS1$ (Equations (10.6) and (10.7)). This process reaches an asymptote when there is just enough firing left during the US to counteract $CS1$ habituation. When training with the compound stimulus $CS1$, $CS2$ starts in the second stage of training, $CS2$ is followed by very little firing in the facilitator neuron and therefore does not become conditioned. Firing of the facilitator neuron at the onset of $CS2$ does not produce activity-dependent facilitation, because that process requires a delay between CS onset and the onset of facilitation (Equation (10.8)).

Blocking illustrates how the model incorporates, in very rudimentary forms, the notions of predictability and internal representation. The predicted effect of $CS1$ is represented internally as the strength of the synapse from $CS1$

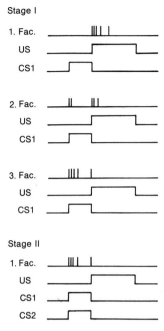

**Fig. 10.8** Proposed cellular mechanism of blocking. As conditioning of CS1 proceeds (Stage I, Trials 1, 2, and 3), the facilitator neuron fires more during the conditioned stimulus (CS) period. This firing produces accommodation which reduces firing during the US period. When compound conditioning starts (Stage II), CS2 is followed by little firing of the facilitator neuron and therefore does not become conditioned.

to the facilitator neuron. The actual consequences of *CS*1 are compared to this prediction through the process of accommodation, which in effect subtracts the associative strength of *CS*1 from the strength of the US that follows it. As these two strengths become equal, *CS*1 can be said to predict the US, which thus loses its reinforcing power, and no further learning occurs. This subtraction process also explains why the response to the CS asymptotes at approximately the level of the response to the US during normal acquisition (see Fig. 10.3)).

Figure 10.9 shows a simulation of blocking. Following Stage II training there is very little conditioning of *CS*2, while *CS*1 retains the associative strength it acquired in Stage I. As control, *CS*2 undergoes substantially more conditioning during Stage II if *CS*1 occurs unpaired with the US in Stage I, or if *CS*1 occurs separately from *CS*2 and the US during Stage II.

In the simulation shown in Fig. 10.9 (with five trials in Stage I and five trials in Stage II) the small increase in responding to *CS*2 is actually due to sensitization which occurs during stage I, and there is *no* increase in

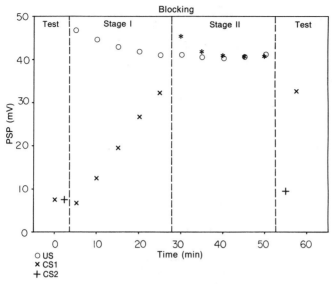

**Fig. 10.9** Simulation of blocking. * = simultaneous occurrence of CS1 and CS2.

responding to *CS2* during Stage II, i.e., blocking is complete. Kamin (1969) noted that blocking is usually less complete if there are fewer training trials in Stage I, and that most of the conditioning that occurs in Stage II occurs on the first trial. In a simulation of blocking with the model described here with only three trials in Stage I and five trials in Stage II, there was some conditioning in Stage II, and approximately 75 per cent of that conditioning occurred on the first trial.

Gluck and Thompson (1987) have reported some difficulty in simulating blocking with a quantitative model based on the ideas suggested by Hawkins and Kandel (1984). Although the Gluck and Thompson model is basically similar to the one described here, it differs in many details. In particular, it is formulated at the level of algebraic synaptic learning rules rather than molecular processes. Gluck and Thompson (1987) note that blocking is much more successful in their model if they assume an S-shaped acquisition function, rather than a decelerating acquisition function (which was their initial assumption). This observation may help to explain why the model described here simulates blocking with little difficulty. An S-shaped acquisition function is a natural consequence of the molecular processes (in particular, calcium priming of the cAMP cascade) upon which this model is based. However, the model described here still produces some blocking if the acquisition function is artificially changed to a decelerating one (by holding priming constant), although in that case blocking is less complete.

*Overshadowing*

Overshadowing is similar to blocking, but involves training with CSs which differ in salience or probability of reinforcement, rather than previous association with the US. As Pavlov (1927) noted, if *CS1* is more salient (stronger) than *CS2* and the compound stimulus *CS1*, *CS2* is paired with the US, there will tend to be little conditioning of *CS2*, even though good conditioning of *CS2* occurs if it is paired with the US by itself. Thus, a strong CS 'overshadows' a weaker CS when they are presented simultaneously, preventing conditioning of the weak CS. Overshadowing of *CS2* when it is part of the compound stimulus *CS1*, *CS2* also occurs if the two CSs have the same salience but *CS1* has a higher probability of reinforcement (i.e. is a better predictor of the US) than *CS2*.

The model described here simulates both types of overshadowing. Figure 10.10 shows a simulation of overshadowing with two different CS strengths (*CS1* = 1.75 and *CS2* = 1.00). The explanation of this effect is similar to the explanation proposed for blocking: *CS1* conditions more rapidly than *CS2* initially (since it has more action potentials and hence greater calcium priming

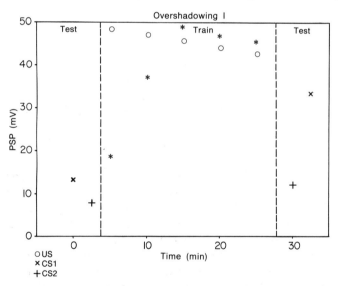

**Fig. 10.10** Simulation of overshadowing by a CS with greater salience: CS1 strength = 1.75; CS2 strength = 1.00; ∗ = simultaneous occurrence of CS1 and CS2.

of the cAMP cascade), and conditioning of both CSs decelerates as their combined associative strengths approach the US strength. In the simulation this occurs by the second paired trial, before there has been much conditioning of *CS2*. As training continues, the CS strengths actually habituate slightly, with the response to *CS*1 remaining near asymptote and the response to *CS*2 remaining at a low level.

Figure 10.11 shows a simulation of overshadowing with two different probabilities of reinforcement. During training, trials on which the compound *CS*1, *CS*2 is paired with the US alternate with trials on which *CS*2 is presented alone. Thus *CS*1 is always followed by the US, whereas *CS*2 is followed by the US for only half of the time. As a result, *CS*1 conditions more rapidly than *CS*2 (see the discussion of partial reinforcement below). Conditioning of both CSs decelerates as the associative strength of the compound *CS*1, *CS*2 approaches

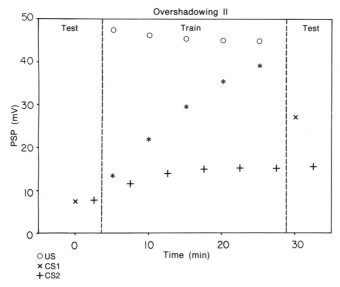

**Fig. 10.11** Simulation of overshadowing by a CS with a higher probability of reinforcement: ∗ = simultaneous occurrence of CS1 and CS2.

the US strength. As in the preceding example, this asymptote occurs before there has been much conditioning of *CS*2, which is thus 'overshadowed' by the more rapidly conditioning *CS*1. In the simulation shown in Figure 10.11, the response to *CS*2 asymptotes at a fairly low level. In similar simulations with a shorter intertrial interval (and consequently more habituation), the response to *CS*2 displays a biphasic learning curve, first increasing and then decreasing to approximately its original level with continued training.

*The effect of contingency*

Like blocking, the effect of contingency illustrates that animals do not simply learn about the pairing of events, but also learn about their correlation or contingency, i.e. how well one event predicts another. Rescorla (1968) demonstrated this effect by showing that adding additional, unpaired CSs or USs to a conditioning procedure decreases learning, although the animals receive the same number of pairings of the CS and US. A similar effect of extra USs has been demonstrated for conditioning of gill- and siphon-withdrawal in *Aplysia* (Hawkins, Carew, and Kandel 1986). Hawkins and Kandel (1984) suggested that habituation of US effectiveness might contribute to the effect of extra USs. Thus, just as CS effectiveness habituates with repeated presentations of the CS, so might US effectiveness habituate with repeated presentations of the US. Adding additional, unpaired USs would therefore cause greater habituation of the US, leading to decreased US effectiveness on the paired trials and decreased learning.

The neuronal model includes US habituation, since the US pathway is not treated any differently than the CS pathways. Figure 10.12 shows a simulation in which additional, unpaired USs are presented during training. This procedure causes extra US habituation and decreased conditioning of the CS.

Rescorla and Wagner (1972) proposed a different explanation for the effect

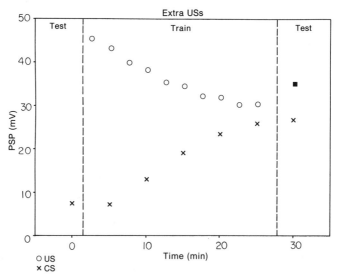

**Fig. 10.12**   Simulation of extra USs (partial warning): ■ = response to the CS at that time if the five extra USs are omitted.

of extra USs, which is that it could be explained by an extension of the argument they advanced for blocking and overshadowing by including in the analysis the stimuli that are always present in the experimental situation (the background stimuli). Thus an experiment with extra USs (alternating trials of *CS*1–US and US-alone) can be thought of as an experiment with alternating trials of *CS*1, *CS*2–US and *CS*2–US, where *CS*2 represents the background stimuli. In this case *CS*2 conditions more rapidly than *CS*1 (since it receives twice as many paired trials) and therefore tends to 'overshadow' conditioning of *CS*1. This explanation of the effect of extra USs and the explanation based on US habituation (Fig. 10.12) are not mutually exclusive, and both may contribute. Thus, if a 'background' stimulus (*CS*2 in the argument above) is added to the simulation shown in Fig. 10.12, degradation of conditioning by the extra USs is more profound.

Presenting additional, unpaired CSs during training (partial reinforcement) also decreases conditioning, as illustrated in the simulation shown in Fig. 10.13. This effect has two explanations: extinction (CS habituation) caused by

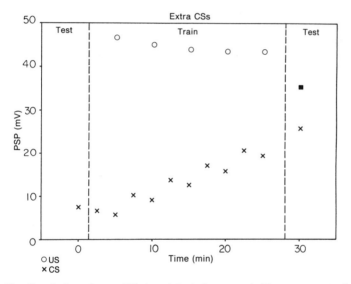

**Fig. 10.13**    Simulation of extra CSs (partial reinforcement): ■ = response to the CS at that time if the five extra CSs are omitted.

the unpaired CSs, and a consequent decrease in calcium priming of the cAMP cascade on the paired trials. As might be expected, presenting both additional, unpaired USs and CSs causes an even greater decrease in conditioning than either procedure by itself.

*Pre-exposure effects*

Learning can be disrupted by presenting extra, unpaired stimuli *before* paired training, as well as during it. For example, presentation of unpaired CSs in

Stage I of an experiment causes a retardation of conditioning during paired training in Stage II. This effect, which is referred to as 'latent inhibition', has a formal similarity to the effect of parital reinforcement described above, and it may have a similar neural explanation. Figure 10.14 shows a simulation of

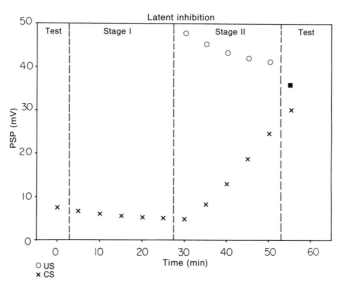

**Fig. 10.14** Simulation of latent inhibition: ■ = response to the CS at that time if Stage I training is omitted.

latent inhibition in which inactivation of $Ca^{2+}$ current during Stage I leads to a decrease in $Ca^{2+}$ priming of the cAMP cascade and hence retardation of conditioning in Stage II. This effect is most evident during the early part of Stage II (compare with Fig. 10.3). With continued training, conditioning eventually reaches the same asymptote as it would have without Stage I training.

For reasons similar to those described above for the effect of extra USs, presentation of unpaired USs in Stage I (US pre-exposure) also decreases conditioning during paired training in Stage II. Furthermore, unpaired presentation of both CSs and USs in Stage I produces an even greater decrease in conditioning than presentation of either stimulus by itself.

## Discussion

In this chapter I have attempted to demonstrate how several higher-order features of classical conditioning might be generated from combinations of the cellular mechanisms used in simpler forms of learning. The model I have described, which is based on known *Aplysia* physiology and neural circuitry, simulates the basic phenomena of acquisition, extinction, differential conditioning, generalization, second-order conditioning, blocking, overshadowing, contingency, latent inhibition, and US pre-exposure.

The model is thus reasonably successful, but it also has several limitations. First, it is simply meant to illustrate what can be accomplished with the mechanisms that have been described in *Aplysia* (in particular, activity-dependent facilitation), and it does not rule out a possible contribution of other cellular mechanisms. A variety of different cellular learning mechanisms have now been described, both in different species and in the same species (for reviews see Carew and Sahley 1986; Byrne 1987; Hawkins, Clark, and Kandel 1987), all of which probably contribute to behavioural learning in some way. Second, several of the behavioural phenomena addressed by the model have not yet been tested in *Aplysia*, so the relevance of *Aplysia* physiology and circuitry to those phenomena is not demonstrated. Third, the model does not explain some of the details of the behavioural phenomena discussed in this chapter, as well as several other important phenomena in conditioning such as conditioned inhibition, sensory pre-conditioning, and the nature of the conditioned response. A virtue of the model is that it should be testable on the neuronal level by recording from the relevant neurons during behavioural conditioning. Whether or not the results of these tests support the details of the model, however, the success of the simulations described in this chapter does support the more general hypothesis that relatively advanced types of learning may result from combinations of known cellular processes in simple neural circuits.

## Comparison with psychological models

The model I have presented is similar in many respects to (and was inspired by) psychological models proposed by modern behaviourists to account for the same behavioural phenomena. In particular, it provides a neuronal version of a concept central to many of those models, which is that learning depends on the degree to which the US is surprising or unpredicted (e.g. Rescorla and Wagner 1972; Wagner 1978, 1981; Mackintosh 1975). Rescorla and Wagner (1972), whose psychological model has probably been the most influential, formalized this idea in the following equation:

$$\Delta V_A = \alpha_A \beta_1 (\lambda_1 - \sum V) \qquad (10.10)$$

where $V_A$ is the associative strength of CSA, $\Delta V_A$ is the change in that strength on a given trial, $\alpha_A$ is a learning rate parameter specific to CSA, $\beta_1$ is another learning rate parameter specific to $US1$, $\lambda_1$ is the maximum learning supported by $US1$, and $\sum V$ is the sum of the associative strengths of all of the CSs present on the trial. In the Rescorla–Wagner model $\alpha$ and $\beta$ are constants, and phenomena such as blocking and overshadowing are explained by changes in the term $(\lambda_1 - \sum V)$. For example, at the beginning of Stage I of a blocking experiment (pairing $CS1$ with the US), the strength of $CS1$ $(V_1)$ is small, $\lambda - V_1$ is large, and the increment in the strength of $CS1$ $(\Delta V_1)$ on each trial is large. As training progresses, $V_1$ becomes larger, $\Delta V_1$ becomes smaller, and $V_1$ gradually approaches $\lambda$. At the beginning of Stage II of the experiment (pairing the compound stimulus $CS1$, $CS2$ with the US), the strength of $CS2$ $(V_2)$ is small, but the sum of $V_1$ and $V_2$ $(\sum V)$ is nearly equal to $\lambda$, so there is little further change in the strengths of either $CS1$ or $CS2$. This is a mathematical representation of the idea that there is little conditioning in Stage II because the US is already fully predicted by $CS1$.

Mackintosh (1975) has proposed an alternative learning rule, which is formalized in the following equation:

$$\Delta V_A = \alpha_A \beta (\lambda - V_A) \qquad (10.11)$$

In this model, phenomena such as blocking and overshadowing are not explained by changes in the term $(\lambda - V_A)$. Rather, they are due to changes in the learning rate parameter specific to the CS, $\alpha_A$, which is postulated to be larger for CSs that are more salient or are better predictors of the US. For example, in Stage II of a blocking experiment the learning rate parameter for $CS2$, $\alpha_2$, becomes smaller because $CS2$ does not predict anything that is not already predicted by $CS1$. This is conceived of as a type of attentional mechanism whereby CSs without predictive value are ignored.

The cellular model I have described has features in common with the psychological models of both Rescorla–Wagner and Mackintosh. These similarities can be seen by comparing Equations (10.10) and (10.11) with my Equation (10.8):

$$\Delta cAMP = C6 \times Spikes \times [1 + (C7 \times Ca(t-1))]$$

In this equation $\Delta cAMP$ is the increase in cAMP level (and hence synaptic output) in a CS sensory neuron, $C6$ and $C7$ are rate parameters, '$Spikes$' refers to the number of spikes in the facilitator neuron, and $Ca(t-1)$ refers to the calcium influx in the sensory neuron during the preceding time unit. The term '$Spikes$' in this equation corresponds to the term $(\lambda - \sum V)$ in the Rescorla–Wagner equation, since accommodation of firing in the facilitator neuron in effect subtracts the combined strengths of all the paired CSs from the strength of the US (Equations (10.5), (10.6), and (10.7)); $C6$, which is a rate parameter specific to the facilitator neuron (and hence potentially specific to the US), corresponds to $\beta$, and $[1 + (C7 \times Ca(t-1))]$, which is a rate parameter specific to the CS sensory neuron, corresponds to $\alpha$. This term acts somewhat like $\alpha$ in the Mackintosh model, since its value changes depending on the previous reinforcement history of the CS (Equations (10.1)–(10.4)).

As these equations illustrate, the model I have described has similarities with psychological models proposed to account for the same behavioural phenomena. It differs from psychological models, however, in that it is formulated at the level of molecular processes rather than algebraic learning rules. The molecular processes result in synaptic plasticity which can be compared qualitatively to the psychological learning rules, as I have done above, but which is too complex to be described quantitatively by simple algebraic equations. The model I have described also differs from most psychological models in that it utilizes a separate mechanism, synaptic depression, for all negative learning (Equation (10.1)). The relative success of the model demonstrates that this mechanism may contribute to a wider range of learning phenomena than has generally been appreciated. However, depression cannot account for conditioned inhibition and related learning phenomena in which CS strengths become negative, since the lowest depression can go is zero. To explain those phenomena, it will presumably be necessary to add inhibitory interneurons to the neuronal circuit shown in Fig. 10.1. Neurons which produce inhibition in this circuit have been identified, and their properties are currently being investigated (Hawkins, Castellucci, and Kandel 1981; Mackey *et al.* 1987).

*Comparison with neural network models*

It is interesting to compare the real nervous system I described in Section I of this chapter with artificial neural network models such as PDP models. Those models are similar to real nervous systems in that they learn to respond differently to different inputs by means of parallel distributed processing in a network of neuron-like elements. They generally differ from real nervous systems, however, in the exact architecture of the networks, in the input–output properties of the neuron-like elements, and in the learning rules which change the strengths of the connections between the elements. For example, network models usually assume that the basic computing unit (the 'neuron') does something fairly simple, whereas real neurons are much more complex. I have reviewed evidence indicating that *single* sensory neurons in *Aplysia* have synaptic plasticity corresponding to behavioural habituation, sensitization, inhibition, and basic classical conditioning. Only the higher-order features of conditioning result from network interactions in the model I have described. The basic types of cellular plasticity in the model are in turn explained by the probabilistic behaviour of millions of ion channels and enzyme molecules which interact in complex ways to determine the behaviour of the neuron. Each neuron is therefore a small computer itself, and the basic computing elements might more properly be considered to be the molecules which make up the ion channels and enzymes.

Neural network models also frequently differ from biological nervous systems in their constraints. For example, real synapses are usually either excitatory or inhibitory, and can't switch from one to the other, whereas some artificial learning rules (such as the Rescorla–Wagner and Mackintosh equations described above) allow such switching. On the other hand, many artificial learning rules are constrained to treat positive and negative learning symmetrically, whereas real synapses use separate mechanisms for positive and negative learning. These seemingly small constraints have important implications for the functional networks which can be built with these rules.

For these and other reasons, most neural network models are not very biologically realistic. This is not a criticism, since most are not intended to advance our understanding of nervous systems, but, rather, are designed to achieve practical goals by any means possible. The biologically realistic approach which I have tried to illustrate has many practical disadvantages compared to a pure artificial intelligence approach, but I believe it also has some advantages. First, it allows physiological tests of the ideas of the model, and intellectual cross-fertilization between the testing and the modelling. In some cases, going inside the 'black box' in this manner is the only way to choose between different models with similar input–output behaviour, and in any case it is potentially a powerful tool for doing so. Second, and perhaps more importantly, nervous systems are still the best computers we have for many tasks, and we can probably learn much more from them. Neural network models have been successful in achieving practical goals by copying biology to the extent of using parallel distributed processing. They might profit further by copying biological 'neurons', learning rules, and network architecture. Although nervous systems have constraints which appear to be (and may actually be) restrictive, using biology as a guide in this manner may none the less turn out to be the best way to create computer models with some of the capabilities of real nervous systems. The model I have described has very modest capabilities, but it represents a first step towards these goals.

## Acknowledgements

I am grateful to Greg Clark and Reid Hastie for their comments and criticisms, Kathrin Hilten and Louise Katz for preparing the figures, and Harriet Ayers and Andrew Krawetz for typing the manuscript. Preparation of this article was supported by a grant from the National Institute of Mental Health (MH-26212).

## References

Abrams, T. W. (1985). Activity-dependent presynaptic facilitation: an associative mechanism in *Aplysia*. *Cell and Molecular Neurobiology*, **5**, 123–45.

Abrams, T. W., Carew, T. J., Hawkins, R. D., and Kandel, E. R. (1983). Aspects of the cellular mechanism of temporal specificity in conditioning in *Aplysia*: preliminary evidence for $Ca^{2+}$ influx as a signal of activity. *Soc. Neuroscience Abstracts*, **9**, 168.

Abrams, T. W., Castellucci, V. F., Camardo, J. S., Kandel, E. R., and Lloyd, P. E. (1984). Two endogenous neuropeptides modulate the gill and siphon withdrawal reflex in *Aplysia* by presynaptic facilitation involving cAMP-dependent closure of a serotonin-sensitive potassium channel. *Proceedings of the National Academy of Science, USA*, **81**, 7956–60.

Abrams, T. W., Eliot, L., Dudai, Y., and Kandel, E. R. (1985). Activation of adenylate cyclase in *Aplysia* neural tissue by $Ca^{2+}$/calmodulin, a candidate for an associative mechanism during conditioning. *Soc. Neuroscience Abstracts*, **11**, 797.

Atkinson, R. C. and Estes, W. K. (1963). Stimulus sampling theory. In *Handbook of mathematical psychology*, Volume 2 (eds. R. D. Luce, R. R. Bush, and E. Galanter), pp. 121–268. Wiley, New York.

Bailey, C. H. and Chen, M. (1985). Morphological basis of short-term habituation in *Aplysia*. *Soc. Neuroscience Abstracts*, **11**, 1110.

Bernier, L., Castellucci, V. F., Kandel, E. R., and Schwartz, J. H. (1982). Facilitatory transmitter causes a selective and prolonged increase in adenosine 3':5'-monophosphate in sensory neurons mediating the gill and siphon withdrawal reflex in *Aplysia*. *Journal of Neuroscience*, **2**, 1682–91.

Boyle, M. B., Klein, M., Smith, S. J., and Kandel, E. R. (1984). Serotonin increases intracellular $Ca^{2+}$ transients in voltage-clamped sensory neurons of *Aplysia californica*. *Proceedings of the National Academy of Science, USA*, **81**, 7642–6.

Bush, R. R. and Mosteller, F. (1951). A model for stimulus generalization and discrimination. *Psychological Review*, **58**, 413–23.

Byrne, J. (1981). Comparative aspects of neural circuits for inking behavior and gill withdrawal in *Aplysia californica*. *Journal of Neurophysiology*, **45**, 98–106.

Byrne, J. (1987). Cellular analysis of associative learning. *Physiological Review*, **67**, 329–439.

Byrne, J. Castellucci, V., and Kandel, E. R. (1974). Receptive fields and response properties of mechanoreceptor neurons innervating siphon skin and mantle shelf in *Aplysia*. *Journal of Neurophysiology*, **37**, 1041–64.

Carew, T. J., Hawkins, R. D., Abrams, T. W., and Kandel, E. R. (1984). A test of Hebb's postulate at identified synapses which mediate classical conditioning in *Aplysia*. *Journal of Neuroscience*, **4**, 1217–24.

Carew, T. J., Hawkins, R. D., and Kandel, E. R. (1983). Differential classical conditioning of a defensive withdrawal reflex in *Aplysia californica*. *Science*, **219**, 397–400.

Carew, T. J., Pinsker, H. M., and Kandel, E. R. (1972). Long-term habituation of a defensive withdrawal reflex in *Aplysia*. *Science*, **175**, 451–4.

Carew, T. J. and Sahley, C. L. (1986). Invertebrate learning and memory: from behavior to molecules. *Annual Review of Neuroscience*, **9**, 435–87.

Carew, T. J., Walters, E. T., and Kandel, E. R. (1981). Classical conditioning in a simple withdrawal reflex in *Aplysia californica*. *Journal of Neuroscience*, **1**, 1426–37.

Castellucci, V. F. and Kandel, E. R. (1974). A quantal analysis of the synaptic depression underlying habituation of the gill-withdrawal reflex in *Aplysia*. *Proceedings of the National Academy of Science, USA*, **71**, 5004–8.

Castellucci, V. and Kandel, E. R. (1976). Presynaptic facilitation as a mechanism for behavioral sensitization in *Aplysia*. *Science*, **194**, 1176–8.

Castellucci, V. F., Nairn, A., Greengard, P., Schwartz, J. H., and Kandel, E. R. (1982). Inhibitor of adenosine $3':5'$-monophosphate-dependent protein kinase blocks presynaptic facilitation in *Aplysia. Journal of Neuroscience*, **2**, 1673–81.

Castellucci, V., Pinsker, H., Kupfermann, I., and Kandel, E. R. (1970). Neuronal mechanisms of habituation and dishabituation of the gill-withdrawal reflex in *Aplysia. Science*, **167**, 1745–8.

Clark, G. A. (1984). A cellular mechanism for the temporal specificity of classical conditioning of the siphon-withdrawal response in *Aplysia. Soc. Neuroscience Abstracts*, **10**, 268.

Colebrook, E. and Lukowiak, K. (1988). Learning by the *Aplysia* model system: lack of correlation between gill and gill motor neurone responses. *Journal of Experimental Biology*, **135**, 411–29.

Colwill, R. M. (1985). Context conditioning in *Aplysia californica. Soc. Neuroscience Abstracts*, **11**, 796.

Dickinson, A. (1980). *Contemporary animal learning theory*. Cambridge University Press.

Duerr, J. S. and Quinn, W. G. (1982). Three *Drosophila* mutants that block associative learning also affect habituation and sensitization. *Proceedings of the National Acadamy of Science, USA*, **79**, 3646–50.

Farley, J. (1987). Contingency learning and causal detection in *Hermissenda:* I. Behavior. *Behavioral Neuroscience*, **101**, 13–27.

Frost, W. N., Castellucci, V. F., Hawkins, R. D., and Kandel, E. R. (1985a). Monosynaptic connections made by the sensory neurons of the gill- and siphon-withdrawal reflex in *Aplysia* participate in the storage of long-term memory for sensitization. *Proceedings of the National Academy of Science, USA*, **82**, 8266–9.

Frost, W. N., Clark, G. A., and Kandel, E. R. (1985b). Changes in cellular excitability in a new class of siphon motor neurons during sensitization in *Aplysia. Soc. Neuroscience Abstracts*, **11**, 643.

Frost, W. N. and Kandel, E. R. (1984). Sensitizing stimuli reduce the effectiveness of the L30 inhibitory interneurons in the siphon withdrawal reflex circuit of *Aplysia. Soc. Neuroscience Abstracts* **10**, 510.

Gingrich, K. J. and Byrne, J. H. (1985). Simulation of synaptic depression, posttetanic potentiation, and presynaptic facilitation of synaptic potentials from sensory neurons mediating gill-withdrawal reflex in *Aplysia. Journal Neurophysiology*, **53**, 652–69.

Gingrich, K. J. and Byrne, J. H. (1987). Single-cell neuronal model for associative learning. *Journal Neurophysiology*, **57**, 1705–15.

Glanzman, D. L., Mackey, S., and Kandel, E. R. (1986). Depletion of serotonin in *Aplysia* interferes with facilitation produced by sensitizing stimuli *Soc. Neuroscience Abstracts*, **12**, 1339.

Gluck, M. A. and Thompson, R. F. (1987). Modeling the neural substrates of associative learning and memory: a computational approach. *Psychological Review*, **94**, 176–91.

Gormezano, I. (1972). Investigations of defense and reward conditioning in the rabbit. In *Classical conditioning* II: *current research and theory* (eds. A. H. Black and W. F. Prokasy), pp. 151–81. Appleton-Century-Crofts, NY.

Hawkins, R. D. and Abrams, T. W. (1984). Evidence that activity-dependent facilitation underlying classical conditioning in *Aplysia* involves modulation of the same ionic current as normal presynaptic facilitation. *Soc. Neuroscience Abstracts,* **10**, 268.

Hawkins, R. D., Abrams, T. W., Carew, T. J., and Kandel, E. R. (1983). A cellular mechanism of classical conditioning in *Aplysia*: activity-dependent amplification of presynaptic facilitation. *Science*, **219**, 400–5.

Hawkins, R. D., Carew, T. J., and Kandel, E. R. (1986). Effects of interstimulus interval and contingency on classical conditioning of the *Aplysia* siphon withdrawal reflex. *Journal of Neuroscience*, **6**, 1695–701.

Hawkins, R. D., Castellucci, V. F., and Kandel, E. R. (1981). Interneurons involved in mediation and modulation of gill-withdrawal reflex in *Aplysia*. II. Identified neurons produce heterosynaptic facilitation contributing to behavioral sensitization. *Journal of Neurophysiology*, **45**, 315–26.

Hawkins, R. D., Clark, G. A., and Kandel, E. R. (1987). Cell biological studies of learning in simple vertebrate and invertebrate systems. In *Handbook of physiology*, Section 1: *The nervous system*, Volume V, *Higher functions of the brain* (ed. F. Plum). American Physiological Society, Bethesda, Md.

Hawkins, R. D. and Kandel, E. R. (1984). Is there a cell biological alphabet for simple forms of learning? *Psychological Review*, **91**, 375–91.

Hebb, D. O. (1949). *The organization of behavior*. Wiley, NY.

Hochner, B., Braha, O., Klein, M., and Kandel, E. R. (1986a). Distinct processes in presynaptic facilitation contribute to sensitization and dishabituation in *Aplysia*: possible involvement of C kinase in dishabituation. *Soc. Neuroscience Abstracts*, **12**, 1340.

Hochner, B., Klein, M., Schacher, S., and Kandel, E. R. (1986b). Additional component in the cellular mechanism of presynaptic facilitation contributes to behavioral dishabituation in *Aplysia*. *Proceddings of the National Academy of Science, USA*, **83**, 8794–8.

Jacklet, J. and Rine, J. (1977). Facilitation at neuromuscular junctions: contribution to habituation and dishabituation of the *Aplysia* gill withdrawal reflex. *Proceedings of the National Academy of Science, USA*, **74**, 1267–71.

Kamin, L. J. (1969). Predictability, surprise, attention and conditioning. In *Punishment and aversive behavior* (eds. B. A. Campbell and R. M. Church), pp. 279–96. Appleton-Century-Crofts, NY.

Kandel, E. R., Abrams, T., Bernier, L., Carew, T. J., Hawkins, R. D., and Schwartz, J. H. (1983). Classical conditioning and sensitization share aspects of the same molecular cascade in *Aplysia*. *Cold Spring Harbor Symposium on Quantitative Biology*, **48**, 821–30.

Kandel, E. R. and Schwartz, J. H. (1982). Molecular biology of learning: modulation of transmitter release. *Science*, **218**, 433–43.

Kanz, J. E., Eberley, L. B., Cobbs, J. S., and Pinsker, H. M. (1979). Neuronal correlates of siphon withdrawal in freely behaving *Aplysia*. *Journal of Neurophysiology*, **42**, 1538–56.

Kistler, H. B. Jr, Hawkins, R. D., Koester, J., Steinbusch, H. W. M., Kandel, E. R., and Schwartz, J. H. (1985). Distribution of serotonin-immunoreactive cell bodies and processes in the abdominal ganglion of mature *Aplysia*. *Journal of Neuroscience*, **5**, 72–80.

Klein, M. and Kandel, E. R. (1980). Mechanism of calcium current modulation underlying presynaptic facilitation and behavioral sensitization in *Aplysia*. *Proceedings of the National Academy of Science, USA*, **77**, 6912–16.

Klein, M., Shapiro, E., and Kandel, E. R. (1980). Synaptic plasticity and the modulation of the $Ca^{++}$ current. *Journal of Experimental Biology*, **89**, 117–57.

Krontiris-Litowitz, J. K., Erickson, M. T., and Walters, E. T. (1987). Central suppression of defense reflexes in *Aplysia* by noxious stimulation and by factors released from body wall. *Soc. Neuroscience Abstracts*, **13**, 815.

Kupfermann, I., Carew, T. J., and Kandel, E. R. (1974). Local, reflex, and central commands controlling gill and siphon movements in *Aplysia*. *Journal of Neurophysiology*, **37**, 996–1019.

Lukowiak, K. (1986). In vitro classical conditioning of a gill withdrawal reflex in *Aplysia*: neural correlates and possible neural mechanisms. *Journal of Neurobiology*, **17**, 83–101.

Mackey, S. L., Hawkins, R. D., and Kandel, E. R. (1986). Neurons in 5-HT containing region of cerebral ganglia produce facilitation of LE cells in *Aplysia*. *Soc. Neuroscience Abstracts*, **12**, 1340.

Mackey, S. L., Glanzman, D. L., Small, S. A., Dyke, A. M., Kandel, E. R., and Hawkins, R. D. (1987). Tail shock produces inhibition as well as sensitization of the siphon-withdrawal reflex of *Aplysia*: possible behavioral role for presynaptic inhibition mediated by the peptide Phe-Met-Arg-Phe-NH$_2$. *Proceedings of the National Academy of Science, USA*, **84**, 8730–4.

Mackintosh, N. J. (1975). A theory of attention: variations in the associability of stimuli with reinforcement. *Psychological Review*, **82**, 276–98.

Mackintosh, N. J. (1983). *Conditioning and associative learning*. Oxford University Press.

Marcus, E. A., Nolen, T. G., Rankin, C. H., and Carew, T. J. (1987). Behavioral dissociation of dishabituation, sensitization, and inhibition in the siphon withdrawal reflex of adult *Aplysia*. *Soc. Neuroscience Abstracts*, **13**, 816.

Ocorr, K. A., Walters, E. T., and Byrne, J. H. (1985). Associative conditioning analog selectively increases cAMP levels of tail sensory neurons in *Aplysia*. *Proceedings of the National Academy of Science, USA*, **82**, 2548–52.

Pavlov, I. P. (1927). *Conditioned reflexes: an investigation of the physiological activity of the cerebral cortex* (Trans. by G. V. Anrep). Oxford University Press, London.

Perlman, P. J. (1979). Central and peripheral control of siphon withdrawal reflex in *Aplysia californica*. *Journal of Neurophysiology*, **42**, 510–29.

Pinsker, H. M., Hening, W. A., Carew, T. J., and Kandel, E. R. (1973). Long-term sensitization of a defensive withdrawal reflex in *Aplysia*. *Science*, **182**, 1039–42.

Pinsker, H., Kupfermann, I., Castellucci, V., and Kandel, E. R. (1970). Habituation and dishabituation of the gill-withdrawal reflex in *Aplysia*. *Science*, **167**, 1740–2.

Piomelli, D., Volterra, A., Dale, N., Siegelbaum, S. A., Kandel, E. R., Schwartz, J. H., and Belardetti, F. (1987). Lipoxygenase metabolites of arachidonic acid as second messengers for presynaptic inhibition of *Aplysia* sensory cells. *Nature*, **328**, 38–43.

Rescorla, R. A. (1968). Probability of shock in the presence and absence of CS in fear conditioning. *Journal of Comparaitive and Physiological Psychology*, **66**, 1–5.

Rescorla, R. A. (1973). Second-order conditioning: Implications for theories of learning. In *Contemporary approaches to conditioning and learning* (eds. F. J. McGuigan and D. B. Hulse). V. H. Winston and Sons, Washington, DC.

Rescorla, R. A. (1978). Some implications of a cognitive perspective on Pavlovian conditioning. In *Cognitive processes in animal behavior* (eds. S. H. Hulse, H. Fowler, and W. Honig), pp. 15–50. Erlbaum, Hillsdale, NJ.

Rescorla, R. A. and Wagner, A. R. (1972). A theory of Pavlovian conditioning: variations in the effectiveness of reinforcement and non-reinforcement. In *Classical conditioning II: Current research and theory* (eds. A. H. Black and W. F. Prokasy). Appleton-Century-Crofts, NY.

Sacktor, T. C., O'Brian, C. A., Weinstein, J. B., and Schwartz, J. H. (1986). Translocation from cytosol to membrane of protein kinase C after stimulation of *Aplysia* neurons with serotonin. *Soc. Neuroscience Abstracts*, **12**, 1340.

Sahley, C., Rudy, J. W., and Gelperin, A. (1981). An analysis of associative learning in a terrestrial molusc. I. Higher-order conditioning, blocking, and a transient US pre-exposure effect. *Journal of Comparative Physiology*, **144**, 1–8.

Siegelbaum, S. A., Camardo, J. S., and Kandel, E. R. (1982). Serotonin and cyclic AMP close single $K^+$ channels in *Aplysia* sensory neurones. *Nature*, **299**, 413–17.

Wagner, A. R. (1978). Expectancies and the priming of STM. In *Cognitive processes in animal behavior* (eds. S. H. Hulse, H. Fowler, and W. Honig), pp. 177–209. Erlbaum, Hillsdale, NJ.

Wagner, A. R. (1981). SOP: a model of automatic memory processing in animal behavior. In *Information processing in animals: memory mechanisms* (eds. N. E. Spear and R. R. Miller), pp. 5–47. Erlbaum, Hillsdale, NJ.

Walters, E. T., and Byrne, J. H. (1983). Associative conditioning of single sensory neurons suggests a cellular mechanism for learning. *Science*, **219**, 405–8.

Walters, E. T., Carew, T. J., and Kandel, E. R. (1981). Associative learning in *Aplysia*: evidence for conditioned fear in an invertebrate. *Science*, **211**, 504–6.

# 11

## Does synaptic plasticity play a role in information storage in the vertebrate brain?
### R. G. M. MORRIS

**Only connect . . .?**

Parallel distributed processing (PDP) models of cognitive function differ with respect to the tasks they are capable of solving, the architecture of their networks of units, and their learning rules. However, common to all PDP models in the idea that 'knowledge is stored in the connections' (e.g. McClelland, Chapter 2, p. 13), this method of storing information being widely claimed as 'neurally inspired' (e.g. Rumelhart and McClelland, 1986, p. 11). There are several ways in which such models might be implemented within the nervous system but the simplest, and the one which provokes the label 'neural-like', is the supposition that the 'units' of PDP models are neurons, that the 'connections' are axons, and that variability in the 'weights' of connections is realized by altering synaptic efficacy. Such a simple isomorphism is almost certainly wrong in detail, but it does have the virtue of capturing the essential metaphor of the connectionist approach: neurons are relatively simple processing units and they are often interconnected in massively parallel circuits. Unfortunately, while it is not obvious how circuits of simple neurons could store information other than by changing synaptic strengths, this central idea has been the subject of relatively few empirical investigations.

The main purpose of this chapter is to describe different strategies and a variety of behavioural experiments explicitly intended as tests of the hypothesis that synaptic plasticity plays a role in learning in the vertebrate brain. Some have pursued the direct route of investigating whether learning gives rise to measurable changes in synaptic morphology or functional efficacy. Others have examined whether the various properties of a well-understood form of synaptic plasticity are of functional significance. My own experiments, described towards the end, fall within the rubric of the second strategy and rest upon a vast foundation of neurophysiological and neuropharmacological research concerning the underlying neural mechanisms of a type of synaptic plasticity called hippocampal long-term potentiation (LTP). More specifically, they employ one of a series of drugs called N-methyl-D-aspartate (NMDA) antagonists, drugs which, in the hippocampal formation (although not necessarily elsewhere), have the remarkable property of blocking the ability of synapses to *change* in strength while leaving *normal* synaptic transmission unaffected. Thus, under the influence of NMDA anatogonists (e.g. the drug 2-amino-5-phosphonopenta-noic acid, or AP5), signals are transmitted normally between neurons but synaptic strength cannot be altered by the very patterns of activity which ordinarily lead to such a change. In the language of PDP modelling, it is as if a network's connectivity were to be temporarily 'frozen' in a given state, irrespective of its dynamic pattern of activation.

The results of experiments pursuing these various strategies include: (1) that learning can give rise to both morphological and functional changes in synapses; (2) that certain properties of LTP are of functional relevance; and (3) that drugs which block LTP also induce a selective anterograde amnesia without effect upon memories established prior to drug adminstration. These findings offer strong neurobiological support for a central tenet of PDP modelling, although, to be sure, in no way distinguishing between different models.

However, in addition to underpinning a central assumption of PDP modelling, it is helpful to cast this work within a broader historical context of ideas about synaptic plasticity, a context which I discuss first and which long predates connectionism. After outlining the two main experimental strategies and work which has followed the first of these, I shall briefly review work on long-term potentiation in order to explain why certain of its physiological properties point to the phenomenon being of functional significance. Behavioural experiments which have explored this possibility will then be described. This will be followed by a review of how recent research on excitatory neurotransmission has yielded important insights into the underly-ing neural mechanisms of LTP. This review provides the essential background for the experiments that I and my colleagues have conducted using NMDA antagonists. I shall then outline one way in which NMDA receptors could be fitted into a realistic neural network model of hippocampal function based on the premise that parts of its circuitry are a type of distributed associative memory. However, in considering (and criticizing) what is missing from this model, particularly the problem of long-term depression of synaptic efficacy, I shall end by discussing how thinking at a more algorithmic level could help neurobiologists search for novel forms of plasticity which would have to exist if the hippocampus is to perform the various computations sometimes ascribed to it.

### Where, when, and how? Conceptual issues in the relation between synaptic plasticity and learning

Interest in the idea that alterations in synaptic efficacy might play a role in learning has a long history. Ramon y Cajal first outlined his view that learning involved an alteration in the connections between neurons in his Croonian Lecture to the Royal Society in 1894. Later, in his treatise on the vertebrate nervous system (Cajal 1911), he distinguished two views about the morphological correlates of learning—Tanzi's (1893) proposal that information was stored as an alteration in the effectiveness of existing connections, and his own idea that new connections were formed from one neuron to another. Despite these differences of detail, which remain debated to this day (Greenough and Bailey 1988), there appears to have been no disagreement that the primary issue was to identify the physical locus of memories, i.e. *where* they were stored. Tanzi and Cajal both believed these were to be found at the minute swellings along dendrites—so-called dendritic spines—visualized using the Golgi histological technique. Dramatic advances in technology over the past century, particularly the use of quantitative electron microscopy, have substantially refined our understanding of the way in which synapse number, density, number per neuron, or morphology might be altered by experience (Rosenzwieg, Bennett, and Krech 1964; Fifkova and van Harreveld 1977; Lee *et al.* 1979; Bailey and Chen 1983; Desmond and Levy 1983; Greenough 1985; Horn, Bradley, and McCabe 1985; Patel, Rose, and Stewart 1988). Thus, the central notion that information is somehow stored at certain kinds of synapses remains with us to this day and is virtually unchallenged (but see Alkon 1987). An important but still unresolved issue has been to identify whether the changes are pre-synaptic (i.e. in the terminal of the axon which is afferent to the synapse), post-synaptic (i.e. in the dendritic spines of the target neuron) or at both pre- and post-synaptic sites. Identifying the locus (or loci) has implications for the types of biochemical events which should be considered likely candidates for giving rise to alterations in synaptic strenth (a list which presently includes: the activation of G-proteins, a conformational change in adenylate cyclase, altered cAMP production, protein synthesis, changing protein kinase C from an activator-dependent to an activator-independent state, and activation of proteolytic enzymes such as calpain leading to structural changes in dendritic spines: Kandel and Schwartz 1982; Lynch and Baudry 1984; Routtenberg, Lovinger, and Steward 1985; Bliss and Lynch 1988; see Abrams and Kandel 1988, and Kennedy 1988, for brief summaries).

Fifty years after Cajal, in his 1949 book *The Organisation of Behaviour*, Hebb addressed a different issue. He pointed out that, in addition to knowing where changes happen, it was also necessary to consider *when* changes happen. In a famous passage, he proposed that an important (although not necessarily exclusive) condition would be the repeated conjunction of pre-synaptic activity and the firing of the cell on to which this activity was afferent (Hebb 1949, p. 62). He wrote:

When an axon of cell A is near enough to excite a cell B and repeatedly or persistently takes part in firing it, some growth process or metabolic change takes place in one or both cells such that A's efficiency, as one of the cells firing B, is increased.

Neither Hebb nor his colleagues of the day had the technology to conduct the necessary physiological study and so were unable to test this proposition experimentally. However, this did not prevent various people exploring its computational possibilities and suggesting modifications that seemed more realistic or efficient in a variety of ways (e.g. Brindley 1967; Stent 1973; Bienenstock, Cooper, and Munro 1982). Meanwhile, and as with the anatomical issue of where memories might be located, advances in technology have helped lead to new discoveries about how synaptic efficacy might be manipulated experimentally. An important discovery was that functional efficacy can be changed in the mammalian brain *in vivo* by stimulating certain fibre bundles with brief high-frequency stimulation. The consequences of such stimulation upon the currents induced near and inside neurons can then be measured and studied using low-frequency stimulation (Bliss and Lomo 1973). More exacting techniques are also available in which mammalian brain tissue is dissected from a sacrificed animal, cut into thin slices and maintained *in vitro* (Skrede and Westgaard 1971). It is then possible to record intracellularly, to stimulate a much smaller number of afferent fibres, and to bathe the tissue in known concentrations of drugs—all techniques which permit a much more detailed analysis of cellular mechanisms. In invertebrates, such as in work on *Aplysia* (Castellucci and Kandel 1974; Kandel and Schwartz 1982), it has proved possible to work with unique, identified neurons and, very recently, to begin the study of the molecular neurobiology of plasticity using isolated neurons in tissue culture. Over the last 15 years or so, research using these and other techniques has revealed that the 'Hebb synapse' is one of a variety of types of synapse in which functional alterations in connectivity are triggered by the conjunction of two different neural events (Abrams and Kandel 1988; Hawkins, this volume; Alkon 1987; Kelso, Ganong, and Brown 1986; Wigstrom *et al.* 1986).

The present re-emergence of ideas about neural networks under the labels of 'parallel distributed processing' (Rumelhart and McClelland 1986) or 'connectionism' (Feldman and Ballard 1982) brings us—40 years after Hebb's book and 100 years after Cajal's lecture—to a third and equally important conceptual issue. After 'where' and 'when' comes the issue of *how* synaptic plasticity enables networks of neurons or neuron-like processing elements to perform various cognitive operations. This very general issue has to be broken down into a number of more tractable questions: There is, first, the need to specify the architecture of any given network—which connections are excitatory, which inhibitory, which are fixed, which are plastic? Second, what local synaptic rule is being used to change synaptic weights, and is the same rule used throughout the network, or are different learning rules used at different stages between the input, hidden and output layers? Third, is the global effect of the application of these learning rules such that the network realizes its computations according to a 'supervised' algorithm (i.e. error-driven) or in an unsupervised (i.e. emergent) manner? A fourth and no less important issue is the problem of how information is to be 'represented' within networks—whether it is in a distributed code and how it is categorized. Many of these and other ideas about the computational implications of synaptic plasticity are currently being debated at a different 'level of explanation' from that of the earlier issues of 'where' and 'when' but, in my view, it would be unfortunate if such debates were ever to be too far removed from neurobiological detail and experimentation (see also Cowan and Sharp 1988). Indeed, as Marr (1982, p. 19) pointed out, it will essential to link the different levels of discourse:

An information processing analysis does not usurp an understanding at the other levels—of neurons or of computer programs—but it is a necessary complement to them, since without it there can be no real understanding of the functions of those neurons.

Answers or assumptions about these issues are essential for building any realistic neural network model of a particular brain area (see Rolls, Chapter 12; Granger and Lynch, Chapter 13). My goal in this chapter is the more limited one of capitalizing upon what we know about mechanisms of plasticity to ask functional questions about their possible roles in learning. PDP theorists may assert that 'knowledge is in the connections' but an assertion, even if it amounts to a widely accepted fact, is not the same as a rigorously established empirical observation. The question at issue, therefore, it 'Does synaptic plasticity play a role in information storage?'

## Two general strategies

Broadly speaking, there are two general strategies for an experimental investigation of the relation between synaptic plasticity and learning. One is to begin with a particular and relatively well-understood type of learning, identify the morphological, physiological and biochemical consequences of training, and then work out which of these consequences is necessary, sufficient and causally related to information storage. The other strategy begins with a particular type of synaptic plasticity whose properties are reasonably well understood and works from there back to the psychological level to establish whether this type is of any functional significance.

Many research programmes have, by the large, followed the former approach. Examples include Kandel's work on habituation, sensitization and classical conditioning in *Aplysia* (Kandel and Schwartz 1982; Hawkins Chapter 10), studies of associative conditioning in *Hermissenda* (Alkon 1987), and work on filial imprinting in chicks (Horn 1985). Equally, many research groups have pursued the opposite approach. Examples include work on proteolytically mediated alterations in receptor sensitivity and its role in olfactory learning (Lynch and Baudry 1984; Lynch 1986), studies of protein phosphorylation and protein kinase C in the up-regulation of synaptic transmission (Routtenberg, Lovinger, and Steward 1985), and the work of Barnes (1979) and McNaughton (1983) exploring the time-course and saturation of long-term potentiation in relation to spatial learning. Of course, as research progresses, the sharp distinction between these two general strategies becomes blurred with experiments moving back and forth between the behavioural and cell-biological levels.

## Imprinting causes changes in synaptic morphology and receptor number

The first of these two approaches is well illustrated by the work on filial imprinting which, although beginning from a very different starting point, is now focusing-in on a similar set of underlying mechanisms of synaptic change as that of my own work described later. If recently hatched, but visually naïve, chicks are exposed to a conspicuous object, such as a moving mother hen or a rotating red light, they will learn to approach it in preference to other objects (Lorenz 1937; Bateson 1966). This imprinting process had been intensively studied in strictly behavioural studies and, capitalizing upon these (e.g. knowledge of optimum training parameters), Horn and his colleagues have gone on to identify a restricted region of the chick forebrain which appears to be intimately involved in the learning process—the intermediate and medial parts of the hyperstriatum ventrale of the left forebrain (IMHV). The work has involved, for example, isolating this as the brain area associated with the greatest increase in protein synthesis during learning (Bateson, Horn, and Rose 1972), establishing that lesions of IMHV impaired the process of imprinting selectively (McCabe, Horn, and Bateson 1981), and discovering that IMHV shows learning-associated changes in electrical activity (Payne and Horn 1982; see Horn, 1985, for review). Recently, Horn, Bradley, and McCabe (1985) have taken the analysis a crucial step further in showing that imprinting is also associated with ultrastructural changes in synapses on dendritic spines in IMHV. Chicks were either undertrained or overtrained using a standard protocol and then compared with dark-reared chicks never exposed to the rotating red light. After training, these and the control birds were sacrificed and their brains prepared for electron microscopy. The authors studied hundreds of ultrathin sections through the IMHV and quantified several measures of synaptic morphology using appropriate stereological techniques. The results, obtained 'blind' with respect to training condition, revealed that the mean length of the post-synaptic densities (PSDs) of dendritic spines in the left IHMV (but not the right) was increased by 17 per cent in overtrained chicks relative to both control and undertrained chicks (Fig. 11.1). McCabe and Horn (1988) have followed up this work with biochemical experiments investigating whether imprinting causes changes in the binding of excitatory amino acids such as L-glutamate and N-methyl-D-aspartate (NMDA) to PSDs. The full significance of such a study will not be apparent until later in this article, but suffice it to say that L-glutamate is the main 'candidate' neurotransmitter for many excitatory pathways in the brain, with NMDA preferring receptors being a particularly important sub-class of excitatory amino-acid receptors. Using a similar training protocol to previous behavioural experiments, they found that imprinting was associated with a 59 per cent increase in NMDA binding (relative to dark-reared controls) and that NMDA binding was highly significantly correlated with the animals' 'preference scores' established in tests where they were required to choose between the training stimulus and a novel object. Thus, the morphological change in the dendritic spine seems to be associated with a functional change in receptor binding (measured biochemically).

These are striking findings. However, a recurring problem with the strategy of searching for the neural correlates of learning is to separate which changes are specifically to do with information storage *per se* and which are causally irrelevant by-products of the training protocol. Horn and his colleagues are acutely aware of this problem and have gone to great lengths to train appropriate control groups (e.g. groups having similar sensorimotor experience but given less or no opportunity to learn about the imprinting stimulus). A second and different worry stems from the supposition that unless the storage capacity of the brain is trivial (which we know it not to be), any change genuinely to do with information storage and arising from a single training experience must surely cause only small changes in perhaps a fraction of the synapses available for change. Such changes would surely be very hard to detect. B. L. McNaughton and I have coined this argument the 'Catch-22' problem of memory, fearing that: 'If you can measure it, it probably isn't memory!' In the case of imprinting, our principle may not hold because the chicks are visually naive, very young (and thus have exceedingly 'plastic' nervous systems) and because they have a very important problem which they must solve in order to survive—namely to learn the identity of their mother. Imprinting many therefore cause massive changes in synaptic morphology and receptor distribution in the process of encoding this information. The attention to detail in both the experimental designs and the analyses of results make Horn's interpretation of the changes he observes particularly convincing. This exception aside, the Catch-22 principle was nevertheless influential in my decision to approach the problem in a different way.

The alternative strategy is to identify a particular type of plasticity and investigate its functional significance. Clearly, this strategy carries with it the

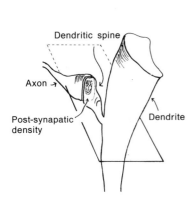
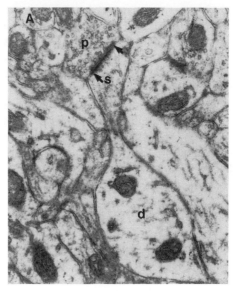

**Fig. 11.1**   An electron micrograph through a spine synapse in IMHV and a cartoon illustrating a possible three-dimensional reconstruction and the plane of section. The darkened area between the arrows on the micrograph is the post-synaptic density—a region lying at the junction of the pre-synaptic terminal (marked p, and containing transmitter vesicles) and the post-synaptic receptors on the spine (s) protruding from the dendrite. Chicks which have been imprinted have a longer post-synaptic density than control birds. (From Horn *et al.* 1985.)

obvious danger of picking the wrong type, with the inevitable consequence that years are wasted studying something of no functional significance (e.g. having only 'homeostatic' or 'repair' functions). However, one now quite well-understood form of synaptic plasticity—hippocampal LTP—seems to possess a number of extremely suggestive properties.

### The physiological properties of LTP are suggestive of a learning mechanism

The physiological phenomenon of long-term potentiation (LTP) refers to a sustained increase in the amplitude of electrically evoked responses in specific neural pathways following brief trains of tetanic stimulation. It was discovered in the late 1960s and first reported in detail by Bliss and Lomo (1973). The original experiments, conducted in anaesthetized rabbits, entailed the bilateral placement of: (1) stimulating electrodes in the perforant path entering the hippocampus; and (2) recording electrodes in the hilus of the dentate gyrus. Their three-phase experiment began with repetitive low-frequency electrical stimulation (at 1 per 30 s) to evoke field-potentials consisting of a mixture of EPSPs, IPSPs and population spikes (the latter reflecting cell-firing). These remained stable throughout the preliminary baseline period. However, when a brief tetanic burst of stimulation was given unilaterally (Phase 2), followed by a return to low-frequency stimulation again (Phase 3), the field potentials recorded on the side of the brain which had received the high-frequency burst were found to be substantially enhanced relative to their pre-tetanic baseline (Fig. 11.2). Bliss and Lomo (1973) showed that this

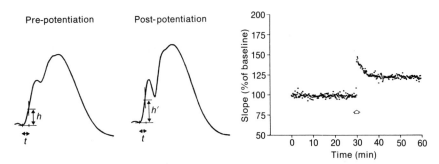

**Fig. 11.2** A repetition of Bliss and Lomo's (1973) experiment conducted in the author's laboratory. The field potentials on the left were obtained in response to a single stimulus given in a series of low-frequency (0.1 Hz). Note that the slope of the early rising phase of the potential has increased as a consequence of potentiation ($h' > h$ at equivalent time $t$). The plot on the right shows: (1) a stable slope during the 30 min baseline prior to the high-frequency burst (arrow); and (2) the resulting post-tetanic (PTP) and long-term potentiation (LTP). PTP has a decay time course of several minutes while LTP appears, in acute experiments such as this, to be relatively nondecremental.

increased responsiveness consisted of both a synaptic component (LTP) and a reduced threshold for cell-firing in response to a given size of EPSP (E–S potentiation). Both components of the increase were found to be very long-lasting. Subsequent work in many laboratories has confirmed and expanded upon these original observations (see Bliss and Lynch 1988; Brown *et al.* 1988a; Nicoll, Kauer, and Malenka 1988, for recent reviews).

The main focus of research on LTP has been to unravel its underlying neural mechanisms and, in the course of this effort, several intriguing properties have been identified indicating that the phenomenon may be a useful synaptic 'model' of memory.[1] Some properties of LTP relevant to its possible role in learning are summarized in Fig. 11.3. First, LTP was discovered and is very prominent in a brain structure—the hippocampus—which has long been implicated in learning and memory on the basis of clinical and experimental studies (Scoville and Milner 1957; O'Keefe and Nadel 1978; Squire and Zola-

Morgan 1983). This circumstantial point about LTP should not be overstressed for at least three reasons: (1) the phenomenon is seen in other brain structures (e.g. Lee 1983; Artolo and Singer 1987); (2) other brain areas and particularly neocortical structures are clearly involved in learning and memory (Mishkin 1982); and (3) part of the reason for the hippocampus being the main area used to study LTP is that features of its anatomy make the analysis of field-potentials relatively easy. However, that LTP was found in a brain area implicated in memory was fortuitous for it encouraged work on the phenomenon at a time when it might otherwise have been disregarded as a laboratory curiousity. Second, LTP develops rapidly over a time-course of about a minute (McNaughton 1983). This property is important because it marks off LTP from certain other forms of neural plasticity whose time-courses of development are much longer (e.g. lesion-induced synaptogenesis). In addition, when LTP is induced, it typically develops during a period when different shorter-lasting forms of potentiation are occurring, including facilitation, augmentation, and post-tetanic potentiation (PTP), all of which decay over time-courses varying from less than 1 s to 3–5 min (McNaughton 1982). Their occurrence masks the time-course of the emergence of LTP. However, by taking advantage of the fact that LTP 'saturates' when repeated attempts are made to induce it, the time-course of its development can be unmasked by subtracting the size of the evoked potentials seen when it is first induced from those seen (at the same times after the tetanus) when a later attempt is made after LTP has saturated. As the amounts of PTP evoked in the two cases are identical, and thus exactly cancel out, the subtraction reveals the time-course of the development of LTP over about 60 s. This time-course suggests that the high-frequency burst (which typically lasts less than 1 s) sets in train a cascade of biochemical events which eventually express and then maintain the altered level of synaptic efficacy. The distinction between events responsible for inducing LTP and maintaining it are stressed by Bliss and Lynch (1988) and, as will become clear later, are of considerable functional significance. A third important property of LTP is that it can be long-lasting. The time-course can only be followed for a few hours in acute and *in vitro* preparations but, in chronic *in vivo* experiments, a decay time-course of hours, days, and in some cases greater than a month, has been reported (Bliss and Gardner-Medwin 1973; Barnes 1979; Racine, Milgram, and Hafner 1983). The longevity of LTP is important because it indicates that the underlying biochemical mechanisms of the phenomenon are at least candidate mechanisms for a long-term storage system. Some have worried that LTP can only serve as an intermediate memory system because it has been seen to decay to baseline in almost every case so far studied. However, new work on long-term depression (see below) puts a different perspective on this problem; LTP may indeed be non-decremental in the absence of specific stimuli which decrement synaptic strength in an associative manner. Fourth, LTP is characterized by a

LTP occurs in a brain structure which has long been implicated in learning—the hippocampus

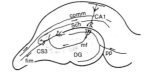

LTP develops rapidly after its induction

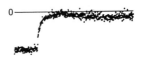

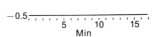

LTP can be long lasting, with a decay time course extending over many days

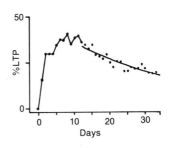

LTP is synapse specific. It only occurs at terminals activated by appropriate stimulation

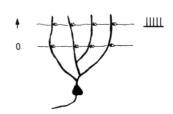

LTP is associative. Weak stimulation may not induce LTP. But, if paired with post-synaptic depolarization (e.g. strong stimulation on other inputs), the weakly stimulated terminals will then potentiate

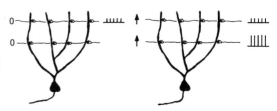

**Fig. 11.3**   A diagrammatic summary of several properties of LTP relevant to the idea that its underlying neural mechanisms may be of functional significance in relation to learning. (Parts of the diagram are taken from papers published by Barnes and McNaughton and reprinted with permission.)

synaptic change which is specific to terminals actually activated by the high-frequency burst or, put formally, it is homosynaptic to the sites of stimulation (Andersen *et al.* 1977). This property could be of significance in relation to information storage capacity: Hippocampal pyramidal cells are believed to have circa $10^4$ synapses. If the induction of LTP on an afferent pathway changed all or most the synapses on a given target cell, the storage capacity would be much less than if only activated synapses were to change (Palm, 1982). Moreover, the ability of individual cells to act as substrates for many independent but overlaid memory traces critically depends on their ability to alter some synapses but not others. Thus, that LTP is homosynaptic to the synapses stimulated is an important property which would permit a parallel distributed processing 'style' of computation. Finally, fifth, the induction of LTP can be associative in the sense that activity at one point on the dendritic tree of an individual cell can influence whether synaptic change occurs at another point. This property was initially deduced from the 'co-operativity' effect, whereby the magnitude of LTP was shown to be dependent upon the number of input fibres stimulated (McNaughton, Douglas, and Goddard 1978). Weak high-frequency inputs to a small number of afferent fibres do not usually induce LTP; strong inputs typically do. However, co-operativity need not necessarily imply true associativity (Brown *et al.* 1988a). Associativity refers to the fact that if a weak input is paired with a strong one, LTP will then be seen on both pathways. Associativity was first seen *in vivo* by Levy and Steward (1979) and *in vitro* by Barrionuevo and Brown (1983). White, Levy, and Steward (1988) have recently shown that, in dentate gyrus, associativity may be restricted to associations between inputs to particular dendritic domains. Associativity is a property of LTP which is highly suggestive of conditioning paradigms (such as Pavlovian conditioning) in which a neutral (i.e. weak) stimulus is paired with a reinforcing (i.e. strong) stimulus and, as a consequence of the pairing, comes to evoke a response corresponding to a 'memory' of the strong stimulus. Tempting as this analogy may be, there is still no unequivocal evidence of a role for LTP in classical conditioning.

### Behavioural studies of the significance of LTP for learning

The discovery of these properties of hippocampal LTP in the late 1970s encouraged a number of people to investigate whether the neural mechanisms of the phenomenon were the same as those involved in learning (Barnes 1979; Ruthrich, Matthies, and Ott 1982; Laroche and Bloch 1982; Berger 1984; Lynch and Baudry 1984; Skelton, Miller, and Phillips 1985; Barnes and McNaughton 1985; Green and Greenough 1986; McNaughton *et al.* 1986). These experiments exploited both the phenomenon and properties of LTP in relation to learning by, for example: (1) investigating its decay time-course; (2) looking for improved signal throughput along potentiated pathways; or (3) studying the behavioural consequences of saturation with repeated activation. The work which particularly influenced my own later efforts was that of Barnes and McNaughton. Barnes (1979) showed that young, middle-aged, and old rats differed with respect to the time-course of the decay of LTP (it lasted longer in young rats) and that these age groups also differed in their ability to learn and remember a circle-maze task involving escape from bright light. Barnes (1979) reported both a significant between-groups correlation and, more interestingly, a weak but significant within-groups correlation between decay of LTP and behavioural performance. Barnes and McNaughton (1985) have replicated and followed up these findings. Recently, in a comprehensive series of experiments, McNaughton *et al.* (1986) have taken advantage of the saturation property of LTP as follows. They reasoned that if subtle but continuous alterations of synaptic efficacy occur in the hippocampus during learning, then saturating LTP to its physiological asymptote *prior* to training should cause anterograde amnesia. Further, if information is permanently stored in the hippocampus as a particular spatial distribution of synaptic weights, saturating LTP should interfere with previously stored traces and thus cause retrograde amnesia also. Accordingly, they implanted rats with appropriate stimulating and recording electrodes, checked that these were working using strictly low-frequency stimulation, and then trained all the rats on the Barnes circle-maze task. Once the animals were performing well (i.e. escaping rapidly with relatively direct paths to the escape tunnel), they were divided into two matched groups. One group (HF) received several bursts of high-frequency stimulation, the other (LF) received equal amounts of electrical stimulation but at low frequency. Relevant recordings were taken to ensure that LTP did not occur in the LF group, but had saturated in the HF group. The rats were then returned to the behavioural task and trained to escape to a goal-tunnel in a *new* spatial location (reversal training). The results were striking. First, the HF group had much greater difficulty than group LF in learning about the new tunnel location—indeed, they barely learned its location at all. However, second, both groups began reversal training by approaching the old tunnel location preferentially—a tendency which group HF continued to demonstrate. Thus, saturating hippocampal LTP had caused a highly effective anterograde amnesia but no retrograde amnesia. Further experiments showed that saturating LTP would also impair new learning by behaviourally 'naïve' rats but was without effect upon short-term working-memory performance (in Olton and Samuelson's (1976) radial-maze). A final study indicated that HF bursts impaired learning if given very shortly (<5 min) after each daily trial in the reversal paradigm. Taken together, these studies indicate that hippocampal synaptic plasticity is involved in some aspect of spatial information processing in the rat and that, while not involved in long-term storage, the hippocampus seems to underly some element of intermediate term memory.

The Barnes–McNaughton studies were the first systematic attempts to investigate the functional significance of LTP. However, decay time-course is neither the easiest property of LTP to measure nor the easiest to manipulate experimentally. Thus only correlational data may be obtained. Similarly, the procedure involved in saturating LTP—repeated induction—may be having effects upon brain electrical activity aside from its single measured consequence of blocking the ability to induce LTP subsequently. This point deserves to be spelled out in a logically formal manner. The independent variable is the application of a high-frequency train of electrical impulses. The measured dependent variables are: (1) a change in behaviour; and (2) the saturation of LTP. Attractive as the hypothesis may be, it is nevertheless logically fallacious to presume that one dependent consequence of a treatment is the cause of any other, and further experiments are required to rule out alternative interpretations. I hasten to add that my own experiments, using a different method to block LTP and described below, are subject to exactly the same logical problem. Recent discoveries about the role of excitatory amino-acid receptors in the mechanism of induction of LTP have, nevertheless, afforded the opportunity to pursue this complementary approach to the problem.

**The induction of LTP depends upon the activation of a particular type of excitatory amino-acid receptor**

A quite separate field of research has its origins in work begun in the late 1950s. Using the then newly developed technique of iontophoresis, Curtis, Phillis, and Watkins (1960) infused minute quantities of the excitatory amino acid, L-glutamate, on to spinal neurons. They found dramatic increases in the rates of cell-firing. While these results indicated that L-glutamate might, therefore, be an excitatory neurotransmitter, much work still had to be done to establish: (1) that glutamate's presence in neurons was not merely because of its well-known metabolic functions; and (2) that it met established criteria for the identification of a neurotransmitter viz. it was present in pre-synaptic terminals, subject to calcium-dependent release, would bind to post-synaptic recognition sites and be subject to high-affinity re-uptake (see Watkins and Evans, 1981, for review). Thirty years of such research have now moved L-glutamate from the status of being a 'candidate' excitatory transmitter to being a definite one in certain pathways.

The most striking advances in our understanding of excitatory amino-acid (EAA) neurotransmission became possible through the development of several potent and selective antagonists of EAA receptors. These compounds, binding to some but not other sites, have led to our current understanding of there being three (or possibly four) main classes of receptor (Watkins and Olverman 1987). These receptors are called the kainate-, quisqualate- and NMDA-preferring receptors, so named after the excitatory amino acid which preferentially activates each site (Foster and Fagg 1984). Certain antagonists (e.g. CNQX, FNQX) bind preferentially to the kainate and quisqualate sites, while others (AP5, AP7, and CPP) bind to the NMDA site. Neurophysiological studies reveal that, in the hippocampus and in certain other CNS structures, the normal activation of kainate/quisqualate (K/Q) receptors on pyramidal neurons mediates fast excitatory transmission, while selective activation of NMDA receptors is usually without any obvious effect. The NMDA receptor does, however, have the unusual property of responding to post-synaptic depolarization (Dingledine 1983) by releasing the voltage-dependent block of its associated ion-channel (Mayer, Westbrook, and Guthrie 1984; Nowak *et al.* 1984). At the resting potential ($c. -80$ mV), the NMDA ion-channel is blocked by the divalent cation magnesium, such that the binding of an agonist (e.g. the endogenous transmitter) to NMDA receptors is unable to open its associated ion-channel. However, if the neuron is partially depolarized (e.g. to $-40$ mV), the magnesium block is released and subsequent activation of NMDA receptors can then open these channels. The conductances mediated by NMDA receptor activation are substantially greater than those mediated by K/Q receptors (Cull-Candy and Usowicz 1987; Jahr and Stevens 1987), but are also much slower.

A particularly important discovery was that NMDA antagonists, while having no effect upon normal fast synaptic transmission in hippocampus (because they do not bind to K/Q receptors), block the induction of LTP (Collingridge, Kehl, and McClennan 1983). Harris, Ganong, and Cotman (1984) extended this finding by showing that AP5 was stereospecific; the D-isomer of AP5 (D-AP5) blocked LTP while L-AP5 was without effect. Our current understanding of why AP5 blocks LTP remains controversial but a widely held view (Collingridge and Bliss 1987) is as follows (Fig. 11.4): Under normal circumstances, pre-synaptic activity causes release of a certain amount of L-glutamate into the synaptic cleft which then binds to both K/Q and NMDA receptors. However, because of the voltage-dependent block of the NMDA-associated ion-channels, only those ion-channels associated with K/Q receptors open and these permit the entry of $Na^+$ into the post-synaptic terminal, giving rise to a fast but quickly decaying EPSP. However, under conditions of sustained pre-synaptic activity, as occurs during a burst of tetanic stimulation, the post-synaptic depolarization mediated via the K/Q receptors is both large enough and long enough to allow the release of the voltage-dependent block of the NMDA-associated ion-channels. The magnesium is released from its binding site in the channel and, in consequence, ions can now move through this channel into the dendritic spine. Importantly, these NMDA-associated channels seem to be particularly permeable to calcium

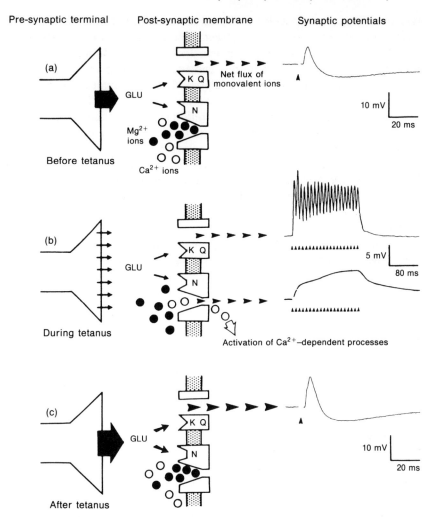

**Fig. 11.4**  The mechanism of induction of LTP in the CA1 region of the hippocampus. (a) Neurotransmitter (e.g. L-glutamate) is released and acts upon both K/Q and NMDA receptors. The NMDA receptors are blocked by magnesium and the excitatory synaptic response (EPSP) is therefore mediated primarily by ion flow through the channels associated with K/Q receptors. (b) During high-frequency activation, the magnesium block of the ion channels associated with NMDA receptors is released by depolarization. Activation of the NMDA receptor by transmitter now results in ions moving through the channel. In this way, calcium enters the post-synaptic region to trigger various intracellular mechanisms which eventually result in an alteration of synaptic efficacy. (c) Subsequent low-frequency stimulation results in a greater EPSP. See text for further details. (Diagram is reprinted from Collingridge and Bliss 1987, by kind permission of the authors.)

(Murphy, Thayer, and Miller 1987), so the sustained tetanic burst has the effect of selectively allowing a *different* ionic messenger to enter the post-synaptic neuron. The calcium then acts upon one or a number of second-messenger systems to set in train a cascade of biochemical events which eventually result in alterations of synaptic efficacy, as alluded to earlier (see Kennedy 1988). According to this account, AP5 blocks LTP by virtue of binding selectively to the NMDA recognition site and so competing with L-glutamate for access. The tetanic stimulation still causes the voltage-dependent magnesium block to be released but, crucially, when the magnesium is released, the channel remains closed because the neurotransmitter agonist is unable to bind to the NMDA receptor to open the channel. Thus AP5 blocks the induction of LTP but it is without effect upon the expression or maintenance of LTP because, once induced, LTP involves an alteration of fast excitatory transmission, i.e. the mediation of EPSPs via K/Q receptors.

This account of the mechanisms involved in the induction of LTP helps to explain several of the properties of LTP referred to earlier. LTP is induced *rapidly* because the calcium signal enters the post-synaptic neuron during the high-frequency burst and the biochemical events set in train take effect rapidly. LTP is *homosynaptic* to the sites of stimulation because the opening of the NMDA-associated ion-channels requires the conjunction of: (1) post-synaptic depolarization; and (2) the binding of neurotransmitter to NMDA receptors. And LTP is *associative* because the post-synaptic depolarization can be caused by neural activation elsewhere on the dendrite than at the site of pre-synaptic activity. NMDA receptors are therefore 'conjunction devices' which endow neurons with the biophysical capacity to detect the co-occurrence of pre-synaptic activity and post-synaptic depolarization, i.e. with the capacity to function as 'Hebb-like' synapses (Kelso, Ganong, and Brown 1986; Wigstrom *et al.* 1986).[2]

NMDA receptors are prominent in a number of regions of the brain and spinal cord (Monaghan and Cotman 1985) and it seems likely that they perform a variety of functions depending on the circuitry into which they are embedded. However, the highest density of NMDA receptors in the forebrain of the rat is to be found in area CA1 of the hippocampus and in the dentate gyrus. The mossy fibre projection from the dentate gyrus to area CA3 has a very low density of NMDA receptors, and it shows an unusual type of 'LTP' which is intermediate in duration (Hopkins and Johnston 1984), non-associative (Nicoll, Kauer and Malenka 1988), insensitive to AP5 (Harris and Cotman 1986) and apparently unaffected by intracellular injections of EGTA into CA3 pyramidal cells (EGTA chelates calcium—Bradler and Barrionuevo 1988). However, the mossy fibre projection aside, LTP in the dentate gyrus, in area CA1 and in the outer layers of area CA3 (where the perforant path and commissural projections terminate) is both associative and sensitive to AP5. This drug is, therefore, a marvellous tool for investigating the functional implications of the main type of hippocampal LTP. Its effects are reversible, it is without toxic effects (on the contrary, it is neuroprotective—Meldrum 1985) and, unlike a lesion, it has the much more subtle effect of leaving almost all aspects of hippocampal electrophysiology unaffected other than the capacity of this circuitry to alter synaptic efficacy.

## The swimming-pool task

All the behavioural experiments involved training rats to escape from water in a large circular swimming pool (2 m diameter). Rats are good swimmers and, as the motor programmes involved in its co-ordination are located in the brainstem, lesions of, or the administration of drugs to the forebrain are without effect upon the motor movements required of the animals in performing the task. By maintaining the water temperature at a constant level (12 °C below body temperature), it is also possible to control the level of motivation to escape.

The simplest task used is that of training rats to find a platform hidden at a fixed place in the pool, its top surface reaching to no higher than 1 cm below the water-surface ('place navigation'). Normal rats readily learn this task such that, from any randomly varied starting point at the perimeter, they are able to swim directly to the platform, even on the first trial of each day (Morris 1981). Presumably the rats build up some internal representation in long-term memory of the layout of the cues in the room and these are sufficient to support appropriate orientation. A variant of this basic procedure is a 'working-memory' paradigm in which the platform is moved from day to day but left in the same position throughout each day's trials. Typically, the rats settle into a pattern of doing poorly on the first trial (when they have no way of knowing where the platform is hidden) but showing a dramatic 1-trial improvement between Trials 1 and 2 (Morris 1983). By varying the interval between Trials 1 and 2, it is possible to probe the efficiency of short-term memory relatively independently of long-term memory. Another variant, but a very different one, is to use platforms which protrude visibly above the water surface. Training with a single platform converts the task from one involving learning to one requiring no more than cue-guided approach to a landmark; it provides a way of checking whether lesions or drugs affect the motivation to escape (Morris 1984). A more demanding version involves two visibly discriminable platforms (e.g. gray v. black-and-white stripes), one of which is rigid and offers escape from the water, the other of which is floating and offers insufficient buoyancy. The rats readily grasp the logic of their predicament and gradually learn to head for the rigid platform.

Using these simple procedures, I and my colleagues have established that aspiration, radiofrequency and neurotoxic lesions of the hippocampus, subiculum and/or entorhinal cortex (the cortical region which projects into hippocampus) impair the performance of the simple 'place-navigation' task (Morris *et al.* 1982; Schenk and Morris 1985). These findings have been corroborated and extended by other investigators (e.g. Sutherland, Whishaw, and Kolb 1983, 1988). However, hippocampal lesions have no effect upon either of the two visible platform tasks (Morris 1983; Morris, Hagan, and Rawlins 1986*b*). Rats with hippocampal lesions swim just as quickly to a single visible platform (showing they have no lack of motivation to escape from the water) and learn to discriminate the gray from the striped platform at the same rate as unoperated controls (I doubt this is because of an inherent insensitivity of these tasks, because high doses of antiocholinergic drugs (e.g. atropine) impair both place-navigation and visual discrimination equally (Hagan, Tweedie, and Morris 1986)). The profile of impairment after hippocampal lesions in the rat is reminiscent of the dissociation between spared and impaired function in human amnesia (Corkin 1968, 1984; Squire and Zola-Morgan 1983; Baddeley 1982; Squire 1987). Indeed, one simple, although far from satisfactory, way of thinking about this, is to consider the place-navigation tasks as analogous to 'declarative' memory tasks, in the sense that we are asking the animal to learn some 'fact' about the world, i.e. where the platform is hidden. Whereas, the visual discrimination task is 'procedural' in the sense that we are merely requiring the animal to build up a disposition to approach one platform but not the other. In any event, the differential sensitivity of these two tasks to hippocampal lesions provides a useful behavioural dissociation against which to assess the effects of AP5 upon learning.

### The NMDA antagonist AP5 causes a selective impairment of learning at doses sufficient to block LTP *in vivo*

The first obstacle to tackle was that AP5 does not cross the blood–brain barrier. Accordingly, the drug was administered in one of two ways: (1) via miniature subcutaneous osmotic minipumps whose contents, discharging slowly over two weeks, were led via a catheter to the lateral ventricle; or (2) via direct injection into the hippocampus or cortex through previously implanted guide cannulae. Each of these procedures involves surgery a few days before the commencement of training. The advantage of the minipump technique is that the animals need not be disturbed further for the period that the minipumps operate, and that the drug levels reach a steady state in brain. The advantage of direct infusion is that particular brain regions can be targeted with AP5 a few minutes prior to daily training.

The first experiment involved giving rats 15 trials to find the hidden platform, followed by a 'transfer' or probe test in which the platform had been removed from the pool (Morris *et al.* 1986). The transfer test lasted for 60 s, during which the animals had an opportunity to search for the now absent refuge. To obtain objective measures of this search behaviour, the animals' movements were tracked using a computerized image-analysing device. Normal rats search in the part of the pool previously occupied by the platform, thereby 'revealing' that they had learned and remembered its location. Three minipump groups were trained: D,L-AP5, L-AP5, and control (the latter consisting of both vehicle-treated and unoperated rats). The results showed that the D,L-AP5 group learned more slowly than the L-AP5 and control groups which, in turn, did not differ. Furthermore, in the transfer test, the D,L-AP5 group showed no evidence of having learned much about the location of the platform (Fig. 11.5). The stereospecificity of these behavioural effects of

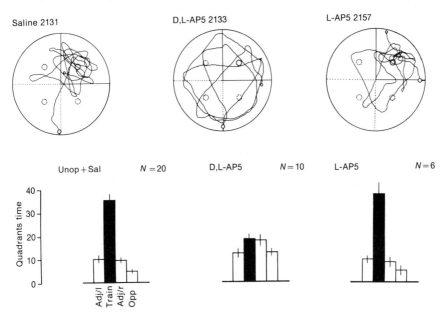

**Fig. 11.5**   The search behaviour of the three median animals in each group during the spatial transfer test. Compare the spatially restricted search of the saline and L-AP5 rats with that shown by the D,L-AP5 rats. The group means are shown in the histograms below. The black bar is the time (s) in the training quadrant during the 60 s test. (From Morris *et al.* 1986.)

AP5 exactly matched that reported by Harris, Ganong, and Cotman (1984) in their study of the induction of LTP, and a subsequent control experiment established that the dose of D,L-AP5 used in the minipumps was sufficient to block LTP *in vivo* without apparent effect upon baseline field-potentials. Both Control and L-AP5 rats showed normal LTP.

This simple result was exciting because it suggested that a dose of AP5 sufficient to block LTP also impaired a task known to be sensitive to hippocampal lesions. However, many issues remained (and still remain) to be sorted out: Was AP5 affecting learning or performance? Does it affect all learning tasks or, by virtue of the high density of NMDA receptors in hippocampus, is it specific to tasks sensitive to hippocampal lesions? Do all tasks sensitive to hippocampal lesions show impairments in the presence of AP5? Does differential task sensitivity reflect a real underlying difference in the neural mechanisms of learning, or could it be due to differential drug distribution to relevant areas of the brain? Does AP5 have side-effects? Might such side-effects account for any or all aspects of the behavioural impairments observed? Is the dose–response function for the impairment of learning in line with that for the blockade of LTP? These and other questions are all of interest, but they are particularly important in so far as they address the crucial logical issue of whether the effects of AP5 upon learning are *caused* by its capacity to block the induction of LTP. AP5 may be, indeed, it almost certainly is, having effects upon brain activity other than just blocking synaptic plasticity (e.g. Leung and Desborough (1988) have raised the possibility that AP5 blocks hippocampal theta activity). Might these 'other effects' be contributing to the behavioural impairments? Resolution of this issue is crucial to establishing whether hippocampal synaptic plasticity is involved in certain types of learning.

Much of this research remains incomplete. However, a recent series of experiments (Morris 1989) have established the following. First, when pumped into the lateral ventricle over 10–14 days via osmotic minipumps, AP5 spreads all over the forebrain in a relatively even manner. HPLC measurements of whole-tissue concentrations show only a slight but non-significant decline in concentration as one moves away from the cannula tip (Butcher, Morris, and Hamberger 1988). Second, AP5 does not affect all types of learning and, in particular, it does not impair visual discrimination learning. Whether pumped into the ventricle or directly into visual cortex, AP5 has no effect upon the rate or asymptotic level of performance of the same two-platform task which was earlier described as unaffected by hippocampal lesions. Thus, AP5 appears to impair at least one type of 'declarative' memory task, but to be without effect upon one 'procedural' task—suggestive of a site of action within the hippocampus. Third, AP5 impairs the performance of other hippocampally sensitive tasks including the non-spatial operant task called 'drl' in which rats must keep track of their behaviour over time (Tonkiss, Morris, and Rawlins 1988). Fourth, minute injections of AP5 (10–100 nanomoles) directly into hippocampus are sufficient to cause a dose-related impairment of the learning and/or reversal of place-navigation in the swimming pool, and a parallel dose-related impairment of LTP *in vivo* (Morris, Halliwell, and Bowery 1988). Companion experiments to this latter study, using radiolabelled AP4 and AP7, established that most of the injected drug remained in the hippocampus throughout the period of testing (20 min).

Other experiments have been designed to exploit our knowledge of the mechanisms of action of AP5 at NMDA receptors more fully. For example, neurophysiological work has established that the drug blocks the induction of LTP but not its expression or maintenance. It follows that if LTP is involved in information storage, AP5 should impair the *acquisition* of place-navigation but be without effect upon the *retention* of previously acquired knowledge. This prediction has been tested in two experiments, both of which involved initial training in the absence of the drug. Only then were the minipumps (containing AP5 or vehicle solution) implanted, this surgery being followed by several days of further training. In the first experiment, all rats were retrained during this final phase to the same platform location as that used in pre-drug training. The results showed that AP5 caused no impairment—drug-treated rats were as fast at escaping from the water as vehicle-treated controls (Morris 1989, Experiment 4). However, proving the null result is hardly the most sensitive test. Accordingly, in a follow-up study being conducted with Roger Hendry, place-navigation training is again being given prior to minipump implantation followed by either: (1) continued training to the same platform location; or (2) training to a new hidden platform location diagonally opposite in the pool (e.g. moving it from NE to SW). The preliminary results show that AP5-treated rats required to learn a new platform location during retraining are impaired, while AP5-treated rats retrained to their original platform location are unaffected (Fig. 11.6). The design of this experiment—and its result—is analogous to the 'saturation' experiment conducted by McNaughton *et al.* (1986). The analogy extends even to the two studies sharing the same logical problem: AP5 administration, no less than repeated induction of LTP, may be having 'side-effects' which are really responsible for the behavioural impairment. However, the burden of proof is surely shifted in as much as two radically different treatments whose only known common consequence is the blockade of LTP have identical behavioural outcomes. In summary, NMDA receptors appear to be involved in the initial acquisition and storage of information into long-term memory but not in the retrieval of such information.

A second experiment guided by neurophysiological considerations concerns the involvement of NMDA receptors in short- or intermediate-term memory. AP5 does not block post-tetanic or paired-pulse potentiation (Harris and Cotman 1983), nor does it affect LTP on the mossy fibres to area CA3 (Harris and Cotman 1986). An intriguing possibility is that the drug may therefore have little effect on tasks which, though impaired by hippocampal lesions, require only the temporary storage of information over short periods. An example of such a task is the 'working-memory' paradigm in which the platform's position remains fixed within each day's set of trials but moves from

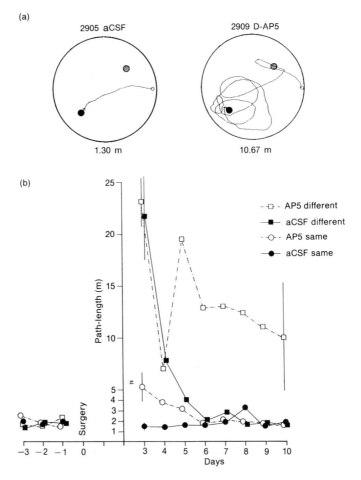

**Fig. 11.6** The paths taken 10 days after the start of 'reversal' training (1 trial/day) by two typical rats given aCSF or D-AP5 in the experiment investigating anterograde and retrograde effects of AP5. The black circle is the current position of the platform, and the striped circle shows its former location during initial training before surgery. While the aCSF rat swims directly to the new location, the AP5 rat approaches the old place preferentially before searching in the general vicinity of the platform's new location. The drug cannot have merely caused a general disorganization of spatial behaviour because AP5 rats retrained to the original platform location show no disruption in performance.

day to day. Recent experiments in Edinburgh by Sabrina Davis indicate that AP5 has no effect upon performance when the interval between Trials 1 and 2 of each day is 30 s, but does impair performance when this interval is lengthened to 2 h. This dissociation supports the earlier conclusion that hippocampal NMDA receptors are particularly involved when information is to be stored in long-term memory.

## NMDA receptors as neural components of distributed associative memories: prospects and problems

How do hippocampal NMDA receptors participate in the long-term storage of information during learning? One possibility is that they detect the conjunction of stimuli presented to a matrix of neurons performing competitive learning and so contribute to pattern separation (see Rolls, Chapter 10). A different possibility is that they enable parts of hippocampal circuitry to instantiate a type of distributed associative memory (such as that described by Willshaw, Bunemann, and Longuet-Higgins 1969), an idea first explored in relation to the hippocampus by Marr (1971) in his theory of 'simple-memory'. This idea has recently been revived by both Rolls (1987) and by McNaughton and Morris (1987) in the light of new anatomical and electrophysiological findings.

The basic idea is that parts of the hippocampus have an intrinsic local circuitry very similar to that required of distributed associative memory networks. Consider, for example, the dentate gyrus. Cortical inputs, arising from layer II stellate cells in entorhinal cortex, project via the perforant path to contact an expanded number of dentate granule cells within transverse strips, called lamellae, which cut across the longitudinal septo-temporal axis of the hippocampus (Andersen, Bliss, and Skrede 1971; Hjorth-Simonsen and Jeune 1972). The terminals of the perforant path, constituting about 70 per cent of the synapses on dentate granule cell dendrites, probably use L-glutamate as their neurotransmitter and have both K/Q and NMDA receptors on post-synaptic dendritic spines (Storm-Mathisen and Ottersen 1988; Monaghan and Cotman 1985). This pathway consists of (at least) two distinct fibre systems in the rat (Wyss 1981). The medial pathway terminates close to the cell bodies, has synapses whose EPSPs are initially more potent than those of the lateral pathway, and terminates topographically in relatively restricted transverse strips. The lateral pathway terminates in a more diffuse way, although in other species (e.g. the cat) a somewhat more specific projection pattern prevails (van Groen and Lopes da Silva 1985). This situation resembles the wiring of a simple one-layered associative network. (Fig. 11.7), with activity on the medial pathway serving as one input (e.g. of an 'event' to be remembered) and activity on the lateral pathway being the other (e.g. as the 'retrieval' cue, or 'context'). Thus, neural activity corresponding to the event ($Y$ inputs in Fig. 11.7) might cause a subset of dentate granule cells to become sufficiently depolarized to release the voltage-dependent block on the NMDA receptors at the terminals of the lateral pathway. Appropriately timed spatial

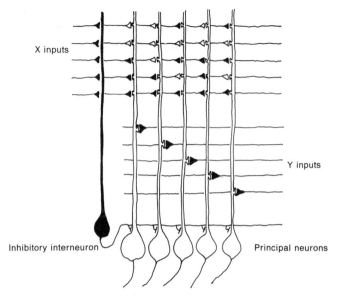

**Fig. 11.7** A simple one-layered associative matrix in the dendrites of an array of neurons consisting of X-inputs synapsing *en passage* (a) onto an inhibitory interneuron; and (b) onto an array of synapses containing K/Q and NMDA receptors, Y-inputs synapsing in an ordered manner onto terminals which are capable of producing a relatively large depolarization. Information about the association of X and Y stimulus events will be stored as a pattern of altered synaptic weights in the X input array. After learning, an appropriate stimulus on the X input array will evoke a 'memory' of the Y event with which it was associated, with feedforward inhibition mediated via the inhibitory interneuron shunting the depolarization of the principal neurons in an appropriate manner to realize the correct pattern of cell firing. Neuronal arrangements not dissimilar to this are found in both the dentate gyrus and area CA3 of the hippocampus. (Based on McNaughton and Morris 1987.)

patterns of activity on the lateral pathway (X inputs) would then cause synapses at which there was a conjunction with post-synaptic depolarization (due to the prior medial pathway activity) to become potentiated. Subsequent presentation of the same lateral pathway stimulus would then cause (at least in a statistical sense) a pattern of depolarization across the dentate granule cells similar to what would have occurred in response to the medial perforant path stimulus during learning. This pattern of depolarization can be translated into an appropriate pattern of cell firing if feedforward inhibition is also considered. Inhibitory interneurons (basket cells) with what appear to be the necessary characteristics to perform this translation are found throughout the dentate gyrus. These cells receive excitatory input from the perforant path afferents in the molecular layer and feedforward inhibition on to the granule cells in proportion to their level of excitatory activation. The inhibitory interneurones are far fewer in number than the granule cells but they have an extensive and diffuse axonal trajectory. Physiological work has shown that the equilibrium potential for the inhibitory transmitter GABA is close to the resting potential of the dentate granule cells and, as a result, inhibition has the effect of dividing the excitation by a variable monotonically related to the number of active afferents. The advance timing of the feedforward inhibition appears to be such that the division operation is in effect before the granule cells would otherwise begin to fire. In this way, the pattern of depolarization induced by lateral pathway activation during recall is translated into the exact pattern of dentate granule cell firing, as would have occurred in response to medial pathway activation during learning (see McNaughton and Morris 1987, for more detailed description).

The dentate gyrus is subject to both regular and irregular electrical oscillations called hippocampal rhythmic slow activity (RSA or 'theta', Vanderwolf 1971) and large-amplitude irregular activity (LIA) respectively. There have been many theories about the behavioural significance of theta activity (Black 1975), but discovery of the mechanisms of action of NMDA receptors suggests a new hypothesis. The regular cycling of voltage at about 7 Hz (varying between 5 and 11 Hz depending upon behavioural state) would cyclically increase and then decrease the probability of the voltage-dependent block of NMDA receptors being released. Appropriately timed neural activity (i.e. timed to maximize the probability of association) should occur on the peak positivity of the intracellular theta wave (Rudell, Fox, and Ranck 1980). Information arriving at other times would be less likely to be associated because it would then be harder to activate NMDA receptors. Theta activity may also provide a way of maintaining information in memory in the absence of either the stimulus event or its retrieval cue. This idea, due to Gary Lynch (personal communication), runs as follows. Dentate granule cells project in a highly specific way onto CA3 pyramidal cells (Blackstad *et al.* 1970), each mossy fibre making relatively few but very powerful contacts close to the pyramidal cell bodies (see Rolls, Chapter 12, where the importance of this point is pursued more fully). As we have seen earlier, these contacts show a non-associative, AP5-insensitive form of LTP (it may even be better described a long-lasting form of PTP). Assume that, at a given moment, the output from the dentate granule cells corresponds to either an event or the retrieved memory of an event, and that this output is projected onto CA3 cells in a pattern which induces LTP of the small subset of mossy fibre terminals which are activated. If the dentate granule cells were thereafter to fire in a synchronous but unmodulated manner (i.e. unmodulated by any *further* stimulus input from entorhinal cortex), the statistical probability of CA3 cells firing would depend upon the previously established spatial pattern of LTP at the mossy fibre terminals. Thus, the dentate and area CA3 could act in tandem as a temporary register of information. Again, in order for there to be good separation between signal and noise, feedforward inhibition would have to shunt the activity of the less well activated CA3 pyramidal cells to prevent inappropriate ones from firing. Such a scheme could work as a limited capacity information-register. However, because (1) the CA3 axons feed back onto their own dendrites and forward to area CA1 with ramifications throughout the longitudinal axis of the hippocampus, and (2) both CA1 and CA3 neurons receive a direct projection from entorhinal cortex via the perforant path, it might be possible to use this circuitry to associate events which are separated in time (Rawlins 1985).

There are, however, a number of problems with this proposal which, in its simplest or literal form, is almost certainly incorrect. First, it is surely a mistake to think of the entire hippocampal circuitry as a series of one-layered associative networks arranged along the trisynaptic circuit. We know that the learning capacities of one-layered nets are limited (see McClelland, Chapter 2), and the connectivity of the hippocampus suggests a more complex arrangement. For example, there are major connections of the perforant pathway to areas CA1 and CA3, and thus the entorhinal input makes contact with transforms of itself processed via earlier parts of the classical trisynaptic circuitry. The computational implications of this 'cascaded feedforward' arrangement have barely been explored (cf. Rolls, Chapter 12), and the timing arrangements for appropriate activation of K/Q and NMDA receptors along the cascade needs to be considered. Second, the idea has little to say about why the density of NMDA receptors should be so high in both the dentate gyrus and area CA1, but so low in the mossy fibre terminals to area CA3. So far, I have hinted that the point of such an arrangement might be to allow the temporary storage of associations between events that may be separated in time (as proposed by Rawlins 1985). However, the idea is not yet expressed in a rigorously testable form. Third, the proposal that even parts of the hippocampus are association matrices does not come to terms with the fact that this structure plays a role in the storage of information but may not be the site of long-term storage itself (cf. Rolls, Chapter 12). This notion is supported by clinical studies indicating that damage to the hippocampus can, sometimes, be characterized by severe anterograde amnesia in the absence of (or a time-restricted) retrograde amnesia (e.g. Scoville and Milner 1957; Corkin 1984; Zola-Morgan, Squire, and Amarel 1986). The LTP-saturation studies of McNaughton et al. (1986) also suggest that the hippocampus is not a site of long-term information storage in rats, although lesion studies in rats (there are no relevant studies on primates) remain ambiguous. Thus, either the hippocampus stores information temporarily (e.g. Marr 1971; Rawlins 1985) and then transfers relevant and useful information into neocortex; or it computes some 'transform' of the input events which is 'backprojected' to neocortex to 'guide' long-term storage there (Rolls, Chapter 12). The problem with my own account is that it is unclear why and how NMDA receptors participate in the process of *long-term* storage (see also Squire, Shimamura, and Amarel 1988).

There is, however, a final problem with the idea that NMDA receptors help instantiate some kind of distributed associative memory. To work properly, such memory systems must have mechanisms for *decreasing* synaptic efficacy as well as for increasing it. LTP is, however, strictly a phenomenon in which synaptic efficacy is increased. There have been a number of reports that LTP is associated with a concomitant heterosynaptic depression (Lynch, Dunwiddie, and Gribkoff 1977; Andersen, Bliss and Skrede 1977; Levy and Steward 1979; Abraham and Goddard 1983), but neither the determinants nor the time-course of this or other types of synaptic depression in hippocampus have been well worked out. One important distinction is between heterosynaptic and homosynaptic depression. Heterosynaptic depression occurs in association with LTP at synapses which are not activated by the tetanic burst. Thus, the local synaptic rule for heterosynaptic depression is a conjunction of post-synaptic activity (possibly post-synaptic depolarization) and pre-synaptic *inactivity*. Since most synapses are, presumably, rarely being activated at any moment in time, heterosynaptic depression constitutes a physiological phenomenon analogous to 'normalization'. It need not be an exact normalization of synaptic weights such that $\sum w_i = 1$ at all times (where $w_i$ is the synaptic weight of the ith synapse on a neuron), but the co-occurrence of a large increase in $w_i$ on a small number of synapses (LTP) and a small decrease in $w_i$ on the larger number of momentarily inactivated synapses will have a similar effect to mathamatical normalization. In comparison, homosynaptic depression would be quite different in that it would involve a selective depression of certain synapses but not others. I can see no obvious way in which homosynaptic depression, if it occurred in hippocampus or elsewhere, could possibly achieve its implicit synaptic selectivity unless the local synaptic rule for its occurrence involved a conjunction with pre-synaptic *activity* rather than, as with heterosynaptic depression, pre-synaptic inactivity. An intriguing possibility is, therefore, that the rule for eliciting homosynaptic depression may be the exact opposite of that studied experimentally in relation to heterosynaptic depression—specifically, that it may require a conjunction of pre-synaptic activity and post-synaptic hyperpolarization. A moment's thought will indicate that these are rather bizarre electrophysiological circumstances because, at excitatory synapses, pre-synaptic activity would normally be expected to depolarize a neuron. It follows that, in order for the necessary conjunction to occur, there must also be some separate post-synaptic inhibition overriding the effects of the pre-synaptic excitatory input, participating in the mechanism through which the excitatory synapses come to be depressed. The essential conjunction may occur during after-hyperpolarization induced by cell firing.

Work on the alteration of ocular dominance and orientation selectivity in visual cortex after reverse eyelid suture in kittens bears upon these ideas. If ocular dominance is measured in kittens reared monocularly, binocularly driven cells in visual cortex show an ocular dominance profile dominated by activation from one eye. Upon reverse suture, the ocular dominance profile reverses such that inputs from the previously inactive eye increase in efficacy while inputs from the previously inactive eye decrease. Various 'rules' have been proposed to describe how this shift in dominance profile is achieved. Specifically, the concept of heterosynaptic depression is, broadly, consistent with the so-called Stent–Singer rule (Stent 1973; Singer 1985), while homosynaptic depression is more consistent with the rule proposed by Bienenstock, Cooper, and Munro (1982) and elaborated physiologically by Bear, Cooper, and Ebner (1987). Both rules differ from the Hebb rule in proposing that both up- and down-regulation of synaptic efficacy can occur. The Stent–Singer rule restricts synaptic plasticity to instances in which post-synaptic activity is above some threshold and asserts that synaptic weights increase when pre-synaptic activity is high, but decrease when pre-synaptic activity is low. The BCM rule involves an adjustable threshold ($\theta$) determined by the time-averaged activity of the postsynaptic neuron (c). The magnitude and direction of the change in synaptic weight is held to be proportional to the product of the amount of pre-synaptic activity (d) and a nonmonotonic function ($\phi(c)$) whose sign is negative for low instantaneous values of $c$ but positive for high values. Bear *et al.* (1987) identify NMDA receptors as the mechanism serving to trigger the transition from a negative value of $\phi(c)$ to a positive value. Thus the product of $d$ and $\phi(c)$ will assume its maximal negative value when $d$ is high and $c$ is low, i.e. when there is a conjunction of pre-synaptic activity and post-synaptic hyperpolarization. Evidence in support of these rules has been reported by Kleinschmidt, Bear, and Singer (1987). A recent study has demonstrated a paradoxical shift in ocular dominance towards the *inactive* eye in a reverse-suture experiment in which visual cortex neurons are subjected to the GABA agonist muscimol during visual experience (Reiter and Stryker 1988). This study would appear to offer evidence in support of the BCM rule.

What are the implications of these ideas for hippocampal synaptic plasticity and its putative role in learning? They do not alter our basic understanding, reviewed earlier, of the role of NMDA receptors in LTP. However, the general form of the equation determining changes in synaptic weights may have to be re-written in expanded form to reflect both Hebb-like (NMDA mediated) and 'non-Hebb-like' components:

$$\Delta w_i = \text{Hebb-type increase} - \text{heterosynaptic decrease} - \text{homosynaptic decrease}$$

There are several points to be made about this expanded function. First, we do not know the relative magnitudes of the heterosynaptic or homosynaptic depression terms, nor even the detailed experimental conditions under which each may occur. Second, the evidence for homosynaptic depression in hippocampus is sparse (Stanton *et al.* 1988) and not wholly convincing. Third, if either hetero- or homosynaptic depression occurs routinely, the concept of a decay time-course for synaptic increases (e.g. of LTP) may be something of a misnomer. LTP may *appear* to decay rapidly because, for other reasons, conditions favouring long-term depression have been inadvertently produced. The issue should be investigated systematically (for example, the BCM rule predicts tht LTP will appear to decay more rapidly in the presence of GABA agonists). Thus, as Lynch and others have long argued, LTP may be non-decremental. Finally, and perhaps more importantly, the addition of these terms to the local synaptic rule gives even a simple one-layered associative matrix added computing power. In addition to learning that stimulus A is associated with stimulus B, such a matrix can also learn that A is no longer associated with B when these two events no longer occur together. In addition, the storage capacity of the network may be substantially improved by both normalization and synapse-specific depression, although this point remains to be established formally.

## Conclusion

The primary purpose of this chapter has been to describe various behavioural experiments conducted to address the limited but important question of whether synaptic plasticity plays a role in information storage. Evidence has been reviewed indicating that learning can give rise to morphological changes in synapses, that certain properties of one well-understood form of plasticity are of functional relevance and that blocking the induction of LTP either physiologically or pharmacologically gives rise to a selective anterograde amnesia.

A final point is that in attempting to bridge the gap between a neuropsychological and neurophysiological account of the mechanisms of learning, it is proving useful to follow both a 'top–down' and a 'bottom–up' strategy. The top–down components to which I have alluded include: (1) capitalizing upon neuropsychological ideas about spared and impaired behavioural function after hippocampal damage; and (2) the conceptual idea of the Hebb synapse. The bottom–up components have been: (1) the way in which information about the voltage-dependency of NMDA receptor action (worked out on neonatal spinal cord neurons grown in tissue culture!) led to thinking about how these receptors might serve as conjunction devices for associative learning; and (2) how a detailed understanding of the neural mechanisms of LTP have led to new pharmacological routes for investigating the role of hippocampal circuitry in learning and memory. The adventure of linking these concepts to the emerging ideas of neural network theory is in its infancy but, like most adventures, is well worth pursuing.

## Acknowledgements

I am grateful to Mark Bear, Tim Bliss, Tom Brown, Gabriel Horn, Gary Lynch and David Willshaw for discussion about aspects of this work, to Edmund Rolls for commenting upon an earlier draft of this chapter, and to Carol Barnes, Philip Bradley, Graham Collingridge, Brian McCabe, and Bruce McNaughton for their premission to reproduce or adapt certain of their figures. My own experiments and preparation of the manuscript were supported by an MRC Programme Grant held jointly with David Willshaw.

## Notes

1. No one seriously believes that LTP *itself* is involved in memory—the synchronous activation of thousands of fibres never happens in the normal functioning brain. Rather, the idea is that the underlying neural mechanisms of LTP may be the same as those recruited during learning and only in this sense is LTP described as a 'model' of memory. This semantic distinction was, incidentally, made at the end of Bliss and Lomo's (1973) original paper.

2. There are two qualifications to thinking of the coupling of K/Q and NMDA receptors as instantiating a Hebb-synapse. First, as discussed by both Kelso, Ganong, and Brown (1986) and Wigstrom *et al.* (1986), the post-synaptic signal is depolarization and not 'activity' as Hebb originally proposed. Thus, Wigstrom and Gustaffson showed that the conjunction of single pulses of afferent stimulation with artificial post-synaptic depolarization (by voltage-clamp) could induce LTP, while Kelso *et al.* showed that blocking $Na^+$ spikes with QX-222 does not block the phenomenon. The pre-synaptic tetanus is not, therefore, a necessary condition for LTP—it being merely one way of releasing the magnesium block of the NMDA associated ion channels. Second, NMDA receptors could act as conjunction devices without setting in motion a Hebbian 'growth process' between the two active cells. For example, Koch (1987) has proposed a model of thalamic function which incorporates NMDA receptors to detect conjunctive neural activation, but the model does not entail synaptic plasticity at the level of the thalamus.

## References

Abraham, W. C. and Goddard, G. V. (1983). Asymmetric relationships between homosynaptic long-term potentiation and heterosynaptic long-term depression. *Nature*, **305**, 717–19.

Abrams, T. W. and Kandel, E. R. (1988). Is contiguity detection a system or a cellular property? Learning in Aplysia suggests a possible molecular site. *Trends in Neuroscience*, **11**, 128–35.

Alkon, D. L. (1987). *Memory traces in the brain.* Cambridge University Press.

Andersen, P., Bliss, T. V. P., and Skrede, K. K. (1971). Unit analysis of hippocampal population spikes. *Experimental Brain Research*, **13**, 208–21.

Andersen, P., Sundberg, S. H., Sveen, O., and Wigstrom, H. (1977). Specific long-lasting potentiation of synaptic transmission in hippocampal slices. *Nature*, **266**, 736–7.

Artola, A. and Singer, W. (1987). Long-term potentiation and NMDA receptors in rat visual cortex. *Nature*, **330**, 649–52.

Baddeley, A. D. (1982). Implications of neuropsychological evidence for theories of normal memory. *Philosophical Transactions of the Royal Society*, **298**, 59–72.

Bailey, C. H. and Chen, M. C. (1983). Morphological basis of long-term habituation and sensitization in *Aplysia*. *Science*, **220**, 91–93.

Barnes, C. A. (1979). Memory deficits associated with senescence: A neurophysiological and behavioural study in the rat. *Journal of Compositive and Physiological Psychology*, **93**, 74–104.

Barnes, C. A. and McNaughton, B. L. (1985). An age comparison of the rates of acquisition and forgetting of spatial information in relation to long-term enhancement of hippocampal synapses. *Behaviour Neuroscience*, **99**, 1040–8.

Barrionuevo, G. and Brown, T. H. (1983). Associative long-term potentiation in hippocampal slices. *Proceedings of the National Acadamy of Science*, **80**, 7347–51.

Bateson, P. P. G. (1966). The characteristics and context of imprinting. *Biological Reviews*, **41**, 177–220.

Bateson, P. P. G., Horn, G., and Rose, S. P. R. (1972). Effects of early experience on regional incorporation of precursors into RNA and protein in the chick brain. *Brain Research*, **39**, 449–65.

Bear, M. F., Cooper, L. N., and Ebner, F. F. (1987). A physiological basis for a theory of synapse modification. *Science*, **237**, 42–8.

Berger, T. W. (1984). Long-term potentiation of hippocampal synaptic transmission affects rate of behavioural learning. *Science*, **224**, 627–30.

Bienenstock, E. L., Cooper, C. N., and Munro, P. W. (1982). Theory for the development of neuron selectivity: orientation specificity and binoculor interaction in visual cortex. *Journal of Neuroscience*, **2**, 32–48.

Black, A. H. (1975). Hippocampal electrical activity and behaviour. In *The hippocampus*, Volume 2 (eds. R. L. Isaacson and K. H. Pribram). Plenum Press, NY.

Blackstad, T. W., Brink, K., Hem, J., and Jeune, B. (1970). Distribution of hippocampal mossy-fibers in the rat. An experimental study with silver impregnation methods. *Journal of Conpositive Neurology*, **138**, 433–50.

Bliss, T. V. P. and Gardner-Medwin, A. R. (1973). Long-lasting potentiation of synaptic transmission in the dentate area of the unanaesthetized rabbit following stimulation of the perforant path. *Journal of Physiology*, **232**, 357–74.

Bliss, T. V. P. and Lomo, T. (1973). Long-lasting potentiation of synaptic transmission in the dentate area of the anaesthetised rabbit following stimulation of the perforant path. *Journal of Physiology*, **232**, 331–56.

Bliss, T. V. P. and Lynch, M. A. (1988). Long-term potentiation of synaptic transmission in the hippocampus: properties and mechanisms. In *Long term potentiation: from biophysics to behaviour* (eds. S. A. Deadwyler and P. Landfield), pp. 3–72. Alan Liss, NY.

Bradler, J. E. and Barrinuevo, G. (1988). Homo- and heterosynaptic expression of LTP in hippocampal CA3 neurons: sensitivity to intracellular EGTA injections. *Soc. Neuroscience Abstracts*, **14**, 255.4.

Brindley, G. S. (1967). The classification of modifiable synapses and their use in models for conditioning. *Proceedings Royal Society, Series B.*, **168**, 361–76.

Brown, T. H., Chang, V. C., Ganong, A. H., Keenan, C. L., and Kelso, S. R. (1988*a*). Biophysical properties of dendrites and spines that may control the induction and expression of long-term synaptic potentiation. In *Long-term potentiation: from biophysics to behaviour* (eds. S. A. Deadwyler and P. Landfield), pp. 210–4. Alan Liss and Co., NY.

Brown, T. H., Chapman, P. F., Kairiss, E. W., and Keenan, C. L. (1988*b*). Long-term synaptic potentiation. *Science*, **242**, 724–8.

Butcher, S. F., Morris, R. G. M., and Hamberger, A. (1988). Measurement of AP5 in rat brain following intraventricular infusion: relationship to impairments in learning. In preparation.

Cajal, Ramon y (1911). *Histologie du Systeme Nerveux de l'Homme et des Vertebres, II.* Maluine, Paris.

Castellucci, V. F. and Kandel, E. R. (1974). A quantal analysis of the synaptic depression underlying habituation of the gill withdrawal reflex in *Aplysia*. *Proceedings of the National Academy of Science*, **71**, 5004–8.

Collingridge, G. L. and Bliss, T. V. P. (1987). NMDA Receptors—their role in long-term potentiation. *Trends in Neuroscience*, **10**, 288–93.

Collingridge, G. L., Kehl, S. J., and McLennan, H. (1983). Excitatory amino-acids in synaptic transmission in the Schaffer collateral-commissural pathway of the rat hippocampus. *Journal of Physiology* **334**, 33–46.

Corkin, S. (1968). Acquisition of a motor-skill after bilateral medial temporal excision. *Neuropsychologia*, **6**, 255–65.

Corkin, S. (1984). Lasting consequences of bilateral medial temporal lobectomy: clinical course and experimental findings in H. M. *Seminars in Neurology*, **4**, 249–59.

Cowan, J. D. and Sharp, D. H. (1988). Neural nets. *Los Alamos Technical Bulletin*, **87**, 4098.

Cull-Candy, S. G. and Usowicz, M. M. (1987). Multiple conductance channels activated by excitatory amino acids in cerebellar neurones. *Nature*, **325**, 525–9.

Curtis, D. R., Phillis, J. W., and Watkins, J. C. (1960). The excitation of spinal neurons by certain acidic amino acids. *Journal of Physiology*, **150**, 656–82.

Desmond, N. L. and Levy, W. B. (1983). Synaptic correlates of associative potentiation/depression: an instrastructural study in the hippocampus. *Brain Research*, **265**, 21–30.

Dingledine, R. (1983). N-Methyl-aspartate activates voltage-dependent calcium conductance in rat hippocampal pyramidal cells. *Journal of Physiology* **343**, 385–405.

Feldman, J. A. and Ballard, D. H. (1982). Connectionist models and their properties. *Cognitive Science*, **6**, 205–54.

Fifkova, E. and van Harreveld, A. (1977). Long-lasting morphological changes in dendritic spines of dentate granular cells following stimulation of the entorhinal area. *Journal of Neurocytology*, **6**, 699–721.

Foster, A. C. and Fagg, G. E. (1984). Acidic amino-acid binding sites in mammalian neuronal membranes: their characteristics and relationship to synaptic receptors. *Brain Research Reviews*, **7**, 103–64.

Granger, R. and Lynch, G. (1988). Rapid incremental learning of hierarchically organised stimuli by layer II sensory (olfactory) cortex, this volume.

Green, E. J. and Greenough, W. T. (1986). Altered synaptic transmission in dentate gyrus of rats reared in complex environments: evidence from hippocampal slices maintained *in vitro*. *Journal of Neurophysiology*, **55**, 739–50.

Greenough, W. T. (1985). The possible role of experience-dependent synaptogenesis, or synapses on demand, in the memory process. in *Memory systems of the brain* (eds, N. M. Weinberger, J. L. McGaugh, and G. Lynch). Guilford Press, NY.

Greenough, W. T. and Bailey, C. H. (1988), The anatomy of memory: convergence of results across a diversity of tests. *Trends in Neuroscience*, **11**, 142–7.

Hagan, J. J., Tweedie, F. and Morris, R. G. M. (1986). Lack of task-specificity and absence of post-training effects of atropine on learning. *Behavioural Neuroscience*, **100**, 483–93.

Harris, E. W. and Cotman, C. W. (1983). Effects of acidic amino acid antagonists on paired-plus potentiation at the lateral perforant path. *Experimental Brain Research*, **52**, 455–60.

Harris, E. W. and Cotman, C. W. (1986). Long-term potentiation of guinea-pig mossy-fiber responses is not blocked by N-methyl-D-aspartate antagonists. *Neuroscience Letters*, **70**, 132–7.

Harris, E. W., Ganong, A. H., and Cotman, C. W. (1984). Long-term potentiation in the hippocampus involves activation of N-methyl-D-aspartate receptors. *Brain Research*, **323**, 132–7.

Hawkins, R. D. (1988). A biologically realistic neural network model for higher-order features of classical conditioning, this volume.

Hebb, D. O. (1949). *The organisation of behaviour*. Wiley, NY.

Hjorth-Simonsen, A. and Jeune, B. (1972). Origin and termination of the hippocampal perforant path in the rat studied by silver impregnation. *Journal of Compositive Neurology*, **144**, 215–32.

Hopkins, W. F. and Johnston, D. (1984). Frequency-dependent noradrenergic modulation of long-term potentiation in the hippocampus. *Science*, **226**, 350–2.

Horn, G. (1985). *Memory, imprinting and the brain*. Clarendon Press, Oxford.

Horn, G., Bradley, P., and McCabe, B. J. (1985). Changes in the structure of synapses associated with learning. *Journal of Neuroscience*, **5**, 3161–8.

Jahr, C. E. and Stevens, C. F. (1987). Glutamate activates multiple single-channel conductances in hippocampal neurons. *Nature*, **325**, 522–5.

Kandel, E. R. and Schwartz, J. H. (1982). Molecular biology of learning: Modulation of transmitter release. *Science*, **218**, 433–43.

Kelso, S. R., Ganong, A. H., and Brown, T. H. (1986). Hebbian synapses in hippocampus. *Proceedings of the National Academy of Science*, **83**, 5326–30.

Kleinschmidt, A., Bear, M. F., and Singer, W. (1987). Blockade of 'NMDA' receptors disrupts experience-dependent plasticity of kitten striate cortex. *Science*, **238**, 355–8.

Kennedy, M. B., (1988). Cellular neurobiology: synaptic memory molecules. *Nature*, **335**, 770–1.

Koch, C. (1987). The action of the corticofugal pathway on sensory thalamic nuclei: a hypothesis. *Neuroscience*, **23**, 399–406.

Laroche, S. and Bloch, V. (1982). Conditioning of hippocampal place cells and long-term potentiation: an approach to mechanisms of post-trial memory facilitation. In *Neuronal plasticity and memory formation* (eds. Ajmone-Marsen and H. Matthies), Raven Press, NY.

Lee, K. (1983). Sustained modification of neuronal activity in the hippocampus and neocortex. In *Neurobiology of the hippocampus* (ed. Siefert, W.). Academic Press.

Lee, K. S., Schottler, F., Oliver, M., and Lynch, G. (1980). Brief bursts of high-frequency stimulation produce two types of structural change in rat hippocampus. *Journal of Neurophysiology*, **44**, 247–58.

Leung, L-W. S. and Desborough, K. A. (1988), APV, an N-methyl-D-aspartate receptor antagonist, blocks the hippocampal theta rhythm in behaving rats. *Brain Research*, **463**, 148–52.

Levy, W. B. and Steward, O. (1979). Synapses as associative memory elements in the hippocampal formation. *Brain Research*, **175**, 233–45.

Lorenz, K. (1937). The companion in the bird's world. *Auk*, **54**, 245–73.

Lynch, G. (1986). *Synapses, circuits and the beginnings of memory*, MIT Press, Cambridge, Mass.

Lynch, G. and Baudry, M. (1984). The biochemistry of memory: a new and specific hypothesis. *Science*, **224**, 1057–63.

Lynch, G., Dunwiddie, T., and Gribkoff, V. (1977). Heterosynaptic depression: a postsynaptic correlate of long-term potentiation. *Nature*, **266**, 737–9.

Marr, D. (1971). A theory of archicortex. *Philosophical Transactions of the Royal Society*, **262**, 23–81.

Marr, D. (1982). *Vision*. Freemans, San Fr.

Mayer, M. L., Westbrook, G. L., and Guthrie, P. B. (1984). Voltage-dependent block by magnesium of NMDA response in spinal cord neurones. *Nature*, **309**, 261–3.

McCabe, B. J. and Horn, G. (1988). Learning and memory: regional changes in N-methyl-D-aspartate receptors in chick brain after imprinting. *Proceedings of the National Academy of Science*, **85**, 2849–53.

McCabe, B. J., Horn, G., and Bateson, P. P. G. (1981). Effects of restricted lesions of the chick forebrain on the acquisition of filial preferences during imprinting. *Brain Research*, **205**, 29–37.

McNaughton, B. L. (1982). Long-term enhancement and short-term potentiation in rat fascia dentata act through different mechanisms. *Journal of Physiology*, **324**, 249–62.

McNaughton, B. L. (1983). Activity-dependent modulation of hippocampal synaptic efficacy: some implications for memory processes. In *Neurobiology of the hippocampus* (ed. W. Siefert). Academic Press, London.

McNaughton, B. L., Barnes, C. A., Rao, G., Baldwin, J., and Rasmussen, M. (1986). Long-term enhancement of hippocampal synaptic transmission and the acquisition of spatial information. *Journal of Neuroscience*, **6**, 563–71.

McNaughton, B. L., Douglas, R. M., and Goddard, G. V. (1978). Synaptic enhancement in fascia dentata: cooperativity among co-active elements. *Brain Research*, **157**, 277–93.

McNaughton, B. L. and Morris, R. G. M. (1987). Hippocampal synaptic enhancement *and information storage within a distributed memory system. Trends in Neuroscience,* **10,** 408–15.

Meldrum, B. S. (1985). Possible therapeutic applications of antagonists of excitatory amino acid neurotransmitters. *Clinical Science,* **68,** 113–22.

Mishkin, M. (1982). A memory system in the monkey. *Philosophical Transactions of the Royal Society,* **298,** 85–95.

Monaghan, D. T. and Cotman, C. W. (1985). Distribution of N-methyl-D-aspartate sensitive L-[3H]-glutamate binding sites in rat brain. *Journal of Neuroscience,* **5,** 2909–19.

Morris, R. G. M. (1981). Spatial localisation does not depend on the presence of local cues. *Learning and motivation,* **12,** 239–60.

Morris, R. G. M. (1983). An attempt to dissociate 'spatial-mapping' and 'working-memory' theories of hippocampal function. In *Neurobiology of the hippocampus* (ed. W. Siefert). Academic Press, London.

Morris, R. G. M. (1984). Developments of a water-maze procedure for studying spatial learning in the rat. *Journal of Neuroscientific Methods,* **11,** 47–60.

Morris, R. G. M. (1989). Synaptic plasticity and Learning: selective impairment of learning in rats and blockade of long-term potentiation *in vivo* by the N-methyl-D-aspartate receptor antagonist, AP5. *Journal of Neuroscience,* in press.

Morris, R. G. M., Anderson, E., Lynch, G. S., and Baudry, M. (1986). Selective impairment of learning and blockade of long-term potentiation by an N-methyl-D-aspartate receptor antagonist. *Nature,* **319,** 774–6.

Morris, R. G. M., Garrud, P., Rawlins, J. N. P., and O'Keefe, J. (1982). Place-navigation impaired in rats with hippocampal lesions. *Nature,* **297,** 681–3.

Morris, R. G. M., Hagan, J. J., and Rawlins, J. N. P. (1986). Allocentric spatial learning by hippocampectomised rats: A further test of the 'spatial-mapping' and 'working-memory' theories of hippocampal function. *Quarterly Journal of Experimental Psychology,* **38B,** 365–95.

Morris, R. G. M., Halliwell, R. F., and Bowery, N. (1989). Synaptic plasticity and learning II: Are different kinds of plasticity involved in different kinds of learning? *Neuropsychologia,* **27,** 41–59.

Murphy, S. N., Thayer, S. A., and Miller, R. J. (1987). The effects of excitatory amino acids on intracellular calcium in single mouse neurons *in vitro*. *Journal of Neuroscience,* **7,** 4145–58.

Nicoll, R. A., Kauer, J. A., and Malenka, R. C. (1988). The current excitement in long-term potentiation. *Neuron,* **1,** 97–103.

Nowak, L., Bregestowski, P., Ascher, P., Herbet, A., and Prochiantz, A. (1984). Magnesium gates glutamate-activated channels in mouse central neurons. *Nature,* **307,** 462–5.

O'Keefe, J. and Nadel, L. (1978). *The hippocampus as a cognitive map.* Oxford University Press.

Olton, D. S. and Samuelson, R. J. (1976). Remembrance of places passed: spatial memory in rats. *Journal of Experimental Psychology Animal Behaviour Proceedings,* **2,** 97–116.

Palm, G. (1982). *Neural assemblies: an alternative approach to artificial intelligence.* Springer-Verlag, Heidelberg.

Patel, S. N., Rose, S. P. R., and Stewart, M. G., (1988). Training induced dendritic spine density changes are specifically related to memory formation processes in the chick, gallus domesticus. *Brain Research*.

Payne, J. K. and Horn, G. (1982). Long-term consequences of exposure to an imprinting stimulus on 'spontaneous' neuronal activity in two regions of the chick brain. *Brain Research*, **232**, 191–3.

Racine, R. J., Milgram, N. W., and Hafner, S. (1983). Long-term potentiation in the rat limbic forebrain. *Brain Research*, **260**, 217–31.

Rawlins, J. N. P. (1985). Associations across time: the hippocampus as a temporary memory store. *Behav. Brain Science*, **8**, 479–528.

Reiter, H. O. and Stryker, M. P. (1988). Neural plasticity without postsynaptic action potentials: less active inputs become dominant when kitten visual cortical cells are pharmacologically inhibited. *Proceedings of the National Academy of Science*, **85**, 3623–7.

Rolls, E. T. (1987). Information representation, processing and storage in the Brain: Analysis of the single neuron level. In *The neural and molecular bases of learning*, (eds. J-P. Changeux and M. Konishi). Wiley and Sons, Chichester.

Rolls, E. T. (1988). Parallel distributed processing in the brain: implications of the functional architecture of neuronal networks in the hippocampus, this volume.

Rosenzweig, M. R., Bennett, E. L. and Krech, D. (1964). *Journal of Compositive Physiology Psychology*, **57**, 438–9.

Routtenberg, A., Lovinger, D. M. and Steward, O. (1985). Selective increase in the phosphorylation of a 47kDa protein (F1) directly related to long-term potentiation. *Behavioural Neural Biology*, **43**, 3–11.

Rudell, A. P., Fox, S. E., and Ranck, J. B. Jr (1980). Hippocampal excitability phase-locked to the theta rhythm in walking rats. *Experimental Neurology*, **68**, 87–96.

Rumelhart, D. E. and McClelland, J. L. (1986). *Parallel distributed processing: explorations in the microstructures of cognition*, Volumes 1 and 2. MIT Press, Cambridge.

Ruthrich, H., Matthies, H., and Ott, T. (1982). Long-term changes in synaptic ex-citability of hippocampal cell populations as a result of training. In *Neuronal plasticity and memory formation* (eds. Ajmone-Marsen and H. Matthies), Raven Press, NY.

Schenk, F. and Morris, R. G. M. (1985). Dissociation between components of spatial memory in rats after recovery from the effects of retrohippocampal lesions. *Experimental Brain Research*, **58**, 11–28.

Scoville, W. B. and Milner, B. (1957). Loss of recent memory after bilateral hippocampal lesions. *Journal of Neurology and Neurosurgical Psychiatry*, **20**, 11–21.

Skrede, K. K. and Westgaard, R. H. (1971). The transverse hippocampal slice: A well defined cortical structure maintained *in vitro*. *Brain Research*, **35**, 589–93.

Singer, W. (1985). In *Synaptic modifications, neuron selectivity and nervous system organisation* (eds. W. B. Levy, J. A. Anderson, and S. Lehmkule), pp. 1–38. Erlbaum, Hillsdale.

Skelton, R. W., Miller, J. J. and Phillips, A. G. (1985). Long-term potentiation facilitates behavioural responding to single-pulse stimulation of the perforant path. *Behavioural Neuroscience*, **99**, 603–20.

Squire, L. R. (1987). *Memory and brain*. Oxford University Press, NY.

Squire, L. R., Shimamura, A. P., and Amarel, D. G. (1988). Memory and the hippocampus. In *Neural models of plasticity* (eds. J. Byrne, and W. Berry) Academic Press, NY.

Squire, L. R. and Zola-Morgan, S. (1983). The neurology of memory: the case for correspondence between the findings for man and non-human primate. In *The physiological basis of memory*, 2nd edn (ed. J. A. Deutsch), Academic Press, NY.

Stent, G. (1973). A physiological mechanism for Hebb's postulate of learning. *Proceedings of the National Academy of Science*, **70**, 997–1001.

Stanton, P., Jester, J., Chattarji, S., and Sjenowski, T. J. (1988). Associative long-term potentiation and depression is produced in hippocampus dependent upon the phase of rhythmically active inputs. *Soc. Neuroscience Abstracts*, **14**, 12.

Storm-Mathisen, J. and Ottersen, O. P. (1988). Localisation of excitatory amino-acid transmitters. In *Excitatory amino acids in health and disease* (ed. D. Lodge). Wiley, Chichester.

Sutherland, R. J., Whishaw, I. Q. and Kolb, B. (1983). A behavioural analysis of spatial localisation following electrolytic, kainate- or colchicine induced damage to the hippocampal formation in the rat. *Behavioural Brain Research*, **7**, 133–53.

Sutherland, R. J., Whishaw, I. Q. and Kolb, B. (1988). Contributions of cingulate cortex to two forms of spatial learning and memory. *Journal of Neuroscience*, **8**, 1863–72.

Tonkiss, J., Morris, R. G. M. and Rawlins, J. N. P. (1988). Intraventricular infusion of the NMDA antagonist AP5 impairs DRL performance in the rat. *Experimental Brain Research*, **73**, 181–8.

Tanzi, E. (1893), cited by Ramon y Cajal (1911).

Vanderwolf, C. H. (1971). Limbic-diencephalic mechanisms of voluntary movement. *Psychological Review*, **78**, 83–113.

van Groen, Th. and Lopes da Silva, F. H. (1985). Septo-temporal distribution of entorhinal projections to the hippocampus in the cat: electrophysiological evidence. *Journal of Compositive Neurology*, **238**, 1–9.

Watkins, J. C. and Evans, R. H. (1981). Excitatory amino acid neurotransmitters. *Ann. Review of Pharmacology and Toxicology*, **21**, 165–204.

Watkins, J. C. and Olverman, H. J. (1987). Agonists and antagonists for excitatory amino acid receptors. *Trends in Neuroscience*, **10**, 265–72.

White, G., Levy, W. B., and Steward, O. (1988). Evidence that associative interactions between synapses during the induction of long-term potentiation occur within local dendritic domains. *Proceedings of the National Academy of Science*, **85**, 2368–72.

Wigstrom, H., Gustafson, B., Huang, Y. Y., and Abraham, W. C. (1986). Hippocampal long-lasting potentiation is induced by pairing single afferent volleys with intracellularly injected depolarising current pulses. *Acta. Physiologica Scandinavia*, **126**, 317–19.

Willshaw, D. J., Bunemann, O., and Longuett-Higgins, H. C. (1969). Non-holographic associative memory. *Nature*, **222**, 960–2.

Wyss, J. M. (1981). Autoradiographic study of the efferent connections of entorhinal cortex in the rat. *Journal of Comparative Neurology*, **199**, 495–512.

Zola-Morgan, S., Squire, L. R., and Amarel, D. G. (1986). Human amnesia and the medial temporal region: enduring memory impairment following a bilateral lesion limited to field CA1 of the hippocampus. *Journal of Neuroscience*, **6**, 2950–67.

# 12

## Parallel distributed processing in the brain: implications of the functional architecture of neuronal networks in the hippocampus
EDMUND T. ROLLS

### Introduction

The form of parallel distributed processing performed by many brain regions is connectionist. In a connectionist system, the computation is performed by a large number of relatively simple neurone-like nodes or units, each of which has connections with many other units in the system. The strengths of the connections between connected units in the system are crucial, and can often be set by simple learning rules, such as that the connection strength is proportional to the conjunctive activity in connected units. At each point in time, each node has a numerical value, called its activation. The operations performed by each unit in the system are typically simple in that they may involve multiplying each input by its connection strength, summing these across all the inputs, and then updating its activation according to a monotonic function of its input to produce its output. In neurophysiological terms, the firing rate or firing probability of each neuron is determined by the firing on each of its afferents weighted by the appropriate synaptic strength of each afferent synapse, often with some non-linearity in the output firing, such as a threshold.

The aim of this paper is to show how some of the advances in connectionism are relevant to understanding the operation of neuronal networks in the brain, and to show that the anatomy and synaptic modifiability of the brain indicate that certain types of model are particularly relevant to understanding brain function. Specifically, it will be argued that neuronal network theories provide a bridge from the anatomical and physiological levels to the computational level, and that they will in this way be crucial to the understanding of brain function, including the complex cognitive operations performed by the brain which have often been the subject of connectionist models (see Rumelhart and McClelland 1986). Some of the ways in which neuronal networks operate in the brain, and the types of computation they could be performing, will be illustrated by considering the functions of neuronal networks in the hippocampus.

## Functions of the primate hippocampus in memory

It is known that damage to certain regions of the temporal lobe in man produces anterograde amnesia, evident as a major deficit in learning to recognize new stimuli (Scoville and Milner 1957; Milner 1972; Squire 1986; Squire and Zola-Morgan 1988). The anterograde amnesia has been attributed to damage to the hippocampus, which is within the temporal lobe, and to its associated pathways, such as the fornix (Scoville and Milner 1957; Milner 1972; Gaffan 1974, 1977; Zola-Morgan, Squire, and Amaral 1986). But it is possible that severe deficits on recognition memory are only found when there is also damage to the amygdala (Mishkin 1978, 1982, 1988; Murray and Mishkin 1984). Memory tasks in which damage to the hippocampus alone produces characteristic impairments in primates, including man, are tasks which require combinations of stimulus attributes with their locations in space to be processed together, such as memory not only for which object was shown but for where it was shown (Gaffan and Saunders 1985; Smith and Milner 1981), and conditional spatial response tasks in which the subject must learn which response to make to each stimulus (Gaffan 1985; Rupniak and Gaffan 1987; Petrides 1985).

## The computational significance of the functional architecture of the hippocampus

The internal connections of the hippocampus, and the learning rules implemented at its synapses will be described first to show how these constrain and help to define the type of parallel distributed processing which can be performed by this part of the brain. This functional architecture provides the basis for a computational theory of the hippocampus.

A schematic diagram of the connections of the hippocampus is shown in Fig. 12.1. One feature is that there is a sequence of stages, in each of which is a major set of input axons which connect with the output neurons of that stage via a form of matrix. The two stages which most clearly exemplify this are the dentate granule (FDgc in Fig. 12.1(b)) and the CA1 stages. It is significant that each of the stages is forward connected with the next stage, and that there are no major back projections within the hippocampus. The type of computation which could be performed by one of these stages is considered first.

The perforant path connections with the dentate granule cells may be taken as an example of one of these stages. A version of this, represented as a simplified matrix, is shown in Fig. 12.2. The perforant path makes one set of

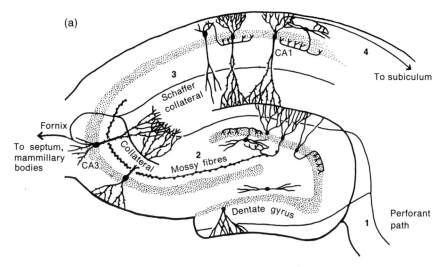

**Fig. 12.1(a)**    Representation of connections within the hippocampus. Inputs reach the hippocampus through the perforant path (1) which makes synapses with the dendrites of the dentate granule cells and also with the apical dentrites of the CA3 pyramidal cells. The dentate granule cells project via the mossy fibres (2) to the CA3 pyramidal cells. The well-developed recurrent collateral system of the CA3 cells is indicated. The CA3 pyramidal cells project via the Schaffer collaterals (3) to the CA1 pyramidal cells, which in turn have connections (4) to the subiculum.

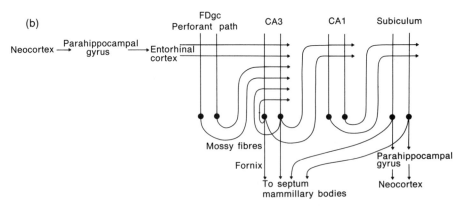

**Fig. 12.1(b)**    Schematic representation of the connections of the hippocampus, showing also that the cerebral cortex (neocortex) is connected to the hippocampus via the parahippocampal gyrus and entorhinal cortex, and that the hippocampus projects back to the neocortex via the subiculum, entorhinal cortex, and parahippocampal gyrus. FDgc—dentate granule cells.

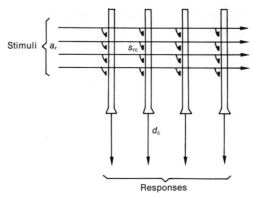

**Fig. 12.2** A matrix for competitive learning in which the input stimuli are presented along the rows of the input axons ($a_r$) which make modifiable synapses ($s_{rc}$) with the dendrites of the output neurons, which form the columns ($d_c$) of the matrix.

synapses with the dendrites of the dentate granule cells, the output neurons of this stage, in the form of a matrix. The synapses are modifiable according to the Hebb rule, i.e. the synapses between active afferent axons and strongly activated post-synaptic neurons increase in strength, as shown by analyses of long-term potentiation in the hippocampus (see Bliss and Lomo 1973; Andersen 1987; McNaughton 1984; Levy 1985; Kelso, Ganong, and Brown 1986; Wigstrom *et al.* 1986). It is important to the style of parallel distributed processing in the brain that this is a 'local' learning rule, in that the modification of synaptic strength is made on the basis of two parameters available locally at every synapse, namely the levels of pre-synaptic activity and post-synaptic depolarization. Other styles of parallel distributed processing in which computed changes in synaptic strength are transported to the correct synapse from a remote site are much more difficult to envisage in the brain because of physical limitations. (This is a difficulty with the neural implementation of back-propagation schemes, e.g. Rumelhart, Hinton, and Williams 1986.) It is notable that the synaptic matrix formed at each stage appears to be different from an association matix memory for pattern association, in that in the hippocampal system there is no pathway for an unconditioned stimulus to act via unmodifiable synapses to force the output neurons to fire (see Rolls 1987), unless a special assumption is made that some of the input fibres happen to act through powerful *unmodifiable* synapses as 'detonators' (McNaughton and Morris 1987). Nor is there a climbing fibre for each output cell, as in the cerebellum, which could act as an error-correcting teacher (see Ito 1984). In the hippocampal circuit there is apparently no teacher, i.e. a signal which can unconditionally set, or correct according to an error, the output firing of each neuron. This appears to be an example of an unsupervised learning system. (It is of course quite likely that some general control of the state of hippocampal neurons which can influence whether they can learn is provided by the cholinergic inputs to the hippocampus, as well as by the noradrenergic and serotonergic inputs.) There are inhibitory inter-neurons present, which synapse mainly on the cell bodies of the output neurons of each stage, where they shunt the membrane and may therefore act to produce division (McNaughton and Morris 1987). The inputs received by the inhibitory neurons are from the preceding stage (e.g. from the perforant path fibres in the dentate gyrus), so that division of the effect of the input fibres on the cell is in proportion to the magnitude of the input received. This feedfoward inhibition thus maintains a constant effect of different strengths of input on the dentate granule cells (McNaughton and Morris 1987), and is equivalent to normalization of the length (magnitude) of the input vector. The inhibitory neurons also receive inputs from the output neurons of each stage (in this case the granule cells), so that mutual inhibition of the output neurons of each stage is effectively produced. This mutual inhibition, if combined with a non-linear (e.g. sigmoid) output activation function of the neurons, can lead to fast firing neurons producing a large inhibition of other neurons, i.e. in a competitive mechanism which enhances the differences in the firing rates of the neurons (cf. Grossberg, 1982).

The type of computation which could be performed by this functional architecture is as follows. Consider a matrix memory of the form shown in Fig. 12.2 in which the strengths of the synapses between horizontal axons and the vertical dendrites are initially random (Postulate 1). Because of these random initial synaptic weights, different input patterns on the horizontal axons will tend to activate different output neurons (in this case, granule cells). The tendency for each pattern to select or activate different neurons can then be enhanced by providing mutual inhibition between the output neurons, to prevent too many neurons responding to that stimulus (Postulate 2). This competitive interaction can be viewed as enhancing the differences in the firing rates of the output cells (cf. the contrast enhancement described by Grossberg 1982). Synaptic modification then occurs according to the rules of long-term potentiation in the hippocampus, namely that synapses between active afferent axons and strongly activated post-synaptic neurons increase in strength (see McNaughton 1984; Levy 1984; Kelso, Ganong, and Brown 1986; Wigstrom et al. 1986) (Postulate 3). The effect of this modification is that the next time the same stimulus is repeated, the neuron responds more (because of the strengthened synapses), more inhibition of other neurons occurs, and there is then further modification to produce even greater selectivity. The response of the system as a categorizer thus climbs over repeated iterations. One consequence observed in simulations is that a few neurons then obtain such strong synaptic weights that almost any stimulus which has any input to one of these neurons will succeed in activating it. The solution to this is to limit the total synaptic weight that each output (post-synaptic) neuron can receive (Postulate 4). In simulations, this is performed by normalizing the sum of the synaptic weights on each neuron to a constant (e.g. 1.0) (cf. von der Malsburg 1973), or by normalizing the vector length of the synaptic weights (Rumelhart and Zipser 1986). This has the effect of distributing the output neurons evenly between the different input patterns received by the network. We (E. T. Rolls, G. Littlewort, R. Payne, and A. Bennett) have found that an extremely powerful competitive network which can separate most different vectors (up to the capacity of the system) is obtained if the length of the synaptic weight vector of each dendrite is normalized after the learning stage, and the length of the input stimulus vector is also normalized before it is applied to the matrix. In the brain the normalization of the synaptic weight vector on each dendrite may be approximated by using a modified Hebb rule which produces some decrease in synaptic strength if there is high pre-synaptic but low post-synaptic activation (cf. Bear, Cooper, and Ebner 1987), and we (E. T. Rolls, G. Littlewort, R. Payne, and A. Bennett) have found that the use of such a learning rule does indeed abolish the need for explicit normalization of the synaptic weight vectors on each dendrite, i.e. for a separate process to implement Postulate 4 above. It is in any case not physiologically unreasonable to postulate that the total synaptic strength onto a post-synaptic neuron is somewhat fixed (Levy and Desmond 1985).

A simulation of the operation of such a competitive neuronal network is shown in Fig. 12.3. It is shown that the network effectively selects different output neurons to respond to different combinations of active input horizontal lines. It thus performs a type of categorization, in which different complex input patterns are encoded economically onto a few output lines. It should be noted that this categorization finds natural clusters in the input events; orthogonalizes the categories such that overlap in input events can become coded on to output neurons with less overlap, and such that many active input lines may be coded on to few active output lines; and does not allocate neurons to events which never occur (cf. Marr 1970, 1971; Rumelhart and Zipser 1986; Grossberg 1982, 1987). It may be noted that there is no special correspondence between the input pattern and which output lines are selected. It is thus not useful for any associative mapping between an input and an output event, and is thus different from associative matrix memories (Rolls 1987). Instead, this type of matrix finds associations or correlations between input events (which are expressed as sets of simultaneously active horizontal input lines or axons), allocates output neurons to reflect the complex event, and stores the required association between the input lines onto the few output neurons activated by each complex input event. It thus acts as a categorizer, which removes redundancy present in the input vectors, and forms new output representations which are more orthogonal to each other than are the input vectors.

There is some evidence that in the hippocampus the synapses between inactive axons and active output neurons become weaker (see McNaughton 1984; Levy 1985). The effect of this in the learning system described would be to facilitate accurate and rapid categorization, in that weakening synapses onto a post-synaptic neuron from axons which are not active when the post-synaptic neuron is strongly activated would reduce the probability that it will respond to a stimulus which must be placed into a different category.

Another feature of the functional architecture of the hippocampus, which is developed in the CA3 pyramidal cells in particular, is the presence of strong recurrent collaterals, which return from the output of the matrix to cross over the neurons of the matrix, as shown in Figs 12.1(a) and (b). This anatomy immediately suggests that it is an autoassociation (or autocorrelation) matrix memory. The autoassociation arises because the output of the matrix, expressed as the firing rate of the CA3 pyramidal cells, is fed back along the horizontally running axons so that the pattern of activity in this part of the matrix (the CA3 pyramidal cells) is associated with itself (see, e.g. Kohonen, Oja, and Lehtio 1981; Rolls 1987). It can be noted here that for this to be the case, the synapses of the recurrent collaterals would have to be modifiable, and the modification rule would require alteration of synaptic strength when both the pre-synaptic fibre and the post-synaptic dendrite were strongly activated. This learning rule does appear to be implemented at these synapses (Ganong

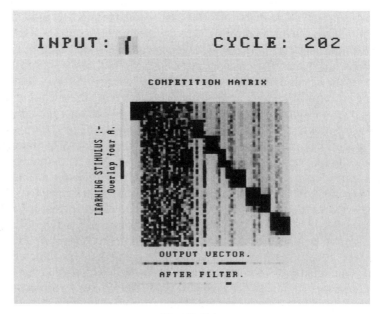

Fig. 12.3(a)

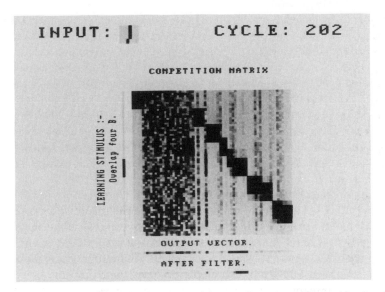

**Fig. 12.3**  Simulation of learning in a competitive matrix memory. The architecture is as shown in Fig. 12.2, except that there are 64 horizongal axons and 64 vertical dendrites which form the rows and columns, respectively, of the 64 × 64 matrix of synapses. The strength of each synapse, which was initially random, is indicated by the darkness of each pixel. The activity of each of the 64 input axons is represented in the 64-element vector at the left of the diagram by the darkness of each pixel. The output firing of the vertical neurons is represented in the same way by the output vectors at the bottom of the diagram. The upper output vector is the result of multiplying the input stimulus through the matrix of synaptic weights. The vector resulting from the application of competition between the output neurons (which produces contrast enhancement between the elements or neurons of the vector) is shown below by the vector labelled 'after filter'. The state of the matrix is shown after 203 cycles in each of which stimuli with eight of 64 active axons was presented, and the matrix allowed to learn as described in the text. The stimuli were presented in random sequence, and consisted of a set of vectors which overlapped in 0, 1, 2, 3, 4, 5, and 6 positions with the next vector in the set. The columns of the matrix were sorted after the learning to bring similar columns together, so that the types of neuron formed, and the pattern of synapses formed on their dendrites, can be seen easily. The dendrites with random patterns of synapses have not been allocated to any of the input stimuli. It is shown that application of one of the input stimuli (overlap four A) or vectors which overlapped in four of eight positions with another stimulus (overlap four B) produced one pattern of firing of the output neurons, and that application of input stimulus overlap four B produced a different pattern of firing of the output neurons. Thus the stimuli were correctly categorized by the matrix as being different.

*et al.* 1986). Further, the probability of contact of the neurons in the autoassociation matrix must not be very low if it is to operate usefully (see Marr 1971). Given that the region of the CA3 cell dendrites on which the recurrent collaterals synapse is long (approximately 11.5 mm), and that the total dendritic length is approximately 15 mm and has approximately 10 000 spines (D. G. Amaral, personal communication; Squire, Shimamura, and Amaral 1988), approximately 7700 synapses per CA3 pyramidal cell could be devoted to recurrent collaterals, which with 180 000 CA3 neurons in the rat makes the probability of contact between the CA3 neurons 0.043. This is high enough for the system to operate usefully as an autoassociation memory (see Marr 1971). It is remarkable that the contact probability is so high, and also that the CA3 recurrent collateral axons travel so widely in all directions that they can potentially come close to almost all other CA3 neurons (D. G. Amaral, personal communication; Squire, Shimamura, and Amaral 1988). It is important to stress that these CA3 recurrent collaterals do run in all directions, including rostro-caudal, so that the lamellar structure of the hippocampus which refers to connections made primarily within a transverse plane does not hold here, with the result that the matrix of connections is not local, and that any CA3 neuron can contact any other CA3 neuron with a probability of 4.3 per cent. This is a key function of the hippocampal circuitry, for it is suggested below that the systems level function of CA3 autoassociation memory is to enable events occurring conjunctively in quite different parts of the association areas of the cerebral cortex to be associated to form a memory which could well be described as episodic. Each episode would be defined by a conjunction of a set of events, and each episodic memory would consist of the association of one set of events. An example of an episodic memory would be where, with whom, and what one ate at lunch on the preceding day. The importance of the hippocampus in episodic memory may arise from the fact that in one part of it, the CA3 region, there is one association matrix with a relatively high contact probability which receives information originating in many different areas of the cerebral cortex.

One reason why there may not be more cells in the CA3 region is that it is important for the connectivity to be kept relatively high so that any event represented by the firing of a sparse set of CA3 cells can be associated with any other event represented by a different set of CA3 cells firing. Because each CA3 pyramidal cell has a limited fan-in or number of synapses (perhaps 10 000, see above), the total number of cells in the autoassociation memory cannot be increased beyond the limit set by the fan-in and the connectivity. The advantages of sparse encoding and a well-interconnected matrix are that a large number of different (episodic) memories can be stored in the CA3 system, and that the advantageous emergent properties of a matrix memory, such as completion, generalization, and graceful degradation (see Kohonen et al. 1977, 1981; Kohonen 1984; Rolls 1987) are produced efficiently. Completion may operate particularly effectively here with a sparse representation, because it is under these conditions that the simple autocorrelation effect can reconstruct the whole of one pattern without interference, which would arise if too high a proportion of the input neurons was active. Another effect of the autoassociation matrix is that the central tendency of a pattern of activity which is noisy is learned, thus achieving useful prototype extraction (McClelland and Rumelhart 1988). It is further notable that these completion and cleaning-up processes may benefit from several iterations (repeated cycles) of the autoassociation feedback effect. It has been suggested (McNaughton and Morris 1987) that one function of hippocampal theta activity may be to allow this autoassociation effect produced by the recurrent collaterals to cycle for several iterations (in a period of approximately 50 ms), and then to stop it, so that the system can operate again with maximal sensitivity to new inputs received on the mossy and perforant path systems by the CA3 cells.

The means by which the efficient (information-rich) yet sparse representation in CA3 neurons which is required for the autoassociation to perform well is, it is suggested, a function of the mossy fibre inputs to the CA3 cells described next, as well as of the orthogonalizing function of competition between the dentate granule cells described above.

The mossy fibre system connects the granule cells of the dentate gyrus to the CA3 pyramidal cells of the hippocampus. In the rat, each mossy fibre forms approximately 14 'mosses' or contacts with CA3 cells; there are $1 \times 10^6$ dentate granule cells and thus $14 \times 10^6$ mosses on to $0.18 \times 10^6$ CA3 cells (D. Amaral, personal communication), and thus each CA3 pyramidal cell may be contacted by approximately 78 dentate granule cells. This means that (in the rat) the probability that a CA3 cell is contacted by a given dentate granule cell is 78 synapses/$10^6$ granule cells $= 0.000\,078$. These mossy fibre synapses are very large, presumably because with such a relatively small number on each CA3 cell dendrite (and a much smaller number active at any one time), each synapse must be relatively strong. One computational effect which can be achieved by this low probability of contact of a particular dentate granule cell with a particular pyramidal cell is pattern separation. This is achieved in the following way. Consider a pattern of firing present over a set of dentate granule cells. The probability that any two CA3 pyramidal cells receive synapses from a similar subset of the dentate granule cells is very low (because of the low probability of contact of any one dentate granule cell with a pyramidal cell), so that each CA3 pyramidal cell is influenced by a very different subset of the active dentate granule cells. Thus each pyramidal cell effectively samples a very small subset of the active granule cells, and it is therefore likely that each CA3 pyramidal cell will respond differently to the others, so that in this way pattern separation is achieved. (The effect is similar to codon formation described in other contexts by Marr 1970.) The advantage of a low number of inputs is that the thresholds of the post-synaptic cell need not be set with great accuracy for pattern separation and sparse patterns to be achieved. The advantage of this low-contact probability is that it achieves by pattern separation relatively orthogonal representations (compared to those on the dentate granule cells, and within the limits set by the relative numbers of dentate granule and CA3 cells shown in Table 12.1), which are required if the autoassociation matrix memory formed by the CA3 cells is to operate with usefully large memory capacity, and with minimal interference (see Kohonen 1977; Rolls 1987). As the neurons have positive firing rates, the only way in which relatively orthogonal representations can be formed is by making the number of active neurons for any one input stimulus relatively low (see, e.g. Jordan 1986), and this sparse representation is exactly what can be achieved by the low contact probability pattern separation effect of the mossy fibres. The advantage of sparse representations is that a large number of different patterns can be stored in the memory, which is likely to be required if the hippocampal CA3 system is one of the few parts of the brain with the appropriate functional architecture and systems level connections to perform this function. An advantage of the modifiability of the mossy fibre synapses may be that CA3 neurons learn to respond to just those subsets of activity which do occur in dentate granule cells, so that cells are used efficiently. Even if these mossy fibre synapses are not modifiable, the mossy fibre system would still achieve pattern separation and form sparse representations.

It is notable that in addition to the mossy fibre inputs, the CA3 pyramidal cells also receive inputs directly from perforant path fibres (see Figs 12.1 and 12.2). This is not a sparse projection, in that each pyramidal cell may receive in the order of 2300 such synapses. (This is calculated using the evidence that of 15 mm of total dendritic length with 10 000 spines, approximately 3.5 mm (range 2.5–4.5 mm) is in the lacunosum moleculare and thus receives inputs from the perforant path, D. G. Amaral, personal communication.) What would be the computational effect of this input together with the very sparse, but strong, synapses from the mossy fibres? One effect is that the mossy fibre input would cause the pattern of synaptic activation (considered as a vector) in each pyramidal cell to point in a different direction in a multidimensional space. However, the precise direction in that multidimensional space could not be well specified by the relatively small number of mossy fibre synapses onto each CA3 pyramidal cell. However, once pointed to that part of space by the mossy fibres, a particular cell would show co-operative Hebbian learning between its activation by the mossy fibre input and the direct perforant path input, allowing the direct input to come through learning to specify the exact direction of that cell in multidimensional space much more effectively than by the coarse mossy fibre input alone. This effect can be seen in Fig. 12.4. The relative weighting in this simulation was that the mossy fibre input had an effect on each neuron which was five times greater than that of the direct perforant path input. Thus it is suggested that the combination of the sparse mossy fibre input and the direct perforant path input is to achieve pattern separation, and at the same time to allow the response of the neuron to be determined not just by the sparse mossy fibre input, but much more finely by making use, in addition, of the direct perforant path input.

**Table 12.1**    *Cell numbers in different parts of the hippocampal formation*

|  | Rat | Monkey | Man |
|---|---|---|---|
| Entorhinal cortex |  | $4.0 \times 10^6$ |  |
| Dentate granule cells | $1.00 \times 10^6$ | $5.0 \times 10^6$ | $8.8 \times 10^6$ |
| CA3/CA2 | $0.18 \times 10^6$ | $0.9 \times 10^6$ | $2.5 \times 10^6$ |
| CA1 | $0.25 \times 10^6$ | $1.4 \times 10^6$ | $6.0 \times 10^6$ |

Contact probability of a granule cell with a CA3 cell $= 0.008\%$ (via mossy fibres)
Contract probability of a CA3 cell with a CA3 cell $= 4.3\%$ (via recurrent collaterals)

It is thus suggested that the sparse, yet efficient (information rich), representation in CA3 neurons which is required for the autoassociation to perform well is produced in two ways by the stage which precedes the CA3 neurons, i.e. by the orthogonalizing function of competition between the dentate granule cells, and by the low contact probability in the mossy fibre–CA3 connections. The function of the CA1 stage which follows the CA3 cells is considered next.

The connections of the CA3 cells to the CA1 pyramidal cells are shown in Fig. 12.1. The connections are of the form shown in Fig. 12.2. It is suggested that the CA1 cells provide a stage of competitive learning which operates as

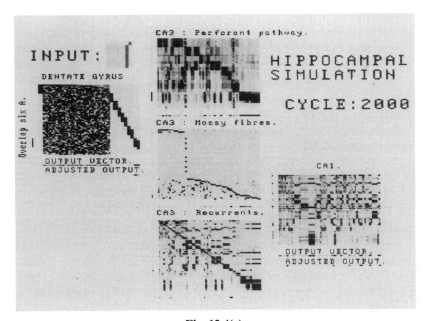

**Fig. 12.4(a).**

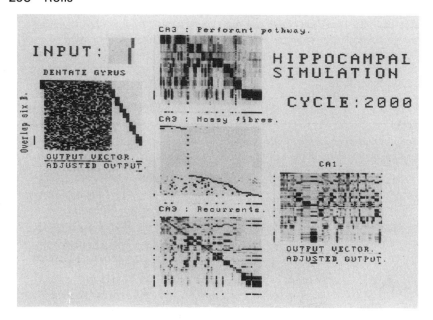

**Fig. 12.4** Hippocampal simulation. Conventions as in Fig. 12.3. The dentate gyrus is shown as a competition matrix at the left, receiving input stimuli from the perforant path. The vertical dendrites of the CA3 pyramidal cells extend throughout the three submatrices shown in the middle. The middle submatrix receives the output of the dentate granule cells via the mossy fibres with potentially powerful synapses and a low contact probability, and operates as a competition matrix. Pattern separation can be seen to operate in that input vectors are converted into output vectors with many elements activated by the inputs about which the submatrix has learned, and in that different output vectors are produced for even quite similar input vectors. The upper CA3 submatrix operates as a competition matrix with a direct perforant path input. The lower CA3 submatrix operates as an autoassociation matrix (formed by the recurrent collaterals). The output of the CA3 cells (summed vertically up and down the dendrite) is then used as the input (via the Schaffer collaterals) to the CA1 cells, which operate as a competition matrix. The states of the matrices after 2000 presentations of the same set of stimuli used for Fig. 12.3 are shown. One point demonstrated is that two very similar stimuli, overlap six A in Fig. 12.4(a), and overlap six B in Fig. 12.4(b), produce output vectors at CA1 which are relatively orthogonal to each other.

follows on the inputs received from the CA3 cells. Consider the operation of the CA3 autoassociation effect. Several arbitrary patterns of firing occur together on the CA3 neurons, and become associated to form an episodic memory. It is essential for this operation that several different sparse representations are present conjunctively in order to form the association. Moreover, when completion operates in the CA3 autoassociation system, all the neurons firing in the original conjunction can be brought into activity by only a part of the original set of conjunctive events. For these reasons, a memory in the CA3 cells consists of several simultaneously active, different ensembles of activity. It is suggested that the CA1 cells, which receive these groups of simultaneously active ensembles, can detect the correlations of firing which represent the episodic memory, and allocate by competitive learning a relatively few neurons to represent each episodic memory. The episodic memory in the CA3 cells would thus consist of groups of active cells, each representing one of the subcomponents of the episodic memory (including context), whereas the whole episodic memory would be represented not by its parts, but as a single collection of active cells, at the CA1 stage. It is suggested below that one role which these economical (in terms of the number of activated fibres) and relatively orthogonal signals have is to guide information storage or consolidation in the cerebral cortex. To understand how the hippocampus may perform this function for the cerebral cortex, it is necessary to turn to a systems level analysis to show how the computations performed by the hippocampus fit into overall brain function. It may be noted that, by forming associations of events derived from different parts of the cerebral cortex (the CA3 stage), and by building new economical representations of the conjunctions detected (the CA1 stage), the hippocampus provides an output which is suitable for directing the long-term storage of information.

**Systems level theory of hippocampal function**

First, the anatomical connections of the primate hippocampus with the rest of the brain will be considered, in order to provide a basis for considering how the computational ability of the hippocampus could be used by the rest of the brain. Then the responses shown by single hippocampal neurons will be described to provide evidence on its systems level function.

The hippocampus receives inputs via the enthorhinal cortex (area 28) and the parahippocampal gyrus from many areas of the cerebral association cortex, including the parietal cortex which is concerned with spatial functions, the visual and auditory temporal association cortical areas, and the frontal cortex (see Fig. 12.5) (van Hoesen and Pandya 1975; van Hoesen 1982; Amaral 1988; Rolls 1989a). In addition, the entorhinal cortex receives inputs from the amygdala. There are also subcortical inputs to the hippocampus, for example via the fimbria–fornix from the cholinergic cells of the medial septum and the adjoining limb of the diagonal band of Broca. The hippocampus in turn projects back via the subiculum, entorhinal cortex, and parahippocampal gyrus (area TF–TH), to the cerebral cortical areas from which it receives inputs (van Hoesen 1982) (see Figs 12.1 and 12.5). Thus the hippocampus can potentially influence the neocortical regions from which it receives inputs. A second efferent projection of the hippocampal system reaches the supplemen-

Afferent connections                    Efferent connections

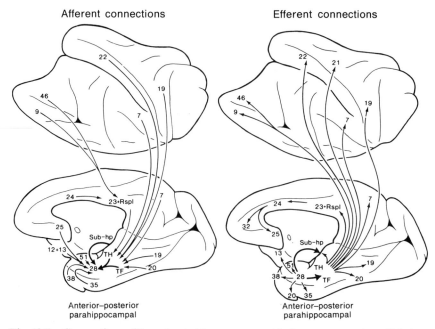

**Fig. 12.5** Connections of the primate hippocampus with the neocortex. A medial view of the macaque brain is shown below, and a lateral view is shown inverted above. The hippocampus receives its inputs via the parahippocampal gyrus, areas TF and TH, and the entorhinal cortex, area 28. The return projections to the neocortex (shown on the right) pass through the same areas. Cortical areas 19, 20 and 21 are visual association areas, 22 is auditory association cortex, 7 is parietal association cortex, and 9, 46, 12 and 13 are frontal cortical association areas. (From van Hoesen 1982.)

tary motor cortex via the subiculum, the fimbria–fornix, mammillary bodies, anterior thalamus, and the cingulate cortex, providing a potential route for the hippocampus to influence motor output (van Hoesen 1982). It is suggested that functions of the hippocampus in, for example, conditional spatial response learning utilize this output path to the motor system.

During the performance of an object–place memory task, for which the primate hippocampus is needed, it has been found that not only do some hippocampal neurons respond to certain positions in space, but that others respond only when novel stimuli are shown in a particular place. These neurons thus responded to a combination of information about the stimulus being shown and about position in space (Rolls *et al.* 1989). Further, in tasks in which the monkeys had to learn which spatial response to make to different stimuli, i.e. to acquire associations between visual stimuli and spatial responses, 14.2 per cent of the neurons responded to particular combinations of stimuli and responses (Miyashita *et al.* 1989). These neurophysiological findings provide support for the computational model described above, for they show that combinations of events received by the hippocampus from different parts of the brain do activate single hippocampal neurons, as predicted from the convergence onto single hippocampal neurons of inputs received from the cerebral cortex. Moreover, particular combinations of events come as a result of learning to activate hippocampal neurons (Cahusac et al. 1988), consistent with the synaptic modifiability which is part of the model. The model is also supported by evidence that during the learning of conditional spatial responses, some hippocampal neurons start, but then stop showing differential responses to the different stimuli, consistent with competitive interactions between hippocampal neurons during learning, so that only some hippocampal neurons become allocated to any one learned conjunction of events (Cahusac et al. 1989).

The analyses above have shown that the hippocampus receives from high-order areas of association cortex; is able by virtue of the large number of synapses on its dendrites and the CA3 autoassociation effect to detect conjunctions of events even when these are widely separated in information space, with their origin from quite different cortical areas; allocates neurons to code efficiently for these conjunctions, probably using a competitive learning mechanism (CA1); and has connections back to the areas of the cerebral cortex from which it receives, as well as to subcortical structures via the fimbria–fornix system. What could be achieved by this system? It appears that the very long-term storage of information is not in the hippocampus, at least in man, in that the retrograde amnesia produced by damage to the hippocampal system in man is not always severe, and in that very old memories (e.g. for events which occurred 30 years previously) are not destroyed (Squire 1986; Squire and Zola-Morgan 1988). On the other hand, the hippocampus does appear to be necessary for the storage of certain types of information (characterized by the description declarative, or knowing that, as contrasted with procedural, or knowing how, which is spared in amnesia). Declarative memory includes what can be declared or brought to mind as a proposition or an image. Declarative memory includes episodic memory, i.e. memory for particular episodes, and semantic memory, i.e. memory for facts (Squire and Zola-Morgan 1988; Squire, Shimamura, and Amaral 1988). How could the hippocampus, then, be involved in the storage of information?

The suggestion which is made on the basis of these and the other findings described above is that the hippocampus is specialized to detect the best way in which to store information, and then directs memory storage there by the return paths to the cerebral cortex. It is suggested that the CA3 autoassociation system is ideal for remembering particular episodes, for, perhaps uniquely in the brain, it provides a single autoassociation matrix which receives from many different areas of the cerebral association cortex. It is thus able to make almost any arbitrary association, including association to the context in which a set of events occurred. This autoassociation type of memory is also what is required for paired-associate learning, in which arbitrary associations must be made between words, and an impairment of which is almost a defining test of amnesia. Impairment of this ability to remember episodes by using the CA3 autoassociation matrix memory may also underly many of the memory deficits produced by damage to the hippocampal system. For example, conditional spatial response learning (see Miyashita *et al.* 1989) may be impaired by hippocampal damage because a monkey or human cannot make use of the memory of the episode of events on each particular trial, for example that a particular stimulus and a particular response were made, and reward was received. Similarly, object–place memory tasks, also impaired by hippocampal damage, require associations to be made between particular locations and particular objects—again a natural function for an autoassociation memory. Further, the difficulty with memory for places produced by hippocampal damage (see Barnes 1988) may be because a place is normally defined by a conjunction of a number of features or environmental cues or stimuli, and this type of conjunction is normally learned by the autoassociation memory capability of the hippocampus (see, further, Rolls *et al.* 1989). (It should be noted that associations to primary reinforcing stimuli do not require the hippocampus. Associations to primary reinforcers seem to require the amygdala—see Rolls 1985). Clearly, the hippocampus, with its large number of synapses on each neuron, its potentiation type of learning, and its CA3 autoassociation system is able to detect when there is conjunctive activation of arbitrary sets of its input fibres, and is able, as indicated both theoretically and by recordings made in the behaving monkey, to allocate neurons economically (i.e. with relatively few neurons active) to code for each complex input event (by the output or CA1 stage). Such output neurons could then represent an efficient way in which to store information, in that complex memories with little redundancy would have been generated. It should be noted that this theory is not inconsistent with the possibility that the hippocampus provides a working memory, in that in the present theory the hippocampus sets up a representation using Hebbian learning which is useful in determining how information can best be stored in the neocortex, and this representation could provide a useful working memory. It may be that by understanding the operations performed by the hippocampus at the neuronal network level, it can be seen how the hippocampus could contribute to several functions which are not necessarily inconsistent.

The question then arises of where the long-term storage occurs, and how it may be directed by the hippocampus. Now, the hippocampus is reciprocally connected via the subiculum and entorhinal cortex with the parahippocampal gyrus which in turn is reciprocally connected with many high-order areas of association neo-cortex (see Fig. 12.5). It is therefore possible that the actual storage takes place in the parahippocampal gyrus, and that this might be particularly appropriate for multimodal memories. However, having detected that, for example, a visual stimulus is regularly associated with an event in another modality (such as a movement) it might be useful to direct the unimodal representation of that visual image, so that it is stored efficiently and can provide a useful input to the multimodal conjunction store. Thus return pathways (via e.g. the parahippocampal gyrus) to unimodal cortex (for example inferior temporal visual cortex, area TE), might, it is suggested, be used to direct unimodal storage also, by contributing to detection of the most economical way in which to store representations of stimuli.

The question of how the hippocampal output is used by the neocortex (i.e. cerebral cortex) will be considered next. Given that the hippocampal output returns to the neocortex, a theory of back-projections in the neocortex will be needed. This is developed elsewhere (Rolls 1989a). By way of introduction to that theory, it may be noted that which particular hippocampal neurons happen to represent a complex input event is not determined by any teacher or forcing (unconditioned) stimulus. Thus the neocortex must be able to utilize the signal rather cleverly. One possibility is that any neocortical neuron which has a number of its afferents active at the same time as the hippocampal back-projecting fibres in its vicinity are active will modify its synapses so that it comes to respond better to these afferents the next time they occur. This learning by the cortex would involve a Hebb-like learning rule. It may be noted that one function served by what are, in effect, back-projections from the hippocampus is some guidance for, or supervision of, neocortical learning. It is a problem of unsupervised learning systems that, while they can detect local conjunctions efficiently, these are not necessarily those conjunctions of most use to the whole system. It is exactly this problem which, it is proposed, the hippocampus helps to solve, by detecting useful conjunctions globally (i.e. over the whole of information space as represented by neuronal activity in many areas of the cerebral cortex), and then directing storage locally at earlier stages of processing (e.g. in unimodal areas of the cerebral association cortex). In this way filters are built locally to provide representations of input stimuli which are useful for later processing.

## Conclusions

In this paper, some of the types of and the constraints on the parallel distributed processing being performed by the brain have been considered using hippocampal function as an example. The following are some of the conclusions which can be suggested.

1. The number of synapses on each neuron (the fan-in), and the number of synapses made by each neuron (the fan-out) is typically large but limited; 10 000 is the order of the number of synapses per neuron in the hippocampus.

This means that the brain, with more than $10^{10}$ neurons is a far from fully connected net. Instead, it is modular, and quite precise figures of the sizes of some of the modules can be given. For example, the numbers of neurons in different parts of the hippocampus are shown in Table 12.1.

2. The learning rules are typically local, in that the modification of the strength of a synapse can be based on the pre- and post-synaptic activity.

3. Because the connections in the neuronal networks can now be specified reasonably quantitatively, as shown above, for example, for the mossy fibre system and for the recurrent collateral system of the CA3 pyramidal cells, and there is evidence on the learning rules for some parts of the brain, the computations capable of being performed by the networks in some parts of the brain can now be investigated, and even specified quantitatively (see also Marr 1971). For example, the functional architecture of the mossy fibre system suggests that it is a pattern-separation device, and of the recurrent collateral system of the CA3 pyramidal cells that it is an autoassociation matrix memory. Moreover, the functional architecture provides constraints on what can be learned.

4. It is possible to proceed from the level of functional architecture (i.e. the anatomy and the learning rules) towards the level of a computational theory, as described above for the mossy fibre and recurrent CA3 systems. A large part of the value of the computational level is that it reveals what may be at first unexpected, i.e., emergent, properties of the networks. An example is that the CA3 autoassociation system almost certainly operates to produce the emergent properties of completion, generalization, and graceful degradation (or fault tolerance) (see, further, Rolls 1987).

5. It is also possible to link from the computational level of analysis to the systems level, so that it is possible to specify, given the computation which can be performed by one module or set of modules such as the hippocampus, how this could contribute to overall brain function considered as a system. This systems level of analysis often involves cognitive operations such as the storage of information, recall, and attention (see, further, Rolls, 1989a,b). Thus an important feature of this approach is that it allows anatomy and physiology to be linked through network computational theory to systems level, often cognitive, functions of the brain. This provides a comprehensive and quantitative approach to brain function which links empirical research with theory, and promises because of this to revolutionize neuroscience. It may also be noted that in so far as connectionism (see Rumelhart and McClelland 1986) is faithful to the principles of operation of the brain, connectionism is likely to continue to be very fruitful, in that it provides one of the ways in which the functions of parts of the brain can be understood. (Of course, connectionism which is not faithful to the principles of operation of the brain may well also be fruitful, by leading to advances in artificial intelligence.)

6. Information is represented in neuronal networks in the brain in a distributed manner in which the tuning of neurons is nevertheless not very coarse, as noted above for hippocampal neurons and as described by Rolls (1987) for neurons in other brain regions. This type of representation of information can be seen as a compromise between storage capacity and the emergent properties of completion, generalization and graceful degradation in neuronal networks (see Rolls 1987).

7. Unlearning, as exemplified by the responses of hippocampal neurons described above, and by the synaptic learning rule discussed by Bear *et al.* (1987), may well be important for ensuring that the representation of information in the brain does not become too distributed so that discrimination and capacity are lost, and may well be used to enhance categorization in competitive networks.

8. Some multilayer neuronal networks in the brain can operate with predominantly forward connections, as shown above for the hippocampus. Such networks are self-organizing, and can operate largely without a teacher. Other systems in the brain, such as connected areas of the cerebral cortex, do have backward connections as well as forward connections, and it is suggested here and developed elsewhere (Rolls 1989*a*,*b*) that the back-projections which originate not only from the next cortical layer in sequence, but also from multimodal structures such as the amygdala and hippocampus, are useful not only in utilizing global information to guide local information storage, but also in recall and attention.

## Acknowledgements

The author has worked on some of the experiments and neuronal network modelling described here with A. Bennett, P. Cahusac, D. Cohen, J. Feigenbaum, R. Kesner, G. Littlewort, Y. Miyashita, H. Niki, and R. Payne and their collaboration is sincerely acknowledged. Discussions with David G. Amaral of the Salk Institute, La Jolla, were also much appreciated. This research was supported by the Medical Research Council.

## References

Amaral, D. G. (1987). Memory: anatomical organization of candidate brain regions. In *Handbook of neurophysiology—the nervous system*. American Physiological Society, Washington, DC.

Andersen, P. O. (1987). Properties of hippocampal synapses of importance for integration and memory. In *New insights into synaptic function* (eds. G. M. Edelman, W. E. Gall, and W. M. Cowan), pp. 403–29. Neuroscience Research Foundation/ Wiley, NY.

Barnes, C. A. (1988). Spatial learning and memory processes: the search for their neurobiological mechanisms in the rat. *Trends in Neurosciences*, **11**, 163–9.

Bear, M. F., Cooper, L. N., and Ebner, F. B. (1987). A physiological basis for a theory of synapse modification. *Science*, **237**, 42–8.

Bliss, T. V. P. and Lomo, T. (1973). Long-lasting potentiation of synaptic transmission in the dentate area of the anaesthetized rabbit following stimulation of the perforant path. *Journal of Physiology*, **232**, 331–56.

Braitenberg, V. and Schuz, A. (1982). Some anatomical comments on the hippocampus. In *Neurobiology of the hippocampus* (ed. W. Seifert), Ch. 2, pp. 21–37. Academic Press, London.

Cahusac, P. M. B., Rolls, E. T., Miyashita, Y., and Niki, H. (1989). Modification of the responses of hippocampal neurons in the monkey during the learning of a conditional response task. In preparation.

Gaffan, D. (1974). Recognition impaired and association intact in the memory of monkeys after transection of the fornix. *Journal of Compositive and Physiological Psychology*, **86**, 1100–1109.

Gaffan, D. (1977). Monkey's recognition memory for complex pictures and the effects of fornix transection. *Quarterly Journal of Experimental Psychology*, **29**, 505–14.

Gaffan, D. (1985). Hippocampus: memory, habit and voluntary movement. *Philosophical Transactions of the Royal Society*, **B308**, 87–99.

Gaffan, D. and Saunders, R. C. (1985). Running recognition of configural stimuli by fornix transected monkeys. *Quarterly Journal of Experimental Psychology*, **37B**, 61–71.

Ganong, A. H., Harris, E. W., Monaghan, D. T., Watkins, J. C., and Cotman, C. W. (1986). Evidence for both NMDA- and non-NMDA-receptor mediated LTP: analysis with D-AP5 and new more potent NMDA antagonist. *Soc. Neuroscience Abstracts*, **12**, 61.

Grossberg, S. (1982). *Studies of mind and brain*. Reidel, NY.

Grossberg, S. (1987). Competitive learning: from interactive activation to adaptive resonance. *Cognitive Science*, **11**, 23–63.

Ito, M. (1984). *The cerebellum and neural control*. Raven Press, NY.

Jordan, M. I. (1986). An introduction to linear algebra in parallel distributed processing. In *Parallel distributed processing*, Volume 1, *Foundations* (eds. D. E. Rumelhart and J. L. McClelland) Ch. 9, pp. 365–442. MIT Press, Cambridge, Mass.

Kelso, S. R., Ganong, A. H., and Brown, T. H. (1986). Hebbian synapses in the hippocampus. *Proceedings of the National Academy of Science*, **83**, 5326–30.

Kohonen, T. (1984). *Self-organization and associative memory*. Springer-Verlag: Berlin.

Kohonen, T., Lehtio, P., Rovamo, J., Hyvarinen, J., Bry, K., and Vainio, L. (1977). A principle of neural associative memory. *Neuroscience*, **2**, 1065–76.

Kohonen, T., Oja, E., and Lehtio, P. (1981). Storage and processing of information in distributed associative memory systems. In *Parallel models of associative memory* (eds. G. E. Hinton and J. A. Anderson), Ch. 4, pp. 105–143. Erlbaum, NJ.

Levy, W. B. (1985). Associative changes in the synapse: LTP in the hippocampus. In *Synaptic modification, neuron selectivity, and nervous system organization* (Eds. W. B. Levy, J. A. Anderson, and S. Lehmkuhle), Ch. 1, pp. 5–33. Erlbaum, Hillsdale, NJ.

Levy, W. B. and Desmond, N. L. (1985). The rules of elemental synaptic plasticity. In

*Synaptic modification, neuron selectivity, and nervous system organization* (eds. W. B. Levy, J. A. Anderson, and S. Lehmkuhle), Ch. 6, pp. 105–121. Erlbaum, Hillsdale, NJ.

Marr, D. (1970). A theory of cerebral cortex. *Proceedings of the Royal Society*, **B176**, 161–234.

McClelland, J. L. and Rumelhart, D. E. (1988). *Explorations in parallel distributed processing*. MIT Press, Cambridge, Mass.

Marr, D. (1971). Simple memory: a theory of archicortex. *Philosophical Transactions of the Royal Society*, **B262**, 23–81.

McNaughton, B. L. (1984). Activity dependent modulation of hippocampal synaptic efficacy: some implications for memory processes. In *Neurobiology of the hippocampus* (ed. W. Seifert), Ch. 13, pp. 233–252. Academic Press, London.

McNaughton, B. L. and Morris, R. G. M. (1987). Hippocampal synaptic enhancement and information storage within a distributed memory system. *Trends in Neurosciences*, **10**, 408–15.

Milner, B. (1972). Disorders of learning and memory after temporal lobe lesions in man. *Clinical Neurosurgery*, **19**, 421–46.

Mishkin, M. (1978). Memory severely impaired by combined but not separate removal of amygdala and hippocampus. *Nature*, **273**, 297–8.

Mishkin, M. (1982). A memory system in the monkey. *Philosophical Transactions of the Royal Society*, **B298**, 85–95.

Mishkin, M. (1989). Neural circuitry and mechanisms for visual recognition and memory. In *Neural models of plasticity: theoretical and empirical approaches* (eds. J. Byrne and W. O. Berry). Academic Press. NY.

Miyashita, Y., Rolls, E. T., Cahusac, P. M. B. and Niki, H. (1989). Activity of hippocampal formation neurons in the monkey related to a conditional spatial response task. *Journal of Neurophysiology*, **61**, 669–78.

Murray, E. A. and Mishkin, M. (1984). Severe tactual as well as visual memory deficits follow combined removal of the amygdala and hippocampus in monkeys. *Journal Neuroscience*, **4**, 2565–80.

Murray, E. A. and Mishkin, M. (1985). Amygdalectomy impairs crossmodal association in monkeys. *Science*, **228**, 604–6.

Petrides, M. (1985). Deficits on conditional associative-learning tasks after frontal- and temporal-lobe lesions in man. *Neuropsychologia*, **23**, 601–14.

Rolls, E. T. (1985). Connections, functions and dysfunctions of limbic structures, the prefrontal cortex, and hypothalamus. In *The scientific basis of clinical neurology* (eds. M. Swash and C. Kennard), pp. 201–213. Churchill Livingstone, London.

Rolls, E. T. (1987). Information representation, processing and storage in the brain: analysis at the single neuron level. In *The neural and molecular bases of learning* (eds. J.-P. Changeux and M. Konishi), pp. 503–40. Wiley, Chichester.

Rolls, E. T. (1989a). Functions of neuronal networks in the hippocampus and neocortex in memory. In *Neural models of plasticity: theoretical and empirical approaches* (eds. J. H. Byrne and W. O. Berry). Academic Press: NY.

Rolls, E. T. (1989b). Visual information processing in the primate temporal lobe. In *Models of visual perception: from natural to artificial* (ed. M. Imbert). Oxford University Press.

Rolls, E. T., Miyashita, Y., Cahusac, P. M. B., Kesner, R. P., Niki, H., Feigenbaum, J., and Bach, L. (1989). Hippocampal neurons in the monkey with activity related to the place in which a stimulus is shown. *Journal of Neuroscience*, **9**, 1835–45.

Rumelhart, D. E. and McClelland, D. (eds) (1986). *Parallel distributed processing.* MIT Press, Cambridge, Mass.

Rumelhart, D. E. and Zipser, D. (1986). Feature discovery by competitive learning. In *Parallel distributed processing*, Volume 1, *Foundations* (eds. D. E. Rumelhart and J. L. McClelland), Ch. 5, pp. 151–193. MIT Press, Cambridge, Mass.

Rumelhart, D. E., Hinton, G. E., and Williams, R. J. (1986). Learning internal representations by error propagation. In *Parallel distributed processing*, Volume 1. *Foundations* (eds. D. E. Rumelhart D. E. and J. L. McClelland), Ch. 8, pp. 318–362. MIT Press, Cambridge, Mass.

Rupniak, N. M. J. and Gaffan, D. (1987). Monkey hippocampus and learning about spatially directed movements. *Journal of Neuroscience*, **7**, 2331–7.

Scoville, W. B. and Milner, B. (1957). Loss of recent memory after bilateral hippocampal lesions. *Journal of Neurology, Neurosurgery and Psychiatry*, **20**, 11–21.

Smith, M. L. and Milner, B. (1981). The role of the right hippocampus in the recall of spatial location. *Neuropsychologia*, **19**, 781–93.

Squire, L. (1986). Mechanisms of memory. *Science*, **232**, 1612–19.

Squire, L. R. and Zola-Morgan, S. (1988). Memory: brain systems and behavior. *Trends in Neurosciences*, **11**, 170–5.

Squire, L. R., Shimamura, A. P., and Amaral, D. G. (1989). Memory and the hippocampus. In *Neural models of plasticity: theoretical and empirical approaches* (eds. J. Byrne and W. O. Berry). Academic Press, NY.

van Hoesen, G. W. and Pandya, D. N. (1975). Some connections of the entorhinal (area 28) and perirhinal (area 35) cortices in the monkey. I. Temporal lobe afferents. *Brain Research*, **95**, 1–24.

van Hoesen, G. W. (1982). The parahippocampal gyrus. New observations regarding its cortical connections in the monkey. *Trends in Neurosciences*, **5**, 345–50.

von der Malsburg, C. (1973). Self-organization of orientation-sensitive columns in the striate cortex. *Kybernetik*, **14**, 85–100.

Wigstrom, H., Gustaffson, B., Huang, Y.-Y., and Abraham, W. C. (1986). Hippocampal long-term potentiation is induced by pairing single afferent volleys with intracellularly injected depolarizing currents. *Acta Physiologica Scandinavia*, **126**, 317–19.

Zola-Morgan, S., Squire, L. R., and Amaral, D. G. (1986). Human amnesia and the medial temporal region: enduring memory impairment following a bilateral lesion limited to field CA1 of the hippocampus. *Journal of Neuroscience*, **6**, 2950–7.

# 13

## Rapid incremental learning of hierarchically organized stimuli by layer II sensory (olfactory) cortex*

### RICHARD GRANGER and GARY LYNCH

### Introduction

Rabbits require dozens to hundreds of trials to learn a nictitating membrane (eyeblink) response to criterion; in contrast, there are forms of learning characterized by extremely rapid acquisition, long retention, and apparently unlimited capacity. For instance, Standing (1973) found that 10 000 photographs, each displayed to subjects just once, for only seconds, were learned to 90 per cent criterion by the subjects; this ability to incrementally learn large numbers of minimally salient stimuli with very little exposure and no opportunity for rehearsal, may be characteristic of human 'everyday learning', i.e. the apparently effortless acquisition and retention of enormous numbers of minute-to-minute environmental cues. Abstract 'neural networks' do not address these abilities: rather, they typically have very limited capacity, require large numbers of learning trials, and learn non-incrementally, i.e. they require all items to be learned to be available at once, in advance of any testing—if stimuli are instead presented one at a time, as in actual experience, early items tend to be lost as subsequent ones are learned, and there will be interference among learned items.

We have studied an olfactory learning task in which animal subjects learn rapidly, incrementally and with long retention and large capacity. We have performed physiological studies of the brain structures underlying these learning and memory abilities, and have constructed a simulation of Layer II sensory cortex (piriform cortex) that empirically reproduces certain of these results, as well as yielding to analytical treatment. As a result, we have been able to construct a mechanism that incrementally generates unique encodings of input stimuli in 1–2 learning trials, with large capacity. This biological network differs strikingly from abstract 'neural networks' not in its learning rule *per se*, but in its performance rules, which enable this single-layer

*This research was supported in part by the Office of Naval Research under grants N00014-84-K-0391 and N00014-87-0838, by the National Science Foundation under grant IST-85-12419, and by the J. Howard Pew Charitable Trust.

threshold network to use timing rules to extract and encode multiple levels of hierarchical information about each stimulus rather than simply generating a single representation of a cue.

Were a human to memorize each incoming stimulus as a completely novel and unique event, then information would be lost about the similarity of various stimuli. This information is critical for learning: without it, no previous learning could ever be brought to bear on subsequent experience, since every experience would be perceived as unique. It is recognition and encoding of the similarities among stimuli that enables generalization to categories of objects and events. Learning the similarities among classes of objects and yet being able to distinguish them from each other are two competing abilities, requiring learning of a hierarchy of information about each object, so as to capture its unique nature without losing information about its relationships with other similar stimuli. The mechanism we have constructed exhibits this ability, and we hypothesize that it is this ability that underlies and may be fundamental to the operation of layer II sensory cortex.

This paper discusses these issues, beginning with the relevant behavioural data, followed by the way in which the behaviour is driven by specific operations of particular biological structures, and leading to empirical and analytical results of our efforts to model layer II of olfactory cortex.

## The behaviours being modelled

Rats actively learning discriminations among large numbers of distinct odours exhibit the ability to acquire novel discriminations in fewer than five trials. The animals are trained in an apparatus in which two novel odours are ejected from randomly chosen loci. One of the two odours leads to a water reward, whereas the other only leads to a mildly aversive stimulus (a flashing light). Each series of trials consists of two different novel odours. The first pair of odours takes these animals roughly 30–40 trials to learn to criterion; the second pair is learned somewhat more quickly. However, by the third or fourth pair of novel odours, the discrimination is learned within the first five trials. The animals thus seem to acquire the equivalent of a 'learning set' (Slotnick and Katz 1974): salient aspects of the overall task are attended to (such as 'there are two odours to be discriminated, one of which leads to water reward'). The rats presumably attend less to other stimuli that are irrelevant to the task, such as the spatial information about which randomly chosen positions contain odours, or other modalities, such as tactile or auditory cues in the environment. Once the set is learned, subsequent trials continue to elicit this nearly immediate learning; strikingly, although these pairs of odours are learned very rapidly, they are also retained by the rat for as long as they have been tested (many weeks), in spite of the fact that the animals are continuing to learn a new pair of novel odours every day. The capacity of the odour memory system must be very large (see Staubli *et al.* 1987 for details of these experiments).

The characteristics of learning in this task stand in contrast to the characteristics of learning in tasks typical in the animal learning literature, such as classical or incremental conditioning: those tasks traditionally do not involve the acquisition of large numbers of distinct cues, and the learning is not rapid, but rather tends to require dozens to hundreds of trials per stimulus (an exception, one-trial avoidance learning, does not involve large numbers of cues). We have argued that this type of olfactory learning in rats resembles 'everyday' recognition learning in humans: perhaps hundreds of marginally relevant environmental stimuli (e.g. coffee machines, co-workers, cars, clothes) are learned without apparent effort during a normal day; these stimuli are readily recognized subsequently, and changes to them can be noticed, even in the absence of salient associations among these stimuli.

## The biology underlying the behaviours

### Electrical stimulation substituted for olfactory stimuli

Direct stimulation of the lateral olfactory tract (LOT) in specific temporal patterns provides as substitute experimental paradigm that allows direct testing of the involvement of olfactory (piriform) cortex in the behaviours. A stimulating electrode giving short bursts of high-frequency (100 Hz) activity, repeated once every 200 ms (i.e. short bursts occurring at the theta rhythm) yields both behavioural learning and measurable long-term potentiation (LTP) of the LOT-piriform synapses. The animals behave as though the electrical stimulation were an olfactory cue: they learn to discriminate between stimulation and a real odour, and they also learn to discriminate between two different stimulating electrodes. In both cases, the learning is quite similar to that observed when two real odours are presented to the animal: learning occurs in five trials or less, is stable for weeks, and shows no apparent interference effects from other learned cues (Staubli *et al.* 1987; Staubli and Lynch 1988; Roman, Staubli, and Lynch 1987). (It is somewhat interesting that upon stimulation, the animals actually sniff as though an odour were present; equally important is the fact that animals presented with real odours in this task (i.e. without electrical stimulation substituted for odours) synchronize their sniffing to the theta rhythm during learning (Macrides, Eichenbaum and Forbes 1982).)

Furthermore, synaptic LTP occurs only in those animals that also show behavioural learning: i.e. LTP is not found in naïve animals (those who have not yet acquired the learning set) who are given an insufficient of trials to learn the odour discrimination.

While this particular activity pattern probably is not the only one that the olfactory bulb (the structure whose primary (mitral) cell axons constitute the LOT) is capable of, nor even the only one that is normally used by the animal in this task, the electrical stimulation none the less is sufficient to substitute for actual bulb activity, in terms of both causing LTP and causing learning of the 'electric odour' by the animal. The same pattern (short (3–4 pulse) bursts at the theta rhythm) induces LTP in hippocampus (Larson and Lynch 1986), and the fact that naïve animals show neither LTP in piriform cortex nor behavioural learning in response to this stimulation strongly suggests that some extrinsic factor is required, such as the cholinergic inputs from basal forebrain that densely innervate the piriform. These might serve to raise inhibitory cell-firing thresholds, thereby rendering the network more excitable, allowing excitatory inputs to depolarize piriform cells beyond a threshold for synaptic potentiation.

*Basic physiology and anatomy of piriform cortex*

Electrical stimulation of afferents in hippocampus elicits excitatory (depolarizing) responses in target cells and, via a collection of interneurons, a complex set of longer-lasting inhibitory (hyperpolarizing) responses. Most of these have also been found in piriform cortex (see Haberly 1973; Haberly and Shepherd 1973; and Haberly 1985, for a review).

1. Excitatory post-synaptic potentials (EPSPs), both monosynaptic, via the feedforward LOT afferents, and disynaptic via layer-II cell axon collaterals synapsing with other layer II cell dendrites; these events depolarize post-synaptic cells and typically last 10–20 ms.
2. Inhibitory potentials (IPSPs), both monosynaptic and disynaptic via collaterals, as above, are chloride-mediated, and last from 50 to 100 ms.
3. Long hyperpolarizing potassium currents (LHP), lasting from 300 to 500 ms.
4. Extremely long (1000 ms) afterhyperpolarization (AHP), also mediated by potassium but in a cell-specific fashion, i.e. causing the equivalent of a refractory period only in those excitatory cells that fire in strong bursts.

In addition, we assume that release is probabilistic and that the size of post-synaptic responses at individual synapses varies according to some probability function.

The rules for learning in the simulation are based primarily on extensive physiological study of the phenomenon of long-term potentiation (LTP). Most of this work has been performed in hippocampal field CA1 (see Larson and Lynch 1986; 1988a,b). The LTP learning rules in the simulation encompass a number of points detailed elsewhere (see, e.g. Lynch and Granger 1989; Lynch et al. 1987; Granger et al. 1987, 1989). The key points are:

1. The post-synaptic depolarization threshold for LTP is distinct from (higher than) the threshold for firing the cell.
2. This threshold is not readily reached, even by high-frequency burst stimulation of the inputs to CA1, due to the effect of feedforward and feedback inhibition (IPSPs) that truncates the EPSP response.
3. The inhibitory process responsible for this truncation exhibits a refractory period for about 200 ms after firing; input burst activity arriving during that period, but after the dissipation of the initial IPSPs, is sufficient to raise the post-synaptic cell to its LTP threshold and cause LTP (Larson and Lynch 1986).
4. LTP is mediated by voltage-dependent N-methyl-D-aspartate (NMDA) receptor channels, which open relatively slowly to admit an influx of calcium into the post-synaptic terminals.
5. LTP occurs in quantal increments, increasing the conductance of the synapse by roughly 10 per cent or less.
6. There is an LTP 'ceiling' of roughly 50 per cent increase in the efficacy of the synapse.
7. While there is evidence for reversibility of LTP by certain types of input given within 15 min of LTP induction (Staubli *et al.* unpublished data), there is no evidence for reversibility of LTP after a longer period than this suggestive 'consolidation period', and no evidence that the conductance of naïve (unpotentiated) synapses can be reduced.

These mechanisms are embedded in an anatomy with a number of salient characteristics:

1. Extremely sparse ($p \leq 0.1$) random connectivity in piriform layer Ia, between the (roughly) 50 000 LOT afferents and the dendrites of the hundreds of thousands of piriform layer II cells.
2. Collateral axons that flow in both rostral and caudal directions, but primarily caudally (Schwob and Price 1978); these axons in fact provide the output of layer II to entorhinal cortex, by flowing caudally into the latter structure. The collateral axons synapse with other cells' apical dendrites in layer Ib, with a sparseness comparable to that of the LOT-piriform synaptic system. These collaterals flow through layer III before rising up (again, primarily in the caudal direction) into layer Ib; the collaterals can form synapses locally with the basal dendrites (in layers II and III) of their neighbouring layer-II cells, and with local inhibitory interneurons.
3. A network of inhibitory cells (of which there are many fewer than excitatory cells), arranged in approximate 'patches', i.e. such that each inhibitory cell's axons affect those primary cells within a certain radius of the inhibitory cell.

Although these are the primary characteristics we have modelled, these physiological and anatomical properties of layer II piriform cortex are part of a larger body of biological parameters embodied in the computer simulation; further discussion of these points will arise later in the paper.

### Identification of algorithms from cortical function

*The physiology re-cast in algorithmic form*

Integrating the various physiological events described above provides for a set of reasonable assumptions about the normal 'operating procedure' of piriform cortex during olfactory learning. The physiological response of layer II piriform cortex to the presentation of an odour (or, alternatively, to the 'electrical odour' stimulation) can be re-cast in terms of a series of hypothetical steps:

1. The animal inspires (sniffs).
2. Bulb mitral cells fire in a short burst, activating the LOT input to pirform.
3. Piriform layer II cells receiving sufficient activation via synaptic connections from the LOT begin firing; in turn, their resulting axonal activity may contribute to the activation of other excitatory and inhibitory cells via the collateral associational system.
4. IPSPs from inhibitory cells activated both by LOT input and by collaterals curtail the firing of layer II cells; the inhibitory process then becomes refractory (see Larson and Lynch 1986) for a period that lasts for about 400 ms and is maximal at about 200 ms.
5. LHP from inhibitory cells lowers the resting potential of excitatory cells.
6. Any excitatory cells that fire sufficiently strongly will become afterhyperpolarized (AHP).
7. The next inspiration (sniff), 200 ms later, will arrive against a hyperpolarized background (due to LHP), but will not activate IPSPs, which are in their refractory period.
8. This combination of hyperpolarization but disabled IPSPs prevents single-pulse EPSPs from providing sufficient depolarization to spike the post-synaptic cells, but, because of the IPSP refractoriness, the pulses comprising high-frequency bursting sum together to an unusual degree; i.e. the response to higher frequency input will be much larger than under normal conditions. If sufficient input converges on a cell during this IPSP refractory period, it will depolarize the cell over its bursting threshold, and over the threshold for opening the voltage-dependent N-methyl-D-aspartate receptor channels that enable long-term potentiation of the cell's active synapses (see Larson and Lynch 1988a).

9. Cells whose synapses have been potentiated will be more likely to fire in response to subsequent sniffs of the same input, since their synapses will contribute more inward current to the post-synaptic cell than naïve synapses will.

10. However, cells that fire sufficiently strongly in response to any given sniff will be refractory, and will not be able to fire again for as long as 1 s, i.e. for the next 4–5 sniffs.

Hence, because of synaptic potentiation, certain post-synaptic cells will become 'recruited' for particular odours; i.e. they will be more likely to fire in response to that odour input. Because of the AHP refractory period, however, precisely those excitatory cells that fire most strongly (i.e. at high frequency) to an input will only do so once (e.g. on the first sniff) and not on subsequent sniffs. What emerges is a series of spatial cell-firing patterns, occurring in short bursts once every 200 ms—due to AHP, a different spatial pattern of cell firing will occur on each of a series of sniffs.

Analysis of the characteristics of the spatial patterns of layer II cell firing reveals that different information about inputs is encoded in different sniff responses; i.e. sniff 1 conveys certain information about the input vector (simulated odour), while, e.g. sniff 3 conveys different information about the same input. In particular, after learning (potentiation) of a number of simulated odours, the sniff 1 response in the simulation tends to be almost identical across a range of relatively similar inputs, whereas sniff 2 and sniff 3 responses exhibit extremely different spatial firing patterns for each individual input. In other words, if the learned odours occur in natural 'groups' or clusters of similarity, such that some of them contain significant overlap with each other (as, for example, a set of distinguishable yet similar odours such as different types of cheese), then the initial sniff response will reflect those clusters, in fact yielding practically the same spatial firing pattern to any members of that cluster, but a quite different response to members of some other group. These responses thus partition the space of input cues into groups according to their similarity. However, later responses (e.g. sniff 3) will yield spatial firing patterns that are unique for each individual odour, distinguishing even among input odours that are quite similar to each other. The emergence of these properties from the algorithms will be described in the following sections.

*Partitioning of experience by the network*

First we will detail the mechanisms by which piriform layer II cells develop first-sniff 'category' responses to groups of similar inputs. Cell firing on the first sniff is determined primarily by the connectivity of the matrix: each layer II cell dendrite only connects with a small proportion of LOT axonal inputs, and, on average, only a relatively small proportion of those input axons are active in response to any particular odour. In rostral piriform, the dominant input to the apical dendrites of layer II cells are LOT axons, since the collateral axons of the layer II cells themselves flow predominantly caudally, and remain in layers II and III (sparsely contacting the basal dendrites of neighbouring excitatory cells) for some distance before rising up to collateralize in layer Ib (see, e.g. Schwob and Price 1978; Haberly 1973, 1985; Haberly and Shepherd 1973). In addition, inhibitory interneurons in piriform layer II receive inputs both monosynaptically from LOT stimulation and disynaptically from collateral stimulation. There are one to two orders of magnitude fewer inhibitory interneurons than there are excitatory layer II cells, with the interneurons arranged in local 'patches', such that each interneuron contacts almost all of the excitatory cells within a given radius.

Of the LOT axons synaptically connected to a given layer II cell dendrite, if enough are active in response to a particular odour, then the cell will receive sufficient total post-synaptic depolarization to enable the cell to spike; if a cell is even more depolarized, it can generate a complex spike: a high-frequency burst. The biophysical additivity characteristics of dendritic conductance provides the constraint that axonal stimulation must all arrive within a relatively short time 'window' in order to sum sufficiently to allow the cell to fire or to burst. Thus the probability of cell firing in piriform layer II will depend strongly on the extent to which its inputs occur synchronously.

For those inputs that occur when the required time window, i.e. occur nearly synchronously, it is relatively straightforward to calculate the probability of any particular post-synaptic cell having a specific number of active axons. Assume that the probabilistic distribution of synaptic connections in layer I is nearly uniform, i.e. there are very nearly a fixed number of synapses per (apical) dendrite. If there are $N$ LOT axons, $A$ of which are active in response to a particular odour, and there are $n$ axons synaptically connected to a given layer II cell dendrite, then the probability that $a$ of those synapses will be active in response to this odour follows the hypergeometric probability density function:

$$p(a \text{ active synapses}) = \frac{\binom{A}{a}\binom{N-A}{n-a}}{\binom{N}{n}} \tag{13.1}$$

That is, there are a particular number of ways of choosing $a$ active synapses from the $A$ active incoming LOT lines; for each of these, each of the remaining $n-a$ (inactive) synapses on the dendrite must be chosen from the $N-A$ inactive incoming LOT lines. The numerator therefore indicates the total number of ways that the LOT axons can be correctly assigned so as to come out with the specified number of active synapses; for each of the possible ways in which the synapses on the dendrite can be chosen (assigned) out of the LOT axons, there are this many ways to achieve $a$ active synapses; hence, the expression is divided by the number of ways these can be assigned, to find out what percentage of these ways (i.e. the probability) of getting $a$ active synapses occur for any particular fixed connectivity of axons to the dendrite.

Before potentiation, all synapses will contribute approximately the same constant amount of conductance, so that, for any cell, post-synaptic depolarization is a simple multiple of the number of active synapses on that cell. Within each patch in layer II dominated by a single inhibitory interneuron, active excitatory cells will excite both their neighbouring primary cells and the inhibitory interneurons, which will in turn tend to inhibit primary cell firing. As a result, the firing of those cells that are most strongly depolarized can continue for a short period of intense firing, yielding a complex spike, while the firing of less depolarized cells will be curtailed by inhibitory activity after only one or two spikes. In other words, these inhibitory patches may take on roughly the nature of a 'winner-take-all' network (Feldman 1982): because of the local interaction of excitatory and inhibitory cells within a patch, only the most strongly depolarized cells in the patch will burst and then succumb to inhibition; those with somewhat less depolarization will fire in a single pulse before falling silent, and other cells in the patch will remain quiescent throughout, having failed to overcome the local inhibition.

The situation then consists of a set of interneuron-defined patches, with a small number of bursting cells in each patch. Overall, the total set of cells that fire reliably in response to a particular input cue define the 'representation' or reliable pattern of response to the input. The question now is how much a response pattern will change as a result of a measured change to the input pattern. That is, if, say, $d$ axons in the LOT are deleted from the input and $d$ different axons are activated instead, how many differences will arise in the set of responding layer II cells? Continuing the simplifying assumption that all active synapses are of the same weight (not that this somewhat problematic assumption will be removed in the following section), then the post-synaptic depolarization is directly related to the number of active synapses on a cell, so we may define a threshold for cell firing in terms of the number of active synapses. Then given two input cues differing by a Hamming distance of $d$ (i.e. as just described, differing by $2d$ axons in the LOT), the expected value of $\hat{d}$, the Hamming distance between the responses to these two inputs is:

$$E(\hat{d}) = \sum_{k=1}^{N_{\mathrm{o}}} \left[ \sum_{\substack{i \geq \theta \\ j < \theta}} S_i I(i, j) + \sum_{\substack{i < \theta \\ j \geq \theta}} S_i I(i, j) \right] \qquad (13.2)$$

Where $N_{\mathrm{o}}$ is the number of post-synaptic cells, each $S_i$ is the probability that a cell will have precisely $i$ active contacts from one of the two cues, and $I(i,j)$ is the probability that the number of contacts on the cell will increase (or decrease) from $i$ to $j$ with the change in $d$ LOT lines; i.e. changing from the first input cue to the second. Hence, the first term denotes the probability of a cell decreasing its number of active contacts from above to below some threshold, $\theta$, such that that cell fired in response to one cue but not the other (and therefore is one of the cells that will contribute to the difference between responses to the two cues). Reciprocally, the second term is the probability that the cell increases its number of active synapses such that it is now over the threshold; this cell also will contribute to the difference in response. As mentioned, this analysis is restricted to rostral piriform, in which there are assumed to be few if any collateral axons. (Analysis of caudal piriform appears in a later section.)

The value of $S_i$, the probability that a cell has precisely $i$ active contacts, is the hypergeometric function given earlier. In changing between the two input cues, we wish to calculate $I(i,j)$, the probability that the number of active contacts on a cell will change (increase or decrease) from $i$ to $j$ as $d$ axons are dropped and another $d$ axons added in the change between the two input cues. Of the cells that fired in response to the first of the two input cues, some will lose some of their previously active synapses due to the input axons that are inactive in the second cue, and some cells will gain some active synapses from the new axons now active in the second cue that were inactive in the first cue. The probability of a cell changing its number of active contacts from $a$ to $\hat{a}$ is:

$$I(a, \hat{a}) = \sum_{g-l=a-a} \left[ \frac{\binom{a}{l}\binom{A-a}{d-l}}{\binom{A}{d}} \left( \frac{\binom{n-a}{g}\binom{N-A-(n-a)}{d-g}}{\binom{N-A}{d}} \right) \right] \quad (13.3)$$

where $N$, $n$, $A$, and $a$ are as above, $l$ is the 'loss' or reduction in the number of active synapses, and $g$ is the gain or increase. hence the leftmost of the two hypergeometric expressions is the probability of losing $l$ active synapses by dropping $d$ axons in the LOT, and the right-hand expression is the probability of gaining $g$ active synapses via the addition of $d$ LOT axons. The product of the expressions are summed over all the ways of choosing $l$ and $g$ such that the net change $g-l$ is the desired difference $a-\hat{a}$. (Granger, Ambros-Engerson, Henry, and Lynch 1987).

*Enhancement of partitioning with LTP*

If synaptic strengthening is now considered, we have shown (Granger, Ambros-Ingerson, and Lynch 1989) that learning will enhance the similarity of spatial pattern responses into categories of such responses. In effect, with learning via synaptic strengthening, inputs that overlap by sufficient amounts (i.e. share sufficient numbers of active LOT axons) will give rise to nearly identical output cell firing patterns, while inputs that differ by more than this amount will give rise to quite different output responses. If training on each cue induces small incremental increases in strength of active synapses ('fractional long-term potentiation'), then over trials, synapses originating from any overlapping portions of the input cues should become stronger than those originating from unique parts of a single cue, since the former will receive more training trials than the latter.

Consider two sets of cues, $x$, $x'$, $x''$, ..., and $y$, $y'$, $y''$, ..., where each member of each group activates 75 per cent of the same axons within categories, whereas the overlap between these categories is less than 40 per cent. Equations (13.1), (13.2), and (13.3) above, together enable the calculation of the probability that a particular number of active synapses will be lost on a dendrite in moving from one cue to another. Assume that a within-category move (from, e.g., $x'$ to $x''$) results in a loss of $l_{(x',x'')}$ active synapses on a particular dendrite. A between-category move (e.g. $x'$ to $y'$) may result in the same number of lost synapses on a dendrite (i.e. perhaps $l_{(x;x'')} = l_{(x;y')}$), but the *strength* of the synapses lost in the former case (within category) should be significantly lower than those lost in the latter case (across categories). Hence, for a given depolarization threshold for firing, the difference $d$ between output firing patterns should be smaller for within-category cues than for cues from two different categories.

Further analysis using these simplifying assumptions led to an optimization formula for producing categorical responses; i.e. cells that respond to any member of a group after several exemplars are learned. This expression takes the form:

$$\frac{\lambda}{\omega_1^\lambda} = \frac{\theta}{\omega_2}$$

where $\lambda$ is the voltage change needed during learning to produce LTP, $\theta$ is the change needed during performance to fire the cell, $\omega_1^\lambda$ is the naïve strength of a synapse during a learning episode, and $\omega_2$ is the strength of the synapses in performance mode, after maximal LTP (Granger, Ambros-Ingerson, and Lynch, 1989). Assuming that $\lambda > \theta$, it would follow that $\omega_2 < \omega_1$ in order for the above expression to hold, which does not accord with biological reality. However, note that the LTP learning rule involves a transient change in strength of naïve synapses during learning, because of the requirement that they occur in a burst plus the refractoriness of the IPSPs, as discussed earlier. That is, the LTP rule distinguishes naïve synaptic strength during learning from that during performance, such that $\omega_1^\lambda = k \times \omega_1$ and we may write

$$\frac{\lambda}{k \times \omega_1} = \frac{\theta}{\omega_2}$$

where $k$ is the multiplicative factor by which naïve synaptic strengths are increased during the learning mode. Using estimates for $\lambda, \theta, \omega_1$ and $\omega_2, k$ was calculated and found to be within the correct range for the percentage amplification actually provided by theta-rhythm bursting of single-pulse responses (Granger, Ambros-Ingerson, and Lynch 1989). In sum, the analysis describes conditions that must be met for optimal partitioning of the input space, and leads to the description of a factor that must be present during learning for this partitioning to take place; this factor is similar to known aspects of LTP-inducing physiological stimulation.

*Development of stable, unique encodings of cues*

Potentiated synapses cause stronger depolarization and firing of those cells participating in a 'category' response (as just described) to a learned cue. This increased depolarization causes strong, cell-specific afterhyperpolarization (AHP), effectively putting those cells into a relatively long-lasting ($\approx 1$ s) refractory period that prevents them from firing in response to the next few sampling sniffs of the cue. Then the inhibitory 'winner-take-all' behaviour within patches effectively selects alternate cells to fire, once these strongly firing (learned) cells have undergone AHP. These alternate cells then activate their caudally flowing recurrent collaterals, activating distinct populations of synapses in caudal layer Ib. Potentiation of these synapses in combination with those of still-active LOT axons tends to 'recruit' stable subpopulations of caudal cells that are distinct from each simulated odour. They are distinct for each odour because first rostral cells are selected from the population of cells that respond primarily to the portions of learned inputs that are not shared across members of a category, after the strongly potentiated cells responding primarily to shared (and thus recurring) LOT inputs have been removed via AHP. We suggest that caudal cells that receive maximal convergence from these selected rostral cells will effectively be responding to the largest proportion of input axons from the LOT, and hence will be the best 'match' to the specific input.

We hypothesize that the probability of a cell participating in the rostral semirandomly selected groups for more than one odour (e.g. for two similar odours) will be lower than the probability of cells being recruited by these two odours initially, since the population consists of those cells that receive insufficient input from the LOT to have been recruited as a category cell and potentiated, yet receive enough input to fire as an alternate cell, more likely in response to the unshared input axons than to those shared across members of a category. The probability of any caudal cell then being recruited by the simulation for more than one odour by these rostral cell collaterals (in combination with weakening caudal LOT lines) is likely to be similarly low. The product of these two probabilities will of course be lower still. Hence, the probability that any particular caudal cell potentiated as part of this process will participate in response to more than one odour should be quite low. As a result, the spatial firing patterns that develop as late-sniff responses to inputs differ markedly from each other in the simulation, even for input cues that are very similar to each other.

*What the algorithms compute: hierarchical encoding of stimuli*

As a result of the above-described operations of the system, as the simulation repeatedly samples an input on successive simulated 'sniffs', the first pattern of cell firing in response to the input indicates similarity among learned odours, whereas later sniffs generate patterns of firing that tend to be quite different for different odours, even when those odours are very similar. Empirical tests of the simulation have shown that odours consisting of 90 per cent overlapping LOT firing patterns will give rise to overlaps of between 90 and 95 per cent in their initial output spatial firing patterns, whereas these same cues give rise to output patterns that overlap by less than 25 per cent on second and third sniffs. The spatio-temporal pattern of output cell firing over multiple samples thus can be taken as a strong differentiating mechanism for even very similar cues, while the initial sniff response for those cues will none the less give rise to a spatial firing pattern that indicates the similarity of sets of learned cues, and therefore their 'category membership' in the clustering sense (Lynch and Granger 1989).

It is important to note that true clustering is an operation that is quite distinct from stimulus generalization. Observing that an object is a car does not occur because of a comparison with a specific, previously learned car. Instead the category 'car' emerges from the learning of many different cars and may be based on a 'prototype' that has no necessary correspondence with a specific, real object. The same could be said of the network. It did not produce a categorical response when one cue had been learned and a second similar stimulus was presented. Category or cluster responses, as noted, required the learning of several exemplars of a similarity-based cluster. It is the process of extracting commonalities from the environment that defines clustering, not the simple noting of similarities between two cues.

An essential question in clustering concerns the location of the boundaries of a given group; i.e. what degree of similarity must a set of cues possess to be grouped together? This issue has been discussed from any number of theoretical positions (e.g. information theory); all these analyses incorporate the point that the breadth of a category must reflect the overall homogeneity or heterogeneity of the environment. In a world where things are quite similar, useful categories will necessarily be composed of objects with much in common. Suppose, for instance, that subjects were presented with a set of four distinct coffee cups of different colours, and asked later to recall the objects. The subjects might respond by listing the cups as a blue, red, yellow and green coffee cup, reflecting a relatively specific level of description in the hierarchy of objects that are coffee cups. In contrast, if presented with four different objects, a blue coffee cup, a drinking glass, a silver fork and a plastic spoon, the cup would be much more likely to be recalled as simply a cup, or a coffee cup, and rarely as a blue coffee cup; the specificity of encoding chosen depends on the overall heterogeneity of the environment.

Any useful clustering device, then, ought to utilize information about the heterogeneity of the stimulus world in setting the heterogeneity of individual categories. Heterogeneity of categories refers to the degree of similarity that is used to determine if cues are to be grouped together or not. Several network parameters will influence category size and we are exploring how these influence the categories formed; one particularly interesting possibility involves a shifting threshold function, an idea used with great success by Cooper and his colleagues (1984, 1987) in their work on visual cortex. The problems presented to the simulation thus far involve a totally naïve system, one that has had no 'developmental' history. We are currently exploring a model in which early experiences are not learned *per se* by the network, but instead set parameters for later ('adult') learning episodes. The idea is that early experience determines the heterogeneity of a representative sample of the stimulus world and imprints this on the network, not by specific changes in synaptic strengths, but in a more general fashion.

### *Other networks, other behaviours*

A number of artificial 'neural networks', using a variety of algorithms, share some basic computational characteristics with each other: in particular, they tend to optimize particular functions. The optimization problem can be translated into a large class of tasks, ranging from classic mathematical problems such as the travelling salesman problem (TSP) to related problems in classification. There is a relatively uniform set of characteristics of these problems: they take as input pre-defined sets of categories and sets of data to be placed into these categories (or, e.g. destinations and order-of-visit information, in the case of TSP). In addition to these performance capabilities, networks can have learning algorithms that enable them to discover regularities in the data as it is presented.

As a special case of these abilities, these networks can, under certain conditions, *discover* categories implicit in the data, rather than having the categories given to them. What is required for the discovery of categories is that second-order properties of the data be extracted and encoded. This cannot be accomplished in a densely connected single-layer network, but it can be performed in either a sparsely connected network (Keeler, 1987, Lynch *et al.* 1987; Granger *et al.* 1987, 1989; Lynch and Granger 1989), or in a network (of any density) with multiple layers (Parker, 1985; Rumelhart,

Hinton, and Williams 1986; Hanson and Burr 1988). The *apparent* discovery of categories can be accomplished in an autoassociative network via careful pre-selection by the experimenter of those data that most prototypically define the intended categories (e.g. phonemes, letters of the alphabet: Anderson *et al.* 1977; Anderson and Mozer 1981). If a simple network (e.g. dense, single-layer) is trained exclusively on such a data set, then in subsequent performance mode, novel inputs will be interpreted as 'degraded' versions of the learned cues, i.e., the net can generate the output corresponding to the learned cue that is most similar (minimum Hamming distance) to the novel input vector. However, if further learning occurs on any of the novel vectors, they will define new categories, just as the original learned inputs did, so that subsequent output responses will not reflect the originally desired (and pre-selected) categories. Indeed, a new category will appear for all inputs on which sufficient learning occurs, so that if all inputs are learned, then each will give rise to its own response, until the capacity of the network is reached, at which point novel inputs will tend to give rise to previously learned outputs, and further learning of unique encodings cannot occur.

Hence, the most common examples of categorization in the artificial neural network literature actually correspond to the learning of unique encodings of cues, up to the network's capacity limits, followed by a performance (non-learning) mode in which any novel cue is treated as a noisy variant of one of the trained exemplars; a category consists of the learned cue and its noisy variants. This noise-reduction ability is achieved by hand in such cases, by the experimenter pre-selecting those data that he or she wishes to form categories around ('prototypes'). The network is trained to criterion on those inputs alone, and then learning is terminated, and the network is then used exclusively as a performance mechanism (not a learning mechanism) from that point forward. The unique encodings generated by these networks have the interesting property that their Hamming distances are a monotonic function of the corresponding distances of their inputs. Kohonen (1984), Grossberg (1976, 1980), and others have made use of this fact to design hybrid mechanisms consisting of (at least) two modules: the first (which can be thought of as a 'novelty detector') tests each novel input for its similarity to those of already learned cues, and if the similarity is within some threshold (which can be set by adjustment of network parameters), then learning is prevented, and the input is interpreted by the second module (in performance mode) as a variant of the prototype that it is similar to; otherwise, the second module learns the novel cue as distinct from other learned cues. In this variant, the experimenter is pre-selecting the radius of similarity required for cues to be categorized together. It should be noted that the process of categorization around a central prototype or exemplar can be viewed either as a process of categorization of individual instances or as a 'noise reduction' or 'error reduction' process that effectively interprets a number of slightly differing inputs as being simply the same cue but accompanied by noise. Learning *both* the individual identities of cues and their natural clusters or categories, as in the network described in this paper, amounts to learning a (two-level or deeper) *hierarchy* of information about each cue. In such a case, then, a principled distinction can be made between noise reduction and categorization: the former can be considered to be performed (on the basis of acuity) in the set of representations of individual exemplars or instances, while the latter is being performed by the cluster representation. When only a single level of representation is learned, as in these other networks, then the two processes accomplish the same effect, as described above; noise reduction, by any method, amounts to a form of categorization at the single representational level.

## Novel physiological results arising from the stimulation

There are a number of specific physiologies whose operation determines aspects of the overall behaviour of the cortical network. We have already described in detail our hypothesis of how a number of relatively well-studied inhibitory currents with different strengths, different durations, and different cell specificity (IPSPs, LHP and AHP) interact in an integrated fashion to give rise to the major 'operating rules' of the system. Such hypotheses are valuable only to the extent that they provide valid views of the integrative action of this cortical system; such view are valid only to the extent that they give rise to testable (and therefore falsifiable) predictions. A number of such predictions have arisen during the course of the integrative modelling effort described here; some of these predictions have since been tested in our laboratory.

One such prediction concerns the asynchronous arrival of multiple afferents converging on a single dendrite. In particular, since LOT axons are myelinated, whereas collateral axons are not, and since the flow of those collaterals is primarily caudal, then by caudal piriform, cells will be receiving inputs from LOT axons many milliseconds (sometimes tens of milliseconds) earlier than those of collaterals from more rostral cells. Assuming this caudal cell fires, the question arises: what will the relative potentiation of the LOT synapses and collateral synapses be? The prevailing mechanisms for induction of long-term potentiation, via long (e.g. 1 s) trains of high-frequency stimulation or 'tetani', suggest that additional depolarization develops as more stimulation enters the cell, and that as a result, later-arriving stimuli will activate synapses on a more-depolarized cell, resulting in increased potentiation. We tested the effect of order of arrival of convergent stimuli within the theta bursting stimulation paradigm we have described, in *in vito* hippocampal (CA1) slices: after an initial 'priming' pulse delivered to three distinct input (Schaffer-collateral) axon pathways converging on a single CA1 pyramidal cell dendrite, each of the pathways was stimulated with a short (four-pulse) high-frequency (100 Hz) burst, at 180 ms, 200 ms and 220 ms after the priming pulse, respectively (therefore, all occurred within the optimal time window for potentiation of their synapses). The initial results indicate the counterintuitive finding that the earlier-arriving inputs showed the most potentiation, and the latest arrivers showed the least; moreover, potentiation of the early arrivers was facilitated by the occurrence of the subsequent stimulation (i.e. this potentiation was greater than that which would have resulted from the early input alone) (Larson and Lynch 1988b).

This implies that post-synaptic cells show an active preference for early arrivers out of a group of nearly synchronous afferents converging on a cell. In computational terms, this result has a large effect on the performance of the system, especially on the development of unique encodings for cues described above. Once an unpotentiated firing rostral cell aids (via its collaterals) in activating a caudal cell, if early arrivers potentiated less than late arrivers, as initially suggested, then the collateral axons on that caudal cell would potentiate more than the LOT afferents to the cell. Then on subsequent exposure to that same input, LOT input alone would remain insufficient to fire that caudal cell (since the LOT synapses would have only weakly potentiated), and activation of the cell would require additional activation of the rostral cells whose collateral inputs to the caudal cell had been potentiated. If, however, early arrivers potentiate more than latecomers, as suggested by the results of the experiments just described, then the LOT lines for the input would be directly tied to the caudal cell, and would be more likely to be able to activate that cell directly, after learning. Hence, the unique learned representations of inputs will be significantly more robust and stable in the latter case than in the former. We are continuing experimentation on this question with intracellular recording, and the results will of course be incorporated into the network simulation. Regardless of the outcome, this is a clear case of integrative simulation raising novel physiological questions which, at least in this instance, may give rise to counterintuitive findings, in turn establishing a computational attribute of the integrated operation of the overall cortical network under investigation.

## Conclusions

The integrated action of the physiological mechanisms of layer II piriform cortex, as embedded in its anatomical structure, give rise to a coherent set of computational functions: with learning, layer II cells robustly generate particular temporal sequences of spatial cell-firing patterns in response to particular olfactory inputs such that the first patterns in the sequence reflect similarity-based 'category membership' characteristics of the input (e.g. foods

v. non-foods; cheeses v. fruits), while the later response patterns constitute unique encodings of individual cues (e.g. Jarlsberg, cheddar). Thus the hierarchical relationships among families of odours are preserved, and an object can be recognized as a unique odour, or a member of some category of odours that are similar to each other. These hierarchical encodings are learned rapidly and incrementally, and are sparsely coded, such that, once learned, future learning offers little interference with extant learning, so that the encodings remain stable. It should be stressed that this form of encoding was not a starting hypothesis of this research; rather, these functions were discerned via observation of the behaviour of a simulation that was fashioned to closely follow the physiological and anatomical characteristics of piriform cortex. But are hierarchical encoding and sequential readout fundamental properties of layer II cortex as suggested by the simulation? Are these properties that emerge due to learning in real cortical networks? The goal of the work reviewed here has been to predict the types of aggregate activities that appear when basic neurobiological properties are expressed in specific cortical circuitries. Success in the endeavour can be gauged by how useful, experimentally testable, and accurate the predictions prove to be. It is worth noting that the idea that organization of memories occurs hand in glove with the encoding of memory has received little attention in animal psychology, focusing as it has on associative learning. It is encouraging that the simulation has produced a behavioural hypothesis that emphasizes an aspect of learning that in fact has been largely ignored in the behavioural neurosciences; the organization of memory has been a major research theme in the cognitive sciences for a number of years.

The simulation and analytical work make predictions at two levels. First, it specified how cells in layer II of piriform cortex should act during certain types of behaviour. The model specifies sparse encoding which would mean that cells would not be broadly tuned. It also predicts that different groups of cells will fire on different sniffs, and that learning will profoundly affect what sensory characteristics the cells will respond to. While the point was not stressed, the simulation also indicates that the anterior and posterior portions of the cortex will be quite different in their selectivity. Second, we can assume that the collective properties of the network will be evident in behaviour. This follows from an unusual feature of olfactory cortex that has been discussed at length elsewhere (Lynch 1986); namely, that it is but two synapses removed from the physical stimulus for smell, and serves as a relay to all higher brain structures involved in olfaction. Because of these properties, it is extremely likely that the cortex participates in and is crucial to all complex olfactory behaviour. Accordingly, fundamental collective activities of the cortex should be detectable in behaviour.

In all, the predictions of the model are testable. Chronic unit recordings are now being collected from layer II piriform cortex in rats engaged in sequential olfactory discriminations. Preliminary results indicate that coding is indeed extremely sparse and is markedly affected by learning in ways compatible with hypotheses based on the simulation and analyses (Larson, McCollum *et al.*, unpublished data). Work is also in progress to test the hypothesis that rats partition their olfactory world and use multiple sniffs to read out information in the manner predicted by the simulation. In closing, it should be noted that the hypotheses resulting from the simulation work concerns a fundamental characteristic of the layer II cortex; there is an enormous number of issues concerning olfaction per se that it does not address. The model is also limited by the extremely simple input signals it processes. Development of an olfactory bulb model simulation, currently under way, will raise new problems but, we hope, expand the range of issues that the cortical model addresses.

## References

Anderson, J. A., Silverstein, J. W., Ritz, S. A., and Jones, R. S. (1977). Distinctive features, categorical perception and probability learning. *Psychological Review*, **84**, 413–51.

Anderson, J. A. and Mozer, M. (1981). Categorization and selective neurons. In *Parallel models of associative memory* (eds. G. E. Hinton and J. A. Anderson), pp. 213–36. Erlbaum, NJ.

Bear, M. F., Cooper, L. N., and Ebner, F. F. (1987). The physiological basis of a theory for synapse modification. *Science*, **237**, 42–8.

Cooper, L. N. (1984). Neuron learning to network organization. In *J. C. Maxwell, the Sesquicentennial Symposium*, pp. 41–90, Elsevier.

Feldman, J. A. (1982). Dynamic connections in neural networks. *Biological Cybernetics*, **46**, 27–39.

Granger, R., Ambros-Ingerson, J., Henry, H., and Lynch, G. (1987). Partitioning of sensory data by a cortical network. *Proceedings of the IEEE Conference on Neural Information Processing Systems*, American Institute of Physics Publications.

Granger, R. H., Ambrose-Ingerson, J., and Lynch, G. (1989). Derivation of encoding characteristics of layer II cerebral cortex. *Journal of Cognitive Neuroscience*, **1**, 61–87.

Grossberg, S. (1976). Adaptive pattern classification and universal recoding: part I. *Biological Cybernetics*, **23**, 121–34.

Grossberg, S. (1980). How does the brain build a cognitive code? *Psychological Review*, **87**, 1–51.

Haberly, L. B. and Shepherd, G. M. (1973). Current density analysis of opossum prepyiform cortex, *Journal of Neurophysiology*, **36**, 789–802.

Haberly, L. B. (1973). Summed potentials evoked in opossum prepyriform cortex, *Journal of Neurophysiology* **36**, 775–88.

Haberly, L. B. (1985). Neuronal circuitry in olfactory cortex: anatomy and functional implications. *Chemical Senses*, **10**, 219–38.

Hanson, S. J. and Burr, D. J. (1988). What connectionist models learn (submitted).

Keeler, J. D. (1987). Capacity for patterns and sequences in Kanerva's SDM. RIACS TR #87.29, NASA Ames Research Center.

Kohonen, T. (1984). *Self-organization and associative memory*. Springer-Verlag, Berlin.

Larson, J. and G. Lynch (1986). synaptic potentiation in hippocampus by patterned stimulation involves two events. *Science*, **232**, 985–8.

Larson, J. and G. Lynch (1988*a*). Role of N-methyl-D-aspartate receptors in the induction of synaptic potentiation by burst stimulation patterned after the hippocampal theta rhythm. *Brain Research*, **441**, 111–18.

Larson, J. and G. Lynch (1988*b*). Theta pattern stimulation and LTP: the sequence in which synapses are stimulated determines the degree to which they potentiate (manuscript in preparation).

Lynch, G. (1986). *Synapses, circuits and the beginnings of memory*. MIT Press, Cambridge, Mass.

Lynch, G., Granger, R., Baudry, M., and Larson, J. (1989). Cortical encoding of memory: hypotheses derived from analysis and simulation of physiological learning rules in anatomical structures. In *Neural connections, mental computations* (ed. L. Nadel).

Lynch, G., Granger, R., Levy, W., and Larson, J. (1988). Some possible functions of simple cortical networks suggested by computer modeling. In *Neural models of plasticity: theoretical and empirical approaches* (eds. J. Byrne and W. O. Berry) (in press).

Lynch, G. and Granger, R. (1989). Simulation and analysis of a cortical network. *The Psychology of Learning and Motivation*, Vol 23 (in press).

Macrides, F., Eichenbaum, H. B., and Forbes, W. B. (1982). Temporal relationship between sniffing and the limbic (theta) rhythm during odor discrimination reversal learning. *Journal of Neuroscience*, **2**, 1705–17.

Parker, D. B. (1985). Learning-logic. MIT TR-47, Massachusetts Institute of Technology, Center for Computational Research in Economics and Management Science, Cambridge, Mass.

Roman, F., Staubli, U., and Lynch, G. (1987). Evidence for synaptic potentiation in a cortical network during learning. *Brain Research* (in press).

Rumelhart, D., Hinton, G. and Williams, R. (1986). Learning internal representations by error propagation. In *Parallel distributed processing* (eds. D. Rumelhart and J. McClelland). MIT Press, Cambridge, Mass.

Schwob, J. E., and Price, J. L. (1978). The cortical projection of the olfactory bulb: development in fetal and neonatal rats correlated with quantitative variation in adult rats. *Brain Research*, **151**, 369–74.

Slotnick, B. M. and H. M. Katz (1974). Olfactory learning-set formation in rats. *Science*, **185**, 796–8.

Standing, L. (1973). Learning 10 000 pictures. *Quarterly Journal of Experimental Psychology*, **25**, 207–22.

Staubli, U., Fraser, D., Faraday, R., and Lynch, G. (1987). Olfaction and the 'data' memory system in rats. *Behavioural Neuroscience* (in press).

Staubli, U. and G. Lynch (1988). Stable hippocampal long-term potentiation elicited by 'theta' pattern stimulation. *Brain Research* (in press).

# Author index

# Subject index